Silvia Bonino • Elena Cattelino • Silvia Ciairano

Adolescents and Risk

Behavior, Functions, and Protective Factors

Foreword by
Richard Jessor

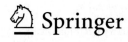 

Silvia Bonino
Department of Psychology
University of Torino, Via Verdi 10
I-10124 Torino

Elena Cattelino
University of Valle d'Aosta
Via dei Cappuccini 2A
I-11000 Aosta

Silvia Ciairano
Department of Psychology
University of Torino, Via Verdi 10
I-10124 Torino

Translation from the original Italian title:
Adolescenti e rischio
© 2003, Giunti Editore S.p.A., Firenze - Milano

Translator: Lindsay Mc Donald

The translation of this work has been funded by SEPS
Segretariato Europeo per le Pubblicazioni Scientifiche

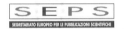

Via Val d'Aposa 7 - 40123 Bologna - Italy
seps@alma.unibo.it - www.seps.it

*The Authors wish to thank the Università della Valle d'Aosta - Université
de la Vallée d'Aoste, Faculty of Science of Education, for the contribution
to the realization and distribution of this volume*

Library of Congress Control Number: 2005927906

ISBN-10   88-470 0290-7 Springer Milan Berlin Heidelberg New York
ISBN-13   978-88-470-0290-6 Springer Milan Berlin Heidelberg New York

Springer is a part of Springer Science+Business Media

springeronline.com

Cover design: Simona Colombo, Milan, Italy
Typesetting: Graficando, Milan, Italy
Printing: Grafiche Porpora, Cernusco s/N, Milan, Italy

Silvia Bonino
Elena Cattelino
Silvia Ciairano
Adolescents and Risk
Behavior, Functions, and Protective Factors

FOREWORD

Over the past several decades, the field of adolescent health and development has undergone a profound and pervasive transformation in the knowledge and understanding of young lives. Popular myths about adolescents - that they are hapless victims of "raging hormones" or risk-takers who see themselves as invulnerable - have been laid to rest. But even more important has been the emergence of a new, scientific perspective about this stage of life. It is a perspective that recognizes that adolescents are active participants in the shaping of their own development; that the influence of context - family, peers, school, media, neighborhood, workplace - is as important in determining the life course as are the attributes of the individual and, indeed, that it is the interaction between context and individual attributes that is really crucial; that there is remarkable diversity in the pathways that can be taken by youth as they traverse between late childhood and young adulthood; and that the adolescent life-stage is, itself, an extended one - a full decade of the life trajectory with very different tasks, opportunities, and challenges in the later years than in the earlier years. It is this new, scientific perspective that so thoroughly informs the present volume by Silvia Bonino, Elena Cattelino, and Silvia Ciairano.

The volume is an impressive contribution to understanding risk behavior among contemporary Italian adolescents, but it goes far beyond that to advance understanding of adolescent behavior and development as a whole. In this regard, it has immediate relevance for American developmental science as well. The reliance of the authors on a theoretical framework that engages both individual and context; their assessment of the multiple contexts in the ecology of daily adolescent life; their insistence that risk behavior - as with all behavior - is meaningful, purposive, and instrumental; and their focus on multiple types of adolescent risk behavior and on their covariation as a life style or a way of being in the world - all of these together give the volume generality beyond youth in Italy and provide a window on adolescence that enables us to look beyond risk behavior alone.

With regard to its particular focus on adolescent risk behavior, the volume is remarkably informative and useful for both scientist and practitioner alike. The data are based on large samples of youth, the analytical methodology is sound, and the presentation of findings is very accessible, relying throughout on graphic representation rather than statistical tables. The chapters deal with each of the key types of risk behavior that are of concern at this developmental stage - drug and alcohol use, delinquency, early sexual experience, risky driving, and unhealthy eating behavior. They show the linkages among them, elaborate the functions served by the various types of risk behavior or the meanings they may have for the adolescent, and examine how they vary with age, gender, and other demographic characteristics.

Important and useful as such descriptive knowledge is, the major contribution of the volume clearly lies in its demonstration of the influential role the theoretical risk factors and protective factors play in adolescent risk behavior involvement. In this regard, the research findings not only strengthen the theory, but they serve as an important guide to the design of intervention efforts to prevent or reduce adolescent involvement in risk behavior.

One comes away from reading this book with a sense of optimism about the usefulness of the knowledge it provides. The emphasis of the authors on the need to strengthen protective factors that can promote positive youth development, and on the need to provide opportunities for behavior that can serve the same purposes that risk behavior does but without compromising health and development, is salutary. This, indeed, is the key challenge for all contemporary societies to accomplish. By meeting that challenge, societies would give young people the kind of protection they probably need most - the protection that comes from a strong sense that they have a viable stake in the future.

Richard Jessor
Institute of Behavioral Science
University of Colorado
Boulder, USA

PREFACE

To all the girls and boys, teachers and principals who, through their receptiveness, enthusiasm, and honesty, made this study possible.

Even the most personal ideas are the fruit of many people's input, whether those people are aware of it or not. This is true all the more so in a study as broad as the one presented here, the authors of which are indebted to the contribution of a great number of people who, in different ways and in different places, have over the years collaborated on this project and still today work on its continuation. It has been an exciting, if at times difficult and exhausting, adventure. For this reason, our acknowledgments are not merely a cold formality but a sincere recognition of those who have been involved in this challenge. Although we are limited by space and cannot here recognize everyone, we would like to mention the people and institutions that have provided the most significant contributions.

Without Richard Jessor's (University of Colorado, Boulder, USA) confidence in our research team, nothing could have been accomplished. To him, we owe an enormous debt of gratitude for having believed in this project. Adam Frączek (University of Warsaw, Poland), who was the first to work in Europe with Jessor's questionnaire and who shared his research process with us, also played a vital role. In more recent years, Sandy Jackson (University of Groningen, the Netherlands) was a patient and thought-provoking interlocutor as well as a tireless organizer; unfortunately, his untimely passing recently brought an end to our collaboration. Michel Born (University of Liège, Belgium) also accompanied us over the course of our research with his receptiveness and open mind.

Nor can we forget the large group of European researchers from the European Association for Research on Adolescence (EARA) whose congresses have served as a platform for the presentation and discussion of this study and some of its results (Liège, Belgium, 1966; Budapest, Hungary, 1998; Jena, Germany, 2000; Oxford, England, 2002; Porto, Portugal, 2004). The congresses, held by the Developmental Division of the Italian Psychological Association (AIP) (Parma, 1999; Alghero, 2000; Palermo, 2001; Bellaria, 2002; Bari, 2003;

Sciacca, 2004) and by the Interuniversity Center for Research on the Origins and Development of Prosocial and Antisocial Motivation (Rome, 1999; Florence, 2000, 2002; Rome, 2003), also provided us with valuable opportunities for exchange with other Italian researchers.

As research cannot be carried out without funding, we are particularly grateful to the institutions that financed and supported this long and broad-reaching study: the J. Jacobs Foundation (Zürich), the Regional Administration of Piemonte (Council for Health, Council for Health Activities, Council for Health Education and Promotion), the Regional Administration of Aosta Valley (Council of Education and Culture, Council of Health), Ministry of University and Research (MIUR, previously MURST, cofinancing 1998 and 2000), National Council for Research (CNR, 1998, 1999), and the European Union (General Directorate XII, Science, Research and Development section - TMR Project "Marie Curie").

A long succession of people, who we are unable to name here, have participated in this research project over the years, including scholarship holders, fellows, technicians, interns, and doctoral and undergraduate students. Our closest collaborators (Tatiana Begotti, Gabriella Borca, and Emanuela Calandri) appear as coauthors in various publications cited in this text. We would also like to recognize the valuable contribution of Manuela Bina, Fabrizia Giannotta, Federica Graziano, Roberta Molinar, Giorgia Molinengo, Daniela Morero, Emanuela Rabaglietti, and Antonella Roggero.

A special thanks to Renato Miceli (Psychology Department, University of Torino, Italy) for his patient and competent statistical consultation.

But our greatest thanks go to all the boys and girls, their teachers and principals who through their receptiveness, enthusiasm, and honesty made this study possible. To them we dedicate this volume, and it is our hope that it may be of use to them in their personal and professional lives.

As it is the fruit of a common effort, the book appears with the names of all three authors. However, we would like to specify that chapters 1, 2, and 8 were written by Silvia Bonino; chapters 3, 4, and 5 by Elena Cattelino; and chapters 6 and 7 by Silvia Ciairano.

Silvia Bonino
Elena Cattelino
Silvia Ciairano

Contents

CHAPTER 1

Risk Behavior in Adolescence

> It depends a lot on the context… what matters it's your intentions when you do a certain thing… what I mean is, it depends on how you personally experience something.
>
> *[Girl, science lyceum, third year]*

1.1 Adolescents and Adolescence

In the most recent psychological literature, the representation of adolescence as an inevitable condition of hardship and suffering has been abandoned although in the mass media this portrayal of adolescents, rooted in nineteenth-century romantic tradition, continues to enjoy widespread popularity. Meanwhile, psychology has also abandoned the idea that adolescence is an absolute process that, due to the fact that it is linked to physiological maturation and the problems that derive from it, it is essentially identical in different historical periods and across different cultures (Koops 1996).

This new vision is the result not only of specific studies on adolescence but of a different way of conceiving human development as a whole. Today, there is consensus in the belief that human development should be viewed from a perspective that considers the entire life cycle: changes and development are not limited to the initial period of life (referred to, in fact, as the developmental phase) in contrast with a period of stability in adulthood and one of decline in old age. Today, we are aware that as our psychological functions continually evolve throughout our lifetime, both change and development affect the entire length of our existence (Baltes et al. 1998). From this perspective, adolescence is neither the conclusion to the developmental phase nor a period of instability that precedes the stability of adulthood. On the contrary, many other times of transition occur over the course of the life cycle that can be difficult and problematic whether encountered in adulthood, maturity, or old age. The adolescent crisis is therefore neither the only nor the most important in a person's life. Moreover, when referring to crisis, at whatever time it occurs in a person's life, we recognize it as a dynamic, positive time of reorganization and a turning point in the process of an individual's development. As a consequence, the term crisis has lost its negative and dramatic connotation, and in the literature on adolescence, it is usually referred to in quotation marks.

In the life-cycle perspective, the temporal dimension plays a central role, as it is throughout the entire lifetime that the interaction between an individual and his or her environment takes place in an incessant flow in which the past is bound to the present and the future. Through this perspective, our attention is no longer focused solely on the past, as was often the case in adolescent and developmental psychology in general; it was believed that the past, constituted by one's first childhood experiences, was capable of strictly determining both one's present and future. It was, in fact, the events and conflicts of childhood - which re-emerged due to the adolescent crisis - that were examined in order to comprehend adolescence. Attention is now focused primarily on the present, the characteristics and specific qualities of which introduce new elements, both negative and positive, that can profoundly affect the development trajectory undertaken (Rutter and Rutter 1992). Therefore, the idea that an influence is much stronger the earlier it occurs has also been discredited, as we have now recognized that development depends both on the type of experience and the ability of each individual to interpret and re-elaborate it in relation to their present experience (Schaffer 2000). The future also gains significance because, although it does not yet exist, it is nevertheless "present" in an individual's mental representations. In adolescence above all, the future, due to cognitive development, becomes an increasingly relevant dimension able to motivate complex plans of action and personal achievement. In short, the present and future development of the adolescent is not imprisoned in his or her past (Ford and Lerner 1992).

At the same time, in contemporary psychology, there is a growing awareness that development is not a linear process and that set paths of development - the same for every individual - do not exist. Development does not occur on a single required route but, rather, across any number of possible, highly individualized, and differentiated paths, which depend on a complex interaction over time between an individual and the context of his or her life. On one hand, individuals continuously affect the world inside and around them thanks to their own unique cognitive abilities affected by changes linked to both biological maturation processes and to experiences that conduct them through life. On the other hand, they are affected by their environment or context, constituted by a plurality of factors of a physical, historical, or cultural type, that they constantly modify and interpret (Fig. 1.1). In this systemic vision, developmental trajectories are highly irregular and cannot be predicted in a deterministic way. This is because of the fact that, depending on the conditions of the system, small influences can in time produce major effects (according to the well-known "butterfly effect") while, on the contrary, major influences can have only minor effects (van Geert 1994) (Fig. 1.2).

The adoption of this holistic, interactionistic, and constructivistic approach, which sees paths of development as probabilistic, is increasingly common in contemporary developmental psychology. The approach also seems to be more consistent with the evolution of other sciences and is the only one that is able to examine and comprehend the complexity of human behavior and development throughout the entire life cycle in relation to different contexts. In this

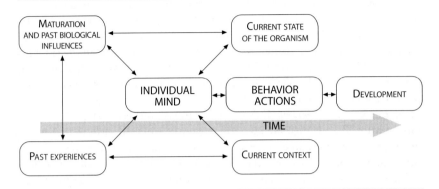

Fig. 1.1. Schematic display of how the individual's mind, over time, acts as a filter to the constant interaction between maturation and experience and is the central variable. Individuals' behavior and actions have a decisive influence on their own development in both neurophysiological terms, as the neuron connections and plastic changes in the brain depend in large part on the type of stimulation the brain is subjected to, and in psychological terms, as experiences and learning can either allow for or prevent future learning (also see Fig. 1.2).

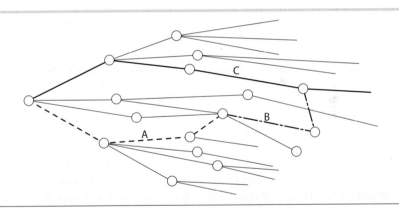

Fig. 1.2. Schematic representation of possible individual development paths. The turning points, identified by *circles*, represent times when choices are made; here, the development path can take different directions, often with lasting effects. Over time, paths that were initially quite similar can have very different outcomes while some trajectories do not lead to developments. Some events, as well as some choices, preclude certain paths in favor of others. For example, having brothers or sisters opens a developmental path that is different than that of an only child. Different, more or less tortuous developmental paths can also lead to the same outcome. For example, an adolescent can build a sufficiently autonomous identity either across a very linear, intentional path or in a more accidental way. While getting back on a given track after a deviation is possible, it may require a great deal of time and effort. For example, the choice to leave secondary school initially leads the adolescent toward a certain path (*A*) that is based on work and blocks access to some professions because of a lack of academic qualifications. Successive events may cause the individual to choose to return to school, returning, although on a longer trajectory (*B*), to an objective and path (*C*) that had previously been barred.

model, individuals and their environment, or context, are considered insepa-
rable elements, forming an integrated, dynamic system and influencing one
another reciprocally (Magnusson and Stattin 1998). The relationship between
the individual and environmental variables is examined through the changes
the individual undergoes over time. Also emphasized is individual action and
the formative role it plays, which is completely unique due to the specific cognitive capabilities of humans.

Adolescence is seen in a different light through this new perspective. Most
importantly, this perspective recognizes that this period of development is
not the same for all adolescents, as was the common conception when the
problems of adolescence were considered to be the necessary consequence of
physiological development and sexual maturation in particular. From that
perspective, only gender differences in adolescent development were acknowl-
edged. Beyond differences between boys and girls, adolescence was described
as a largely similar experience that did not differ based on culture, life context, opportunities offered by the individual's environment (most importantly, those related to family and school), or individual differences. Missing from
that view was the concept that sexual maturation is an important, even critical, event because of the social and psychological effects it has on adolescents
and for the profound structural changes it imposes. Adolescents in Western
society today find themselves with adult bodies capable of procreating while
at the same time they still have many years ahead before they can achieve stable, generative relationships - an often confusing, ambiguous, and conflictual
future objective in a society characterized by a wide range of varied and contradictory behavior models.

On a cognitive level as well, the development of formal reasoning, a characteristic of the last of Piaget's stages, is not the necessary result of neurophysiological maturation; maturation alone, at any age, cannot determine but
only makes possible the acquisition of certain cognitive capacities. Abstract reasoning abilities, therefore, are achieved within an appropriate environmental
context, which in Western cultures is the school. Here, students use the tools
of reading and writing in a systematic way, the means by which higher cognitive capabilities are acquired. Also in this context, the adolescent's developmental process may unfold in a variety of ways. This is contrary to the once commonly held view of development in terms of a rigid stage model where the
appearance of hypothetical, deductive reasoning was the consequence of neurophysiological development and thus characteristic of all adolescents. On the
contrary, in Western culture where there is a period of mandatory schooling,
developmental paths are quite varied in relation not only to family background
but to different opportunities and types of schools. Piaget himself (1972) pointed out that in adults, the achievement of formal reasoning is not uniform
across different areas of cognitive functioning but is, rather, related to professional specialization; therefore, some significant horizontal décalages can also
exist. When we consider that mediation and cognitive re-elaboration also play
an important part in affective and social experiences, it is clear how differ-

ences and lack of uniformity in cognitive development are connected to different levels of self-awareness, different ways of resolving problems, different ways of expressing emotion, different social competencies, different abilities to plan for the future and set goals, and different representations of identity.

For all these reasons, adolescence cannot be described as a uniform experience (Zazzo 1966). Major differences exist between individual developmental paths, although, in Western society, adolescence is increasingly characterized by a sort of "in-between" state where boys and girls are sexually and cognitively adults but do not yet participate in life as adults. As Margaret Mead (1928) pointed out almost a century ago, adolescence does not exist in primitive societies where the social organization is simple, highly stable over time, and ruled by unchanging, undisputed, social norms. In these cultures, puberty signals the passage, often marked by a ritual, from childhood to adulthood and an official entrance into working life and marriage. Adolescence in Western society, on the other hand, is an increasingly lengthy period of transition. Children in these cultures grow up in a highly complex social context in which the entrance into adulthood is postponed to an increasingly late age and there is no single set of norms or values. The greater opportunities offered by Western culture in terms of individual freedom and personal achievement, combined with the lack of clear points of reference, make this "in-between" age, in which adolescents are not yet full participants in society, problematic on one hand while, on the other hand, it consents the development and elaboration of values and personal objectives. Today, even more so than in the past, adolescence is a time full of opportunities, challenges, and risks. However, along with greater individual freedom and increased social resources, adolescents are also faced with rapidly changing models, values, lifestyles, and professional and family roles, which require a greater degree of autonomy and decision-making abilities.

However, although the unique quality of the social environment is stressed in the interactionistic model, the roles of environment and socialization processes are not overemphasized at the expense of the ever-important role of the individual. In reality, there is a mutual and reciprocal interaction between individual and environment (Fig. 1.3). Conceptions that focus on the determinism of the environment, such as those commonly reflected in the media, are now considered outdated. While these conceptions lead to the assumption that adolescents in Western society inevitably suffer due to the social conditions in which they live - and in particular due to the inadequacies of school and transformations of family - in reality, adolescent developmental paths are actually quite varied and prevalently nonproblematic (de Vit and van der Veer 1991). Individual developmental paths are determined by a complex interaction between the individual, who is equipped with certain capabilities and personal characteristics, and the individual's unique social context, which, apart from some basic similarities, differs widely from that of other adolescents. In short, interactionistic and constructivistic models in modern psychology do not explain adolescent development in terms of physiological growth or through environmental influence but, rather, through the interaction between individual and environment. Due to the specific cognitive capabilities each individual possesses, that individual plays an active role in this interaction.

This perspective has directed a great deal of attention in recent years to cross-cultural comparisons, particularly in areas where major changes have occurred due to immigration, for instance, or the collapse of the communist regime in eastern Europe (Noack et al. 1995; Crockett and Silbereisen 2000a). These studies offer interesting insight into the complexity and variety of adolescent developmental trajectories and are also useful in understanding adolescence in situations of less rapid and less dramatic change.

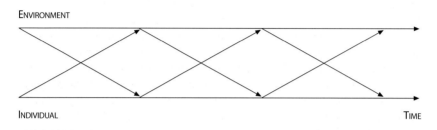

ENVIRONMENT

INDIVIDUAL   TIME

Fig. 1.3. Schematic representation of the continuous reciprocal interactions between individual and environment over time. The relationship between reciprocal influences represented here as equivalent is never so in reality. Over the course of development, the change in cognitive capacities and the potential for autonomous action modify the way in which the individual and environment interact. It is precisely for this reason that adolescents perceive an increase in their ability to influence the environment with which they interact.

1.2 Development as Action in Context

Within the framework of this systemic, interactionistic, and constructivistic conception, some authors have defined development as "action in context" in order to stress the importance of the individual's actions when interacting with an environment that offers limits and restrictions as well as opportunities and resources (Silbereisen et al. 1986; Silbereisen and Noack 1988; Silbereisen and Todt 1994a). This conception, which is becoming prevalent in contemporary psychology, views individuals not as mere reactive organisms moulded by the events of their environment or moved by internal instincts but, rather, as active subjects capable of self-organization, self-regulation, and self-reflection. The ability to exercise broad forms of control on one's thought processes, motivation, affectivity, and action allows adolescents to be active builders of their own environment and not simply "products" of it; therefore, they are able to influence nature and the course of their existence (Bandura 1986, 1997).

Action can be defined as intentional, voluntary behavior subjected to personal control, albeit to widely varying degrees. Actions are based on a system of values, beliefs, norms, goals, evaluations, and meanings that the individual formulates within the context of a certain culture. These actions are put into effect in order to reach certain objectives, resolve certain problems, affirm the values that are important to the individual, and make plans that are significant for the individual's identity (Brandstädter 1997). From this interpretation, behavior is defined as actions that, as opposed to reflexes or automatic reactions, imply a decision and a choice: an individual may act in a certain way but could have acted differently. In short, the concept of action refers back to the combination of symbolic systems that humans utilize to construct their identities and their relationships to the world. The individual's mind knows and interprets reality by using and constructing symbols and signs within a certain cultural system; in this process of mediation, cognitive, emotional, affective, and social spheres are closely connected and interact reciprocally (Bruner 1986). An action based on these processes is not a simple response to environmental stimulus or a biologically determined, automatic reflex; it is, on the contrary, significant, intentional, and reflexive and serves a specific purpose. The action, in short, refers back to a system of the Self that integrates and coordinates its functions in its relationship with the world in order to create the best-possible relationship, to lend meaning to experiences, and to guarantee a sense of unity and continuity. It is worth noting that in the last decades, neurophysiology - an entirely different theoretical perspective - has also focused a great deal of attention to complex, goal-oriented behavior in the framework of studies on executive functions and on the activity of the frontal lobe of the cerebral cortex (Dubois 1995).

The individual always acts within a precise context. On one hand, there is the environmental context filled with both resources and limitations. It can be defined as the immediate environment in which the individual is in direct contact: family, school, neighborhood, and peer groups are examples of these immediate environments. They represent, according to Bronfenbrenner (1979; Bronfenbrenner and Morris 1998), "microsystems" within the ecological environment in which each of us is immersed (Fig. 1.4). On the other hand, there is the individual with his or her own physical characteristics and personal history, which form a framework of possibilities and personal limitations. Thanks to their unique cognitive capabilities - it is precisely during adolescence that the development of formal reasoning is made possible - individuals constantly elaborate stimuli, evaluate their experiences, attribute meaning to themselves and the world, make plans for the future, and develop self-reflect. All of this is manifested in precise actions that are not determined by biological factors, environmental stimuli, or personal background. Consequently, the actions of adolescents are not meaningless and are not the result of simple environmental pressures; they are self-regulated, they have aims, and they are carried out in order to meet these aims to express certain values and convictions, to resolve problems, and to construct an identity. In other words, the majority of adolescent behavior results from a choice between various alternatives, is based on beliefs and values, and is regulated by a personal control that is related to the rules of society.

Because they have a return effect, which can be either positive or negative on both the individual who carries them out and the environmental context, these actions are capable of directing the course of development. As a result, development is based not only on the interaction between individual and environment but also on the interaction between these two aspects and the individual's actions. Development is defined as "action in context" precisely for this reason: to underline the fact that development is also a result of the individual's actions, which are intentional, oriented toward a particular objective, and seek to adjust objectives and individual potential to the requirements and opportunities of one's context. For example, an active, intelligent adolescent may find himself in a school that has very little to offer on a social and cultural level. His decision to continue in this school, to change school, or to drop out would have considerable consequences for his development both in the near and distant future.

By affirming that an individual action is intentional and directed toward an aim that has a particular meaning for the individual, we certainly do not intend to claim that the individual is always aware of all the elements involved in that decision. As individuals are unable to represent in a complete way both the complexity of the meaning, aims, and consequences of their actions and the interrelationship of the contextual and internal conditions that limit them, such awareness is always necessarily partial. The fact that the processes involved in intentional actions are never entirely conscious and can, on the contrary, be

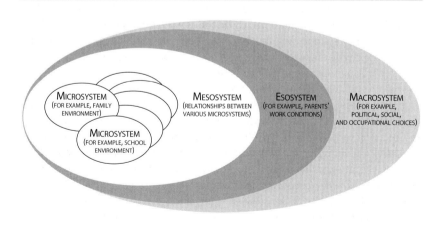

Fig. 1.4. Different environments considered in Bronfenbrenner's ecological model. With the term "ecology," the author refers to the environmental structures in which the individual lives and to which he or she is directly (microsystem and mesosystem) or indirectly (esosystem and macrosystem) tied.

in some cases almost totally unconscious, does not invalidate the affirmation that the majority of human actions are not at all reflexes or automatic reactions. Intention and willingness concern, indeed, the agency of a being, such as the human who is able to self-regulate and direct his or her behavior toward reaching meaningful goals (Silbereisen et al. 1986; Bandura 1997). In reality, there is a constant synergy between the conscious and unconscious, as the psychological phenomena that escape awareness are essential for the construction of the consciousness itself, for the self-regulation of actions, and the disclosure of intention. In other words, there is a reason for the existence of unconscious activity in terms of adjustment in the existence of an individual who is self-aware and self-regulated and whose actions are intentional.

An individual's degree of awareness changes constantly throughout development and is tied to the exercise of metacognitive reflection. Even though the gradual development of formal reasoning allows adolescents to achieve a higher degree of self-awareness, many limitations can be caused both during adolescence and after by a difficulty in decentralizing, by a lack of experience in exercising metacognition and by emotional interference. Due to its characteristics, action, as it is the product of "limited rationality," can provoke unexpected and unwanted effects. These experiences, although painful, serve as powerful stimuli to revise and readjust one's beliefs and objectives, leading individuals to seek a balanced relationship between potential and individual goals on one hand and opportunity and environmental limitations on the other (Brandstädter 1997). In this attempt, individuals are able to choose the "ecological niche" that best fits them.

The goals that propel actions are not necessarily rational in the common sense of the word; in fact, an action that seems absolutely irrational to others may make perfect sense to the individual. Returning to the previous example, the adolescent may choose to leave school indefinitely to achieve the objective of immediately pursuing a successful professional life. However, when analyzed objectively, these goals would prove to be unrealistic so that the adolescent's choice is, in fact, a loosing choice.

In a culture like today's, where our points of reference are more and more diversified, contradictory, and in constant evolution, it is to be expected that the process of "constructing meaning," while similar in people belonging to the same culture, is in reality widely varied, depending both on the individual and the cultural subgroup to which he or she belongs. In fact, the personal process of constructing meaning, which is the foundation of goal-oriented intentional actions, always occurs in relation to the social context in which the individual lives (Bruner 1990).

From what has been said up to now, it is clear that the action referred to is not omnipotent although at times individuals tend, quite childishly, to believe that it is so. As the control exercised by an individual - both by his or her own internal processes and his or her environment - is always partial, action is subject to obligations and limitations. However, within the range of these limitations, the action can make use of resources and opportunities that stem from both the individual and his or her context (Fig. 1.5). In the example that was just made, the adolescent's decision is linked most importantly to limits and individual resources that stem from the individual's biological characteristics. These characteristics may be stable (such as intellectual capacity) or contingent (for example, a momentary situation such as an illness); they might stem from the individual's past (in which he or she may have had a successful or unsuccessful school experience and have developed capabilities or, rather, incompetence, on a cognitive, affective, or relational level) or from the individual's present reality (for example, a sense of self-efficacy). All of these variables do not, however, determine the individual's decision. A decision is the result of a personal evaluation, with varying degrees of awareness and freedom, based on what is most important to the individual, what his or her expectations are for the future, and how he or she feels these objectives can be achieved.

At the same time, the context in which the adolescent interacts is also relevant. Constraints and opportunities, not always balanced, are part of the context. Referring back again to the previous example of the student suffering in an unsatisfactory school environment, this adolescent's decision may by limited by his family's lack of financial means or by the fact that in the small town where he lives, not all types of schools are present. Other more dramatic examples might be adolescents who grow up in war-torn countries, in a period of major economic recession, or in a family where one of the parents has passed away. It is important, in any case, to remember that apart from the objective characteristics of the context, what actually makes the difference is each person's subjective representation of his or her environment, experience in that environment, and ability to confront it. In other words, there is no direct correspondence between the objective constraints and possibilities provided by one's environment (for example, a lower-than-average income) and what one personally experiences (feeling that he or she lacks resources for a successful future). Once again, what is important is the meaning that the individual attributes to his or her relationship with the world around him or her. The model of development as action in context can be considered "useful fiction" with a great deal of heuristic value (Silbereisen et al. 1986) because it recognizes the central role of the individual and his or her actions, which are meaningful and oriented toward different objectives although subject to numerous limitations.

The degree of complexity of actions carried out can also vary. At higher levels, we find long-term plans of action, such as deciding to enroll in a lyceum following middle school, for example, thus planning to pursue a university degree instead of joining the workforce immediately following secondary school. [In Italy, secondary school - which adolescents enter at 14 years - lasts five years, and at the end of this, they take a final examination. There are different paths for secondary school, with diverse specializations. Secondary schools can generally be divided into lyceums (classical, scientific, linguistic, psychopedagogic, artistic), technical institutes (for accountants, surveyors, industrial technicians), and professional institutes (with different specializations ranging from artisan or secretarial and tourism to social care). Lyceums

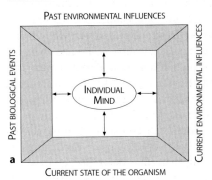

PAST ENVIRONMENTAL INFLUENCES

PAST BIOLOGICAL EVENTS

INDIVIDUAL MIND

CURRENT ENVIRONMENTAL INFLUENCES

a

CURRENT STATE OF THE ORGANISM

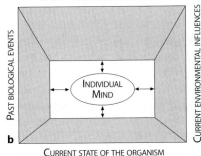

PAST ENVIRONMENTAL INFLUENCES

PAST BIOLOGICAL EVENTS

INDIVIDUAL MIND

CURRENT ENVIRONMENTAL INFLUENCES

b

CURRENT STATE OF THE ORGANISM

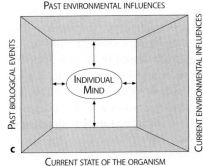

PAST ENVIRONMENTAL INFLUENCES

PAST BIOLOGICAL EVENTS

INDIVIDUAL MIND

CURRENT ENVIRONMENTAL INFLUENCES

c

CURRENT STATE OF THE ORGANISM

☐ AREA OF RESOURCES

▨ AREA OF LIMITATIONS

Fig. 1.5. Schematic representation of the area of resources and limitations. The figure shows how the individual must act within an area of opportunities and resources (both personal and contextual) surrounded by an area of limitations and obstacles. Panels **b**, **c** show how the size of this area can be different for every individual at a given moment in their development. The action of each, at a specific time of life, is carried out by drawing from certain personal or contextual resources while some other resources are unavailable. Panel **b** may represents an adolescent with a troubled, conflict-ridden family life during childhood, which in turn leads to greater limitations and less opportunity in the present. Panel **c** may be representative of an adolescent who attends a very unsatisfactory school. The opportunities and limits to the adolescent's development can increase, decrease, or disappear over time based on the actions of the individual. The individual can alter the dimensions of the area, although not without constraints, in the following ways: acting on the consequences of past environmental influences; acting on the current environment; acting on the current state of the organism; acting on the consequences of past biological events. For example, the use of psychoactive substances influences the present neurophysiological conditions, reducing the area of available resources and, as a consequence, causing greater limitations to cognitive elaboration. At the same time, this action also affects the adolescent's present environment due to the strain it causes in relationships with family members. Again, it is the individual's representations that mediate the action. These representations can change over time, contributing to the expansion or reduction of resources and obstacles that originate from past experiences. For example, a different representation of a long-past experience, re-elaborated through memory, can lead to a change in the emotional value placed on it and its potential to influence the present; memory is not a photographic reproduction of the past but, rather, a constant reconstruction (Schacter 1996). An example of this might be the different representation a woman can have of her ambivalent attachment to her mother, allowing her to be a good mother to her children despite a negative past experience.

offer a wider general education giving more emphasis to Italian and foreign literature, history, and philosophy; technical and professional institutes mostly emphasize practical subjects and focus on preparation that aims for a faster insertion into the workforce.] At an intermediate level, we find less-complex and less-lengthy sequences of action that can either facilitate a plan of action or make it more difficult. An example might be the decision to attend a language course to make better marks both in secondary school and at university. At a lower level, we find the single instrumental acts that can either facilitate or hinder the reaching of intermediate and long-term goals: for example, deciding whether or not to go out with friends in the evening when tired of studying but still having English homework to finish for the following day. These levels can be considered in a hierarchical sequence but in adolescence, there is actually a complex interrelationship between them. While on one hand the adolescent's newly acquired cognitive capacities make it possible to formulate long-term plans of action, the future often appears vague and distant and can hardly be considered important. At the same time, the effective capacity to postpone satisfaction conflicts with the trend - so strongly emphasized in Western culture - to favor immediate gratification.

As already noted, an action has the important consequence of producing changes both in an individual and in his or her surrounding environment. Precisely because of these changes, development itself is seen as a self-regulated process in which an individual's choices can either modify the course of developmental in a positive or negative way or else maintain the development path that has been undertaken. For example, an adolescent's decision, whatever the motivation may be, to do volunteer work might change his or her values and world view and seriously alter his or her future choices. Numerous studies have shown that competent adolescents who are able to plan for their future and make choices that will be useful for their future are better able to acquire and maintain social supports and to reach their objectives. The outcome for these adolescents is that in adulthood and with maturity, they achieve positive results that in turn build their self-esteem, triggering a virtuous cycle of success (Clausen 1991). Another case of adolescent action that has a profound influence on future development is the precocious assumption of an adult role. An example of this might be early initiation in the workforce or marriage at a young age, both of which often compromise personal and social development in the long term and limit richer or more advanced future achievements.

At the same time, an individual's actions also alter his or her social context. While in a more traditional perspective the environment's effect on the individual was particularly emphasized (for example, the influence of peer-group models on the behavior of adolescents), today it is recognized that individuals also exert an important influence on the environment in which they live. First of all, individuals select the environments with which they interact; for example, when they choose to spend time with a particular peer group or make friends with one person instead of another. Furthermore, their behavior within a certain environment alters the environment itself. For instance, a particularly creative, extroverted adolescent who is able to involve a group of friends in various activities and to establish quality relationships with others in turn contributes to creating a positive environment that he or she benefits from. The ability to select and mould one's environment in such a way as to influence one's own development improves throughout childhood to adolescence (Lerner 1998). In fact, it is in this age group that individuals acquire the cognitive and relational capabilities that allow them to have a greater impact on themselves and their environment and, consequently, on their own development. Although enormous individual differences exist, it has been shown that some particular processes allow adolescents to exert such an influence: these processes have been identified as personal objectives, identity, a sense of self-efficacy, and ability to plan (Crockett and Silbereisen 2000a).

1.3 Developmental Tasks

One of the most interesting aspects of the interaction between individual and context concerns the developmental tasks that, little by little, the individual is confronted with. As individuals progress gradually through the life cycle, they find that they have to resolve a series of specific tasks characteristic of each stage of existence. These tasks derive from an interaction between physiological maturation, new cognitive and relational capabilities, and individual aspirations, on the one hand, and the combination of influences, requirements, and societal norms, on the other hand. According to the definition by Havighurst (1952, 1953), who introduced this concept, overcoming the developmental tasks that characterize each stage of life leads to a state of well-being and a harmonious, well-adjusted relationship between the individual and his or her social context; heightened self-esteem; and a foundation laid to successfully reach the developmental tasks of future stages. One example of a developmental task that is characteristic of our society is learning to read and write in the early years of childhood.

With regard to adolescence, the general and universal developmental tasks are identified as follows (Palmonari 1997):
- Developmental tasks related to puberty and sexual maturation
- Developmental tasks related to the broadening of personal and social interests and the acquisition of hypothetical and deductive reasoning
- Developmental tasks related to identity construction and the reorganization of the concept of self

This description offers a general framework on which to base a more precise identification of the specific developmental tasks that adolescents are faced with at a given moment of their personal development. The primary developmental task that an adolescent must face in relation to sexual and cognitive development clearly rests in the formation of his or her own clear and distinct identity, which allows the individual to face the world in an autonomous, coherent, and responsible way. The ability to do so is recognized as an adult characteristic; thus, we consider adolescence to be terminated when these capabilities have been at least sufficiently acquired (Box 1.1). Today, there is consensus in the life-cycle perspective on the fact that identity development occurs throughout the entire existence of the individual and that it is therefore appropriate to discuss construction rather than acquisition of identity in adolescence. Even the concept of crisis between identity and role confusion, characteristic of Erikson's conception (1950, 1958), has been substituted by the more neutral concept of exploration (Marcia 1996). In fact, there is a growing awareness, which has matured based on empirical evidence, that for the majority of adolescents the development of identity does not involve particularly conflictual situations as much as times of exploration of varied length related to different areas that can be resolved or not through the construction of various aspects relevant to individual identity. Identity is no longer defined as a single construction but as a dynamic, complex, and not necessarily uniform system that is continuously reorganized by the individual.

As they originate from the confrontation between a precise social context and an individual at a precise moment of that individual's physical and psychological development, developmental tasks, especially in a rapidly changing society, are not unalterable over time. As both the requirements of society and the opportunities it offers have changed, being an adolescent today is quite different from being an adolescent at the beginning of the 20th century. Even tasks

Box 1.1. **Developmental Tasks in Adolescence**

In 1953, Havighurst identified the following developmental tasks typically accomplished during adolescence:
- Establish new and more mature relationships with peers of both genders
- Prepare for marriage and family life
- Develop intellectual competencies and knowledge necessary for civic competence
- Have a desire to be and to behave in a socially responsible way
- Acquire a system of values and an ethical conscience that guide behavior
- Gain emotional independence from parents and other adults
- Aim and prepare for an occupation or profession
- Acquire a masculine or feminine social role
- Accept one's own body and use it effectively.

This list clearly shows that developmental tasks depend both on historical period and social context. In fact, the above-listed developmental tasks relate to white, middle-class North American adolescents in the 1950s. Since that time, attempts have been made to redefine and update the developmental tasks while the concept has been criticized for its generic nature and for lack of empirical criteria for evaluation (Koops 1996). Instead of attempting to make an exhaustive list of developmental tasks, which would inevitably be incomplete and his-

that can be considered universal, such as the ability to establish heterosexual relationships, can vary widely within the same Western society in relation to the specific family, school, and social contexts that the adolescent has been raised in. This developmental task is carried out in different ways in European society, depending on the educational background of the family and the different school paths, within the different national cultures (for example, the Nordic as opposed to the Mediterranean model). Both the moment (for example, age of leaving the family home, age of maternity and paternity) and the way in which certain tasks are carried out (for example, marriage, living together, stable relationship without living together, no stable relationship) can vary greatly.

In particular, it has been noted that the additional requirements placed by today's society on adolescents are both more complex and less clearly defined. One example is the ambiguity of professional and personal goals to be achieved in a society that is filled with contrasting values and in which professional profiles change rapidly. This lack of clarity is combined with the requirement to make a precise decision about the type of school to attend, a decision that can have major consequences on the adolescent's future.

In other words, the universal task of constructing an identity and, consequently, of gaining autonomy and adult responsibilities can occur in very different ways depending on the individual and his or her context. An individualized developmental path is defined based on the different developmental tasks and the different solutions that each individual chooses. It has been shown

Box 1.1.

torically dated, it would be better not to reify developmental tasks but to apply the notion to analyze the different and multiple problems that every adolescent, boy or girl, must face and overcome in order to construct an identity and gain autonomy from adults (Palmonari 1997), both on an individual as well as an interpersonal and institutional level. It is the construction of an autonomous adult identity that can truly be considered the fundamental developmental task of adolescence. This task, however, can be carried out in different ways based on the historical setting and specific sociocultural context that the individual belongs to.

In Western culture, adolescents are given the opportunity to develop their identity in a condition of "social suspension," meaning that while they already have many of the characteristics of adults, they are free from the responsibilities of adulthood. While this state of suspended social status may cause some difficulty for adolescents - as it can signify a lack of participation in society, marginalization, and separation in a world of school and leisure time - it also allows adolescents to use their personal resources in the process of constructing their identity and forming new relationships with the world around them without rush. The literature indicates that assuming adult roles precociously in adolescence, for example by entering the workforce, often compromises personal and social development in the long-term and can place limitations on more advanced future achievements.

that having the opportunity to face demanding developmental tasks in a sequence and not at the same time serves as an important protective factor (Coleman 1989). The majority of adolescents do well when facing even complex developmental tasks because they are able to confront them one at a time. When adolescents are requested to confront many tasks at the same time, they can have serious difficulties. For example, an adolescent may successfully confront the tasks that involve exploration of the social world outside the family and be progressing in the ability to establish significant friendships. The next task to overcome would be preparing to enter the workforce. If a tragic event, such as the death of the family breadwinner, forces the adolescent to start working prematurely, the demands of this task could make resolving the first task more difficult, and the adolescent could suffer as a result.

The concept of developmental tasks allows us to identify the social expectations that apply to adolescents. These expectations form a point of reference for the development of an adolescent's individual objectives. As we have seen, these objectives in turn guide the actions of that adolescent. It is based on developmental tasks that adolescents carry out self-regulated actions aimed at achieving personally significant objectives. From this it can be inferred that it is necessary to go beyond the exterior appearance of behavior to comprehend which objectives the adolescent aims to reach with a particular action in relation to one or more of the developmental tasks characteristic of his or her culture or social context. This means that types of behavior that appear similar may have very different motivations. For example, some students who are still dependent on their parents and eager to seek their approval may work hard in school mainly to please their parents while for others, working hard in school may be a way to reach greater autonomy from their parents through the academic success. On the contrary, very different types of behavior can also have similar objectives; for example, while dangerous behavior such as using drugs can serve the objective of affirming one's self and identity, this objective can also be reached through socially productive behavior such as, for example, working to help others.

1.4 Risk and Well-Being

The various individual paths to development during adolescence are therefore the result of actions oriented toward objectives that have a specific meaning for each individual adolescent. The adolescent, with his or her own unique biological characteristics and history, responds differently to the developmental tasks posed by the particular context in which he or she lives. The action carried out in turn has an influence on both the individual and his or her context. These different developmental paths, although quite varied, are not as pervasively problematic and maladjusted as is often thought. As already noted, empiric research has demonstrated that the situation is quite the opposite; only a minority of adolescents experience major difficulties while the majority make the transition from youth to adulthood without seriously jeopardizing their health and well-being (Koops 1996). Adolescence is undoubtedly a time of transition that, along with a certain degree of continuity with the past, also presents strong discontinuity. It is often these elements of discontinuity, which are certainly numerous compared to previous ages, that attract the attention of many parents, teachers, and adults, giving the impression that the condition of adolescents is generally one of suffering and danger. Examples of this discontinuity apply not only to the physical appearance and physiological and sexual maturation of adolescents, but also to the way they think, the way they behave, and the way they interact with adults and their peers. The mass media, trying to capture the attention of an audience who has become used to all the "noise," emphasizes the most shocking, negative events involving adolescents, contributing to creating the erroneous impression that a very large number of adolescents are involved in risky or criminal activities. Based on a common error in judgment caused by the availability heuristic, we tend to believe that those types of behavior we hear talked about the most, and that we remember most easily, are the ones that occur most frequently. For this reason, many adults lack the more realistic view of adolescence as a time when the majority of boys and girls are gradually constructing, through often trying personal elaboration, a balanced and differentiated relationship between themselves and the world around them (Verhofstadt-Denève et al. 1996). Once again, it is important to remember that development, throughout the entire life cycle, experiences times of imbalance from which a new, more differentiated, and more complex psychological organization emerges; it is this, in fact, that distinguishes development from simple change.

It is important to note that our vision of adolescence began to change when all adolescents began to be studied and not only those suffering from various pathologies or involved in delinquency or drug abuse. The methodological error of moving from an analysis of a pathological condition to explain normal behavior occurred in the past not only with adolescence. Just consider for example how, for years, the normal behavior of children was interpreted based on models drawn from studies of pathological behavior in adults who were asked to reconstruct backward the phases of their own development based on their memories. While for the study of infancy and childhood these conceptions have become obsolete, for adolescence, they have persisted more easily as, indeed, at this age, a significant number of adolescents show problematic or risky behavior that can surprise, disturb, or worry adults (Jessor and Jessor 1977). The visibility and exaggeration of many types of adolescent behavior has led us to confuse normal development in which this conduct is transitory, with pathological development in which, on the contrary, these types of behavior persist over time. Thus, it was erroneously believed that all these adolescents could be grouped together and that the behavior of normal adolescents could be interpreted based on that of pathological adolescents. Today, it is evident to all scholars that the development of all adolescents cannot be explained through an analysis of only those developmental trajectories that have led to a failure (Jessor et al. 1991), as the processes involved are different. We will return to this topic shortly (Fig. 1.6).

The challenge of development is experienced in adolescence jointly with the adolescent's parents, peers, and teachers within a precise community; therefore, it is an undertaking that involves not only adolescents but many other people and social contexts that constitute the fabric within which growth is achieved. In this sense, adolescence is an effort that involves not only the family but also the school and even the community that the adolescent belongs to, despite the fact that this community is not always aware of the role it plays and often considers the adolescent more as a foreign or damaged element than a vital part of the social fabric (Box 1.2).

It is precisely this relationship between the adolescent and his or her context that must be referred to in order to comprehend risk behavior in adolescence. These are types of behavior that appear at this age and that can, in a

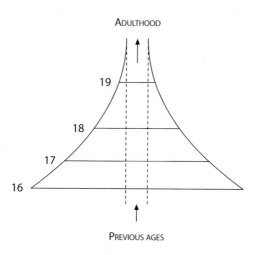

ADULTHOOD

19

18

17

16

PREVIOUS AGES

Fig. 1.6. A dual trend can be found in some types of risk behavior, such as deviant behavior (discussed in detail in Chap. 5). This type of conduct is more common in adolescents between the ages of 16 and 17 and tends to decrease with age in the great majority of adolescents. For this reason, they have been defined as "desistent." For these adolescents, deviant behavior can perform, in Western society today, functions related to identity development and social participation, such as transgression, self-experimentation, and the sharing of actions and emotions with friends. Some adolescents, mostly boys, continue, however, to manifest deviant behavior even in the later years of adolescence and into adulthood. These subjects have been defined as "persistent" (Moffit 1993; Moffit et al. 2001); not only were they deviant at 16-17 years of age, but their behavior was already irregular at earlier ages. In these adolescents, deviant behavior does not perform the functions mentioned above but is related to other processes and has other origins. An analysis restricted to only these adolescents would not allow comprehension of deviant behavior of the large majority of adolescents and would risk offering a wrong explanation of the motivations behind these adolescents' behavior.

direct or indirect way, jeopardize social and psychological well-being as well as physical health in the present and future. Thus, a little girl who had always up to that moment obediently followed the dietary habits of the family, might suddenly decide to refuse these habits in exchange for a dangerous diet or unhealthy eating habits. Other adolescents show curiosity and interest in psychoactive substances and begin to experiment with their use. This use can then stabilize, becoming a habit that carries over into adulthood, such as cigarette smoking, for example, the harmful effects of which on one's physical health cannot be perceived in the short term. Other behavior that appears at this age, such as risky driving, for example, can have immediate negative effects on one's physical health and survival; in Italy, car accidents are the primary cause of death for young people. Still other behavior, such as precocious or unprotected sex, can involve psychological and social risks, such as early pregnancy or physical risks tied to sexually transmitted diseases. In the case of other behavior, such as vandalism or theft, the risks involved are mainly psychological and social, as it undermines the peaceful relationship between the individual and the society in which he or she lives. The majority of boys and girls give up in later years some of the risky behavior that emerged during adolescence: this is generally the case for marijuana use as well as many other types of deviant behavior (Jessor and Jessor 1977; Silbereisen et al. 1986; Silbereisen and Noack 1988).

The few examples stated here illustrate that these are different types of behavior that have, however, the common characteristic of being able to compromise the physical, psychological, and social well-being of the adolescent in the present as well as in the long term. In a more restrictive theoretical perspective than the one used today, based largely on the norms and expectations of society, this type of behavior was defined in the past as "problem behavior." Today, in a broader theoretical perspective that takes into consideration the physical, psychological, and social well-being of the adolescent, we commonly refer to risk behavior (Jessor 1998), as it can compromise both physical health and psychosocial well-being. These types of behavior vary widely and hence have often been examined separately in literature; smoking marijuana is not evidently the same as being involved in a sexual relationship. In reality, however, these types of behavior, although very different in the way they are carried out and in their consequences, are linked to common problems characteristic of adolescence. For this reason, in order to comprehend them, it is necessary to go beyond an analysis that is limited to each single, specific behavior. Instead, we must take a broader, more in-depth view of the interactions between various types of behavior, what they have in common, and what causes them to appear - often they are not isolated but associated in the form of a syndrome - at this time in the life of an individual (Jessor and Jessor 1977).

The widespread nature of risk behavior during adolescence in Western culture and the fact that many types tend to disappear or diminish successively in the majority of young people and adults clearly demonstrates that it is impossible to interpret them in terms of individual psychopathology, a theoretical and methodological error which has often been made in the past. Neither is it possible to interpret risk behavior as an expression of social psychopathology, as the term used in a metaphorical sense assumes a generic meaning that lacks heuristic value and is disparaging when applied to large groups of otherwise well-adjusted adolescents. Just consider that roughly one fourth of adolescents today in Italy between the ages of 16 and 17 have smoked marijuana at least once. Some decades ago, Jessor wrote - quite provocatively at that time - that these types of behavior are not necessarily irrational, perverse, or pathological; for adolescents, they can fulfill important functions and can be essential aspects of psychosocial development (Jessor and Jessor 1977). With regard to the functions carried out by alcohol consumption, he also pointed out that maturation and the process of separation from the family occurred later in nondrinkers.

Just as they cannot be interpreted in terms of psychopathology, these types of behavior also cannot be explained as being the result of the mechanical repetition of the environmental models offered by their peers (Engels 1998).

Box 1.2. **Adolescence as a Conflict and Problem: An Adult Projection**

Developmental psychologists today agree that the representation of adolescence as a period of drama and conflict, which dates back to the Romantic period and the study of Stanley Hall (1904), does not correspond with reality. Today's more positive vision of adolescence is based on empirical evidence gathered from numerous studies. Nevertheless, the belief that adolescence is a time of storm and stress remains strong in Western society's popular psychology and is loudly sustained by the media. Those who seek to present more realistic data, related to suicide or crime, for example, are often accused of having an overly simplistic, superficial view of the problem and of a guilty unwillingness to own up and take care of the drama of adolescent suffering.

In an attempt to explain the pervasiveness and insistence in maintaining a negative cultural representation of adolescence, Meeus (1994) advanced the hypothesis of a reversed generation gap. His analysis was based on studies of the opinions of adolescents and adults on their own and the other generation. The results of these studies show that adults have a more negative opinion of the next generation than of their own while adolescents, on the other hand, have a more positive view of adults than of their own peers. Therefore, it is inaccurate to speak of adolescents harboring hostility toward adults; in reality, it is the adult generation who has a hostile attitude toward adolescents. Nevertheless, adults are convinced that adolescents have an attitude of opposition toward them, a belief, claims the author, that results from a projection mechanism through which adults attribute their own negative attitudes to the younger generation. This projection by adults forms the basis for their belief in the generation gap and the diversity, in a negative sense, between themselves and adolescents. The emphasis on the discord and negativity of adolescence as opposed to adulthood is therefore the result of a defense mechanism used by adults to deal with the successive generation, which they both envy and view as a threat. This would explain both the persistence in public opinion and in mass media of the negative view of adoles-

Individuals, in fact, are not externally regulated and do not act in an entirely passive way toward others of their age. Quite on the contrary, they actively select their peers, as we will see in greater detail in the chapter dedicated to psychoactive substances. Our research findings on this topic confirm that peer influence is much weaker than is commonly believed and does not necessarily counteract the influence of parents although peer influence is stronger where family relationships are lacking or are conflictual (Cattelino and Bonino 1999, 2000; Bonino 2000, 2001; Cattelino et al. 2001).

In summary, these actions must be considered as a means, used by numerous adolescents at a specific time of their lives and in a particular context, of reaching personally and socially meaningful objectives. The model of development as action in context allows us to understand these types of behavior as self-regulated and oriented toward reaching significant objectives concerning individual development; these actions actually express an attempt to overcome difficulty. In no other case than in risk behavior has it been so clear

Box 1.2.

cence as a period of opposition, difficulty, and conflict, as well as the resistance to change this representation despite much evidence to the contrary.

This defense mechanism also seems to be quite common in various historical periods, attested to by this passage from a 3,000-year-old Phoenician text that many today would agree with: "Today's youth are devoted to the devil, godless and lazy. They will never again be like the youth of the past and they will never succeed in lending continuity to our culture." It is not difficult to find other proof of similar prejudices toward youth from many other more recent time periods and in many different cultures. It appears that there is nothing new in the attitudes of adults in today's Western society if not the fact that modern media have given adults of our era much more powerful tools to convince themselves - and, unfortunately, teenagers as well - of the drama of adolescence. Consider, for instance, how frequently we hear degrading terms used in the news to refer to adolescents, such as "gang" instead of "group". The result is the formation of a deep-rooted negative attitude toward the young generation, which runs the risk of initiating a vicious cycle in which adolescents, in a kind of perverse self-fulfilling prophecy, actually do become a problem and cease to be a positive resource for the community.

Because the elderly population in the Western world is steadily increasing due to better living conditions and the widespread availability of advanced medicine, this negative prejudice toward youth may worsen in time. The increasingly strong tendency to separate individuals by age group may also serve to accentuate this prejudice. Although not as marked in Italy as in North America, there are many signs of this negative tendency, supported by the consumer industry, to separate the experience of adolescents and emerging adults from that of adults and the elderly (Csikszentmihalyi and Schneider 2000). For these reasons, situations that allow for interaction between different generations, involved in common activities and projects, should be seen as valuable opportunities for both individual and community development.

how greatly individual action can affect the development of an adolescent. Just think of the devastating, often irreversible, consequences that a risk behavior such as dangerous driving can have on the life of an adolescent. Similarly, involvement, even if temporary, in the use of psychoactive substances can have serious consequences. In addition to the direct effects it has on the functioning of the nervous system, drug use can also lead to marginalization from society, which can in turn limit the social and cognitive development of the adolescent. Especially in the case of drug use, behavior can become automatic, following an initial phase in which the behavior is carried out for the positive functions it seems to serve.

This phenomenon of becoming automatic, a clear example of which is cigarette smoking, does not apply to all adolescents but only to a small minority of heavy users and becomes more evident in adults (Engels 1998). Even so, it can limit the development of an individual's full potential and make it more difficult to discontinue use of the substance.

1.5 Functions of Risk Behavior

Adolescents act within a certain context, not by casual manner but in order to reach precise, personally significant aims related to the developmental tasks of a certain culture. Therefore, cognitive processes of evaluation, mediated by the symbolic systems provided by the culture, play a central role; in fact, it is the individuals' representations that guide their actions and give meaning to their emotional and affective experiences. For example, a biological occurrence, such as sexual maturation, common in all boys and girls can take on very different meanings for different adolescents, depending on both their past and present and the particular values and expectations of their cultural context. Their experience of this process may be positive, seen as a sign of development but not yet as a real initiation into adult life; it can be seen as a clear division between childhood and adulthood and therefore signify the start of adult life; it can be experienced in a negative way, seen as a condition that exposes one to the risks of pregnancy or unwanted behavior. The way in which boys and girls then choose to act, for example to have sex or not to have sex, is a result of the meanings, which are widely varying and often contradictory, that they attribute to the action in a particular moment of their development and the objectives that they aim to reach.

Thus, it becomes evident that the actions of adolescents, whether they are dangerous or healthy, have a precise function, as they serve adolescents in reaching personally and socially meaningful objectives for growth during the adolescent transition. Affirming this implies the necessity to go beyond the simple description of a behavior and to comprehend what meaning this behavior has for the particular adolescent who acts it out. Very different types of behavior, both risky and otherwise, can actually be carried out to serve similar aims for growth and are therefore "functionally equivalent" (Silbereisen and Noack 1988). For example, the goal of achieving one's autonomy from adults can be reached either through risk behavior, such as smoking cigarettes or marijuana, or through more socially advanced and competent behavior that is life expressing and supports the individual's own opinion. The choice of one or the other of these ways depends on both personal characteristics and the opportunities offered by the social context. Inversely, similar or identical behavior can actually be motivated by very different aims. For example, adolescents might choose to have sex in order to behave like their friends and therefore be accepted by their peers, or it might serve to show adults that they are "grown up." The personal significance attached to the behavior can differ between genders, as is the case with eating-related behavior (Spruijt-Metz 1999). The same behavior can have different meanings for different cultural groups. For example, it has been demonstrated that for German adolescents, alcohol consumption has mainly the function of raising self-esteem while for adolescents from Turkish families who have emigrated to Germany, the same behavior displays an opposition to traditional values (Silbereisen et al. 1990). Also, the relationship between developmental tasks and risk behavior is not unequivocal. A particular risk behavior may reflect an attempt to tackle different developmental tasks and therefore be "multifunctional" while a specific developmental challenge might lead to different behavior (Silbereisen et al. 1986).

The functions of all the different types of risk behavior fall into two main, tightly connected areas related to identity development on one hand and participation in society on the other. As we saw earlier when discussing developmental tasks, the fundamental developmental task in adolescence, which can be achieved through specific and differing tasks based on the culture, is to construct one's own identity, which is at the same time individual and social (Box 1.3). People construct their identities through social interaction that begins with a physical body to which both the individual and others assign an identity. This means that in adolescence, the construction of one's identity occurs through the redefinition and construction of new relationships with adults and peers. The functions of various types of risk behavior in adolescence are closely associated precisely because they are all connected to the construction of an autonomous adult identity.

As already mentioned, both risky and healthy behavior can carry out the same functions in the process of constructing one's identity and redefining one's relationships. As we will see more clearly in the chapters to follow, the major differences in the degree or lack of involvement in various types of risk behavior can be traced back to the fact that some adolescents choose nonrisk behavior to reach growth objectives while for others, the developmental tasks characteristic of this age are overcome through behavior that entail varying degrees of risk. These differences are linked both to differences in the development of individual capabilities as well as different opportunities offered by the social context. An individual's actions contribute to increasing or decreasing both individual and social resources. For example, the use of psychoactive substances can diminish one's cognitive elaboration as well as reduce participation in groups performing a wider variety of activities. Involving adolescents in healthy, productive activities that are meaningful in terms of carrying out developmental tasks is the foundation for strategies that prevent risk behavior, which will be discussed at length in this book.

Although the different functions of risk behavior are strongly associated and, at times, partially overlapping, it is useful for clarity of presentation to consider them in a more analytical way. Let us consider, first of all, the functions that are most closely linked to identity development:

Box 1.3. **Identity Development: Continuity and Change**

Although the process of constructing an identity unfolds throughout the entire life of an individual, one of the crucial steps in this process occurs during adolescence and is prompted by both sexual and cognitive development as well as the demands of society. Identity can be defined as the relational and temporal quality of the experience of the Self. The Self, as recent research has shown, develops very early on (Stern 1985) and results from a dynamic relational process that refers to the validation of others and the personal elaboration of a sense of unity, coherence, and continuity over time. Therefore, cognitive, emotional, and social aspects are closely connected to the development of both Self and identity.

Identity is related to the social roles, beliefs, and values imposed by society. If on a personal level identity is experienced by each of us as a coherent sense of unity with the Self, even when we take on different roles at different times (phenomenological aspect), identity appears to others as a belief in certain values and an orientation toward a profession, role, or vocation (behavioral aspect). From a structural point of view, identity results from the dynamic interaction between the needs and competencies of an individual and the requirements or pressures of a particular society (Marcia 1980).

With this brief side note, we certainly do not intend, nor would it be possible, to offer a summary and discussion of the various theories that have been proposed on the concept of identity and its development during adolescence. For this we must refer to the literature on adolescents and on this specific topic. Here we mention just a few relevant points from the most recent developments in the research. In Erikson's classic theory, the "life conflict" that applies specifically to adolescents is the conflict between the two poles of identity and identity diffusion, where the acquisition of identity is defined as the dynamic equilibrium between involvement in and confusion about one's roles in society. The revision made by Marcia was focused on the possible identity statuses, which are defined as the interrelationship of two dimensions: exploration of alternatives (in the field of work, sexuality, family, values, religion, etc.) and commitment to the prechosen alternative. Marcia identified four identity statuses: the achievement of identity occurring when, through a process of exploration, a personal, original identity is elaborated; foreclosure, when this exploration does not occur and one is limited to imitating the models provided by significant adults; the diffusion of identity, when exploration leads only to momentary and dispersive identity development without a lasting commitment; moratorium, when the explo-

Adulthood. This entails the precocious acting out of behavior considered normal in adults, such as cigarette smoking, alcohol consumption, or sexual behavior. As stated previously, adolescents in Western society live in an "in-between" status where their entry into the adult world is delayed. Despite the advantage of a period that is free from obligations during which adolescents can dedicate themselves to experimentation and the construction of personal identity, this condition can be a source of difficulty and can stimulate some adolescents to assume some of the exterior, visible behavior thought to signify adulthood

Box 1.3.

ration concludes without results and the attempt is postponed due to a difficulty in finding a point of equilibrium between one's ambitions and reality.
The critical analysis of these theories has led to an understanding that the construction of identity does not occur in absolute, "all or nothing" terms but, rather, in relative terms; in other words, identity is constructed in different ways in different areas of life. This means that the commitment and involvement in significant areas of life varies and can occur at different times, be more or less critical, and can have different resolutions (Bosma and Jackson 1990). The concept of imperfect identity (Palmonari et al. 1979; Palmonari 1997) refers to the statement that identity construction in adolescence is a prolonged and differentiated process during which different conflicts and critical moments can be faced and resolved at different times and in different areas in relation to the construction of the various components of identity. It must be added that in today's social context, defined as postmodern, the difficulty in constructing a stable, coherent identity persists even after adolescence in a growing number of people.
The most recent research redirects our attention from the definition of typologies to a comprehension of the processes involved in the evolution of identity in order to better understand different individual developmental paths. The interaction between the cognitive, social, and emotional aspects of identity has been studied in order to disprove the conception that identity is, more or less explicitly, a synonym for self-concept and to try to comprehend which processes safeguard our sense of the stability of identity over time in a life cycle perspective (Bosma and Kunnen 2001). By adopting a systemic view, we are able to understand the continuity of the sense of identity - despite the incessant changes that characterize the biological and psychological life - through the process of self-organization. In dynamic systems, this process allows order to emerge from disorder, with the structuring of first simple then gradually more complex forms into a higher level of organization (Lewis and Ferrari 2001; van Geert 2001) through a change in the relationship between the components of the system. Identity in particular comes out as the result of a continual and recurring self-evaluation in which narration - a powerful tool of construction and coherence - plays a central role. It has been shown that identity is a stable system that changes over time in a discontinuous, although regulated, way. Emotion and context are the conditions from which identity arises through a process of self-organization: identity is rooted in emotion, emerging in relationships and developing as a dynamic, self-organizing system (Bosma and Kunnen 2001).

(Silbereisen and Noack 1988). Acting out certain risk behavior allows adolescents to feel like adults by doing things that adults do, hence reinforcing their identity at a time when other essential aspects of adulthood are not achievable. Other adolescents, although they feel the same need, thanks to the different personal or environmental resources they possess, are able to find other less outwardly visible, superficial ways of experiencing adulthood, for example, by assuming responsibility or participating in the community by doing volunteer work. It must also be noted that in Western culture, young people are pushed by the mass media to develop adult consumer habits very early on because of huge economic interests seeking new markets to target - not only in adolescents but even in prepubescent children. Just think of the tobacco industry's advertising campaigns, first launched in the United States and then in Europe, designed to appeal to the very young.

Acquisition and affirmation of autonomy. Involved in the process of constructing an adult identity, adolescents must overcome their condition of dependence, characteristic of childhood, in order to acquire autonomy. This process is a lengthy one due to the fact that some aspects of autonomy, for example the economic aspect, occur quite late. Under this condition, the adolescent often acts out behavior that has the function of achieving autonomy in choices made regarding the norms, values, and advice of adults - and parents above all. This kind of autonomy is achieved essentially through greater participation in peer groups and the acceptance of its new rules as well as through the renegotiation of family relationships and the norms that govern those relationships in order to gain a greater degree of reciprocity. Autonomy, first conquered through the small decisions made in daily life, increasingly extends to include more important aspects, such as major life choices. The achievement of autonomy is often signaled, both to adolescents themselves and to others, in an obvious, highly externalized way in order to ensure that it will not go unnoticed. Insecurity in their ability to be truly autonomous can cause adolescents to act in a showy and, at times, ostentatious way. Even involvement in risk behavior often serves the function of demonstrating to themselves and others that they possess the ability to make decisions in an autonomous way unaffected by the opinion of parents or other adults; this can be the case for drug use, sexual behavior, distorted eating behavior, or even antisocial behavior (Silbereisen and Kastner 1986). Many other types of nonrisk behavior can also be used in order to affirm one's autonomy, such as supporting an opinion, developing personal values, or making decisions about the future.

Identification and differentiation. Adolescents therefore have the dual task of identifying themselves as individuals with particular characteristics and differentiating themselves from adults in general and first and foremost their parents, who were their first role models. Identification is achieved therefore by acting in a way that defines the adolescent and draws a distinction between the adolescent and adults. Many types of risk behavior, such as norm violation, fulfill this function, which naturally can also be carried out by safe behavior such as wearing eccentric clothing or showing unconventional ideas. In this process, the adolescent seeks the support of his or her peers who are also experiencing the same developmental processes. Consequently, identification and differentiation are achieved through group actions, both risky (for example, smoking in groups) and nonrisky (for example, going to concerts). These types of behavior cannot be interpreted, as often occurred in the past, solely in terms of peer influence and passive imitation. As many studies have recently demonstrated (Engels 1998), adolescents actively select their peers, seeking out those groups in which they find others who think and act like they do, thus reinforcing their own identities and their own inner consonance. This selection also responds to adolescents' need to differentiate themselves not only from their parents but also from people of their same age; for this reason, quite often, both individual adolescents and especially groups of adolescents openly declare their diversity and superiority compared with the behavior of other adolescents.

Self-affirmation and experimentation. This function deals mainly with the new and diverse physical, psychological, and social possibilities offered by cognitive and sexual development. Self-affirmation is achieved by testing oneself and one's abilities; very often this implies acting in a way that is different from what adults expect and from how one acted as a child. Self-affirmation and experimentation are tightly linked to the search for autonomy because the adolescent seeks to affirm autonomy from others, especially from adults. Because of the insecurity surrounding it, self-affirmation and experimentation often occur in a showy, exaggerated way through actions that can be extremely physically dangerous, such as being involved in risky games. Carrying out these strong and extreme actions is a way of declaring that childhood has been overcome. For these reasons, all risk behavior can serve the function of allowing adolescents to affirm themselves and experiment. In this case as well, it is evident from advertising messages that the current cultural context strongly approves of affirming one's identity and putting one's self to the test in a variety of fields, even through extremely risky behavior as in the case of dangerous driving. Many other types of nonrisk behavior could be used instead to carry out the self-affirmation and experimentation function, not only through physical activity but also in intellectual and school activities as well.

Transgression and surpassing limits. This function consists in going against the rules and laws of the adult world in order to declare, in a more obvious way, autonomy, independence, decision-making capacity, and a life style that conforms to adolescent needs. Deviant behavior and the use of illegal drugs are the types of risk behavior that most clearly express transgression. The use of legal drugs can perform the same function if the adolescent's environmental context regards it as inappropriate for the adolescent's particular age and gender. Transgression is also emphasized by the "in-between" condition in which adolescents live, relegated to a carefree dimension that is entirely separate from the adult world (Crockett 1997) in which rules may be seen as arbitrary and incomprehensible. Transgression can even be achieved through different means, such as violating the conventions and traditions of the family surrounding vacations or the celebration of holidays.

Exploration of sensations. Here the aim is to investigate and experience not only the new possibilities that result from sexual maturity but also those that can come from a different, more personal and autonomous way of living one's identity. The exploration of sensations is strongly associated with both self-affirmation and experimentation and seeking to achieve autonomy because in the process of constructing ones identity, the adolescent finds herself or himself wanting to experiment with new states of consciousness, explore different physical sensations, and feel new, previously unknown emotions. This adolescent need is reinforced in Western culture today by a strong pressure to experience new things and explore anything and everything that is different or unusual. The exploration of new sensations is particularly evident in the use of psychoactive substances, in sexual behavior, in risky driving, and in dangerous actions. Also in this case, many nondamaging types of behavior can perform the same function; think, for example, of the rush of energy that comes with playing sports, the emotion that is stirred by music or poetry, or the sensations provoked by traveling to a new place.

Perception of control. The moment adolescents put their identity to the test and explore their possibilities by seeking out new sensations, they must also try to overcome the fear that can come with these new sensations by seeking to have control over their own actions rather than being governed by adults. This can lead adolescents to carry out risky actions in order to demonstrate that they are capable of resisting, that they cannot be overcome, and that they are in charge of the situation and can leave it when they want to without any damage. Many types of risk behavior, such as those related to diet, aim to demonstrate an ability to control their own reality at a time when they have a great deal of uncertainty about who they are. Naturally this perception of control and invulnerability is at the most illusory and can have severe, even deadly, consequences because the ability to avoid dependence is overevaluated (for example, in the case of psychoactive substances), as is the ability to effectively control the situation (for example, in the case of risky driving or dangerous actions in general).

Coping and escape. Coping methods are the sociocognitive strategies that allow individuals to deal with the difficulties, personal problems, and relationship problems of daily life in a healthy, well-adjusted way. In adolescence, the most common problems that must be dealt with are linked to redefining relationships with parents, resolving school-related difficulties, socializing with peers, and friendships and relationships with members of the opposite gender (Frydenberg 1997). When the adolescent is not able to effectively deal with the task itself, meaning the identification and resolution of the problem, emotional strategies are employed that seek to bring an immediate emotional resolution to the problem (Labouvie 1986; Bosma and Jackson 1990). Some types of risk behavior - for example the use of marijuana and other drugs, alcohol abuse, disordered eating, and comfort eating - can also be used as coping strategies to deal with the failure to meet the requirements of family, school, or social environment (Silbereisen and Noack 1988). These attempts at dealing with problems, however, are illusory and lead to further failures. Such behavior not only fails to resolve adolescents' problems, it adds to them and make them worse, creating even greater cognitive and relational difficulties. In the most serious cases, heavy involvement in risk behavior acts as an extreme form of defense - an actual escape from reality and all of the difficulties that the adolescent feels unprepared to resolve and at times even to express.

Now let us consider the main functions linked to the redefinition of social relationships, both with adults and others of the same age:

Communication. The need to communicate with others of the same age is very important for adolescents, as it constitutes the first step toward getting to know others and establishing deeper, more meaningful relationships. Some types of risk behavior are used precisely because they encourage communication and contribute to creating an atmosphere of relaxation, openness, and well-being in social situations. This is the case with some psychoactive substances, such as marijuana and moderate alcohol consumption, which give a pleasant sense of fluidity to social situation, eliminating inhibitions and providing an atmosphere of closeness and intimacy. Other types of behavior create an opportunity to communicate with peers by doing something similar, relying on actions more than words. This is the case with cigarette smoking, which is used often to overcome embarrassment in social situations or as a way to start conversation with another person, for example, by offering or asking for a cigarette (Silbereisen and Noack 1988). The greater the difficulty in communicating, the more adolescents rely on actions to communicate.

Sharing of actions and emotions. As was already pointed out in the discussion of identification and differentiation, individual identity is not constructed in a vacuum. The individual achieves and expresses individuality through the sharing of experiences, feelings, and emotions with others in the same age group. Many types of risk behavior, because they imply concrete, visible actions carried out with others, offer easy, tangible ways for adolescents to express their identity as part of a group in order to gain recognition, reputation, and popularity. This is the case with the use of psychoactive substances as well as deviant or dangerous actions. The sharing of such actions reinforces individual identity in that "the private claim of an identity depends upon public acceptance of that claim and the social support for expressing that claim" (Emler and Reicher 1995). Many actions that adolescents carry out individually are actually acted out so that they can tell their peers about it later on. These actions also allow the group to gain the kind of visibility and attention, even if negative, that adolescents generally do not receive. When the context offers opportunities to participate in society in a positive way (for example, sharing in activities enjoyed by the community), adolescents can achieve the same objectives through nonrisk behavior.

Bonding rituals and rites of passage. Many types of risk behavior carried out with peers are aimed at forming a bond with others of the same age through ritualized behavior characterized by repetition, redundancy, and exaggeration of particular actions (Eibl-Eibesfeldt 1974); the ritual of sharing a cigarette or a joint is a clear example. Such behavior is also often at the same time a rites of passage; it marks the transition from childhood to a group of older kids who are not afraid to act decisively and at times to transgress. This function is expressed not only through the ritual use of tobacco, alcohol, or marijuana but also through aggressive behavior by the group or through sexual behavior. These actions serve as a marker signaling that these adolescents are no longer children. It should be noted that in Western culture, few emotionally charged and collectively significant bonding rituals, rites of initiation, and rites of passage exist although involvement in athletics and religious affiliation does offer some ritual.

Emulation. Within a group of peers, adolescents not only feel the need to conform to the actions of others and imitate them, they often also feel the need to enter into a sort of race, whether they make it known or not, in which every individual or every group tries to emulate and surpass the others. Out of this competition can come a progressive intensification in the gravity of involvement in risk behavior, the results of which can be dramatic. An illusion of control, which was mentioned previously, contributes to altering the realistic perception of risk and exposes the adolescent to hazards that cannot be controlled. This progressive increase in risky behavior, both in terms of quantity and quality, can involve such behavior as dangerous driving and dangerous games, deviant actions, the use of psychoactive substances, and dangerous sexual and eating behavior. In this case as well, school-related activities, for example, can also offer opportunities to compete with peers in nonrisk activities.

Exploration of reactions and limits. The adolescent, who is involved in the process of identification and differentiation and therefore in the affirmation of himself or herself as an autonomous individual, often carries out certain actions in order to test the reactions of adults, be it parents or teachers. Many transgressive types of behavior, involving varying degrees of danger to the individual or society, are acted out in order to observe the reactions of adults, to understand how attentive and interested they are in the behavior of the adolescent, to test the limits put in place by adults, to see what they can get away with, and to understand whether the rules are actually enforced. The age of adolescence demands that adolescents and adults take part in a continual, flexible process of redefining their relationships with one another, which must result in the adolescent's achievement of greater autonomy. Adults can facilitate this process by adopting authoritative, instructive attitudes that combine rules with dialogue and support. As with the other functions outlined, the exploration of reactions and limits can be achieved through actions that are harmful to the individual and social well-being (disordered eating, drug use, or deviant behavior, for example) or through other, less-risky methods (dressing in an unconventional way, for example).

Differentiation and opposition. As we have seen, the fundamental developmental task of adolescence is the redefinition of one's identity. In this process, adolescents seek identity models that are different from their parents and from adults in general. As a consequence, they seek new models among their peers and struggle against parental models, focussing on the aspects of difference and opposition. The passage from an all-powerful, unrealistic vision of one's parents, which is characteristic of childhood, to a more realistic vision that recognizes the limitations and imperfections of one's parents, is certainly not linear, nor is it painless. It takes place in phases of opposition and negativity where differences between adolescent and parent are emphasized. Only later on in young adulthood or as adults when identities are more solid is it possible to recognize the similarities between one's self and parents. For these reasons, many displays of opposition (for example, refusing the religious or political models of one's parents) and many types of risky behavior are acted out because of adolescents' needs to differentiate themselves by acting in a way that is contrary to the desires or beliefs of their parents.

The chart below summarizes the main functions that have been identified here related to the development of identity and the redefinition of relationships with adults and peers. Again, it must be noted that these aspects are tightly interrelated, and we have separated them here for clarity of presentation. Identity formation in reality does not occur in social isolation and is not an entirely intrapsychic process. On the contrary, it is an interpsychic process that is played out through social relationships within a certain culture.

Identity	Relationships
- Adulthood	*With peers:*
- Acquisition and affirmation of autonomy	- Communication
- Identification and differentiation	- Sharing of actions and emotions
- Self-affirmation and experimentation	- Bonding rituals and rites of passage
- Transgression and surpassing limits	- Emulation
- Perception of control	- Exploration of reactions and limits
- Exploration of sensations	*With adults:*
	- Exploration of reactions and limits
- *Coping* and escape	- Differentiation and opposition

CHAPTER 2

The Study

> Any major undertaking runs the risk of producing nothing or of having nothing interesting to say. Those who come into contact with that which has been produced don't care about the author's hard work; they want only to find something that expands their horizons and that provides them with a bit of knowledge.
>
> *[A. Palmonari, Foreword to G. Tonolo,*
> *Adolescence and Identity, 1999]*

2.1 Theoretical Framework and Objectives

The following chapters report the main findings of a wide-reaching study of risk behavior in adolescents. The study, based on a large sample of secondary school students between the ages of 14 and 19 years, examined different types of behavior that can pose risks, both immediately and in the long term, to the physical, psychological, and social well-being of adolescents: cigarette smoking, the use of marijuana and other drugs, heavy alcohol consumption, precocious and unprotected sex, antisocial behavior, dangerous driving, risk-taking behavior, and disordered eating. This research project was based on an interactionistic, constructivistic, theoretical model (discussed at length in the previous chapter) that considers individuals and their context as a system in which there is a constant and reciprocal interaction. In this model, the central focus is placed on individual action. Jessor's interpretive framework (Jessor and Jessor 1977) was used as the operational point of reference for the research conducted. This framework, which was highly innovative at the time of its development, has proven to maintain its validity over time (Jessor et al. 1991) and serves as the foundation for the methodological instrument - the questionnaire - used in our research. The study takes into consideration four areas (see Fig. 2.1) that constitute the four main variable systems, each of which interacts with the others: the behavior system, the personality system, the perceived environment system, and the social environment system.

First of all, risk is studied through an analysis of behavior, as it is, in fact, behavior that constitutes a problem: it can be harmful, dangerous, or disturbing. Certain types of behavior are organized in a systemic structure in which each one influences the other. Furthermore, the different types risk behavior rarely occur in an isolated manner; more often they form constellations that shape a person's lifestyle.

In terms of research, an analysis on two levels is required in order to comprehend the interaction between behavior types. On the one hand, the study must consider the interaction between various types of conduct, as different types of behavior can serve similar psychological functions and be oriented toward reaching common personal and social objectives. On the other hand, a more specific analysis is necessary, which considers all the differences existing between various behavior types. Hence, in studying the similarities and differences between the types of risk behavior, a delicate balance must be maintained in the analysis of both single aspects and their reciprocal interactions.

Within the behavioral system, other factors are also considered in addition to risk behavior: daily activities of adolescents, their participation in different kinds of groups, and other types of behavior that can counter, diminish, or increase the effects of risk behavior. In accordance with the theoretical model, all these behavior types are considered as significant actions that express a specific mode of interaction between the individual and his or her environment. An analysis of these behavior types is essential in order to comprehend the functions of each type of risk behavior and protective factors.

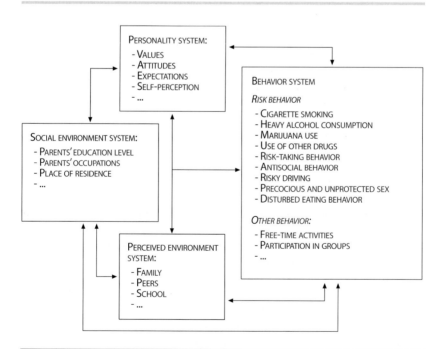

Fig. 2.1. The variable systems. Four reciprocally interacting systems considered in the questionnaire utilized in this study based on Jessor's conceptual model (modified by Jessor et al. 1991).

Within the personality system, in keeping with the constructivist model, particular attention has been dedicated to the processes of evaluation, elaboration, and construction of meaning of the world and of the individual's personal experiences with the conviction that it is impossible to comprehend human action without focussing on its specific symbolic meaning. Only by referring to this symbolic activity are we able to comprehend the complexity of human action and its emotional, affective, and social value. For these reasons, particular attention has been directed toward how adolescents interpret their external realities and their own experiences, how they evaluate the possibilities offered by their environment and their actions, how they anticipate the consequences of their own and others' actions, and what their interests and expectations are.

Because of the importance attributed to these aspects, the variables related to the environment system are mediated by the adolescents' individual representations. For this reason, the system has been defined as "perceived environment." For example, when we speak about "parental support," we are not referring to an objective evaluation of the parents' ability to provide support but rather an evaluation of the adolescents' perception of their parents' ability, or lack thereof, to provide support. As was clarified by Jessor, this choice is based on the conviction that the perceived environment - in the logic of explanation - is causally closer to behavior (Jessor et al. 1991). Recent literature has confirmed the effectiveness of this constructivist approach, showing that from a methodological standpoint, the evaluation of subjective "perception" is preferable to other, apparently more objective, measures (such as direct observation or assessment by parents, peers, and teachers) because perceived environment has a greater influence on the behavior of adolescents (Aunola et al. 2000). It is the personal experience of adolescents that they use to construct their attitudes and regulate their behavior. The system of perceived environment includes variables that can be grouped into three main areas in the life of the adolescent: family, and particularly parents; peer group and friends; and school. The daily experiences of adolescents unfold within these three contexts, and it is in these areas that adolescents are presented with developmental tasks to overcome (Palmonari 1997) as well as opportunities, proposals, and requirements.

Naturally, the social environment system is also considered, which consists of "objective" or sociodemographic variables, which have been examined previously to varying degrees, particularly in the sociological and epidemiological literature. The variables considered here include type of school attended, place of residence, composition and integrity of the family unit, and parents' education level.

The aim of this study was not only to discover the kinds of risk behavior adolescents are engaging in but primarily to begin to shed light on the functions of these behavior types and the protective and risk factors that can increase or diminish adolescents' involvement in them. A description of adolescent behavior is therefore not the main scope of this study but rather a preliminary objective, as it supplies us with some necessary, although alone insufficient, knowledge. The description is followed by an analysis of the main sociodemographic variables (in particular, gender, age, place of residence, type of school attended) and an analysis of the relationship between the variables connected to the various systems examined in the theoretical model and in the questionnaire that is based on this model (see Fig. 2.1). In reality, the functions carried out by certain types of risk behavior cannot be examined directly but can be comprehended by analyzing the relationships between different behavior types and between the various systems examined in the study. Based on this foundation, and always in light of our theoretical model, we can identify the main functions of risk behavior in this period of life, as well as the protective factors that allow the same positive functions to be fulfilled in terms of developmental tasks through nonrisk behavior or through involvement in risk behavior that is neither lasting nor serious.

This knowledge in turn provides the general methodological indications that can be useful in designing and executing effective prevention programs. In terms of prevention, an analysis of functions and protective factors is essential. The former allows us to understand why risk behavior is so alluring and provides an indication of which other types of behavior can substitute for risk behavior; the latter directs the intervention in a positive way, even where the risk factors, as is often the case, cannot be eliminated or altered.

This vast research project is cross-sectional in design. We are aware of the limitations of a cross-sectional design that does not allow an understanding of the changes and the processes involved in them: changes of behavior, of functions, of protective and risk factors. Within these limitations, a theoretically well based, cross-sectional design, can provide useful information about the variables that are related to risk behavior in the different age cohorts. To overcome this, we are conducting a longitudinal analysis on a part of the sample, which has not yet been finished. Also, cross-national comparisons (Ciairano 2004) and in-depth analyses of some of the topics based on interviews are currently in progress (Giannotta et al 2004). Some of the quotations found at the beginning of the chapters in this volume, which pertain to the various types of risk behavior considered, were extracted from these interviews. In addition, based on the results presented in this book, other research projects have been designed and are currently being conducted in order to study the specific role of school in the prevention of risk behavior.

2.2 The Instrument

The instrument utilized for this study is the specially designed questionnaire, *Io e la Mia Salute* (Me and My Health) (Bonino 1995, 1996), which is the Italian version of an analogous questionnaire developed at the University of Colorado (Boulder, USA) by Jessor (Health Behavior Questionnaire, 1992) and previously adapted in Europe in Poland (Frączek and Stepien 1990). The questionnaire was adapted for the Italian context through a lengthy process of revision and expansion, which lasted almost one year, carried out directly with adolescents in different secondary schools. Particular care was taken to ensure the print quality of the questionnaire in order to produce a text that was clear, legible, and aesthetically pleasing.

The questionnaire examines the four systems indicated in Fig. 2.1: the personality system, the social environment system, the perceived environment, and the behavior system. It is structured in such a way as to engage the adolescent gradually, starting with neutral questions related mainly to sociodemographic characteristics and leading up to increasingly personal and emotionally charged themes. As a result, the questions are not grouped according to the various systems identified; their sequence does not appear to have any kind of logical order, with different topics being touched upon and returned to in different places. Questions concerning different types of risk behavior are presented in blocks and are scattered throughout, always interspersed with neutral questions. The reason for this sequence was to keep the adolescents from becoming tired or losing interest and to avoid provoking defensive or insincere responses. The questionnaire contains a total of almost six hundred questions.

The "Appendix" includes a description of the variables used in the research made up of single questions or of scales formed from multiple questions. These are organized based on the conceptual framework displayed in Fig. 2.1 and are not in the order in which they appear in the questionnaire. For each question in the questionnaire, the contents and possible responses are reported, and for each scale, the statistical properties are reported. In the "Appendix," some of the particular procedures used for the description of data are also reported; these are indicated in each chapter.

The questionnaire was administered in schools by carefully selected and trained researchers in the absence of teachers; completed individually, anonymously, and in its entirety; and turned in immediately upon completion by 100% of the students sampled. Questionnaire administration was preceded by a presentation of the study to the schools and students and was followed by a presentation of some of the general results. The care dedicated to the presentation of the study and the conditions under which the questionnaire was completed, along with the assurance of anonymity, motivated the interest of the adolescents, who regarded the study with great interest, willingness, and seriousness, ensuring that the questionnaire would be completed with accurate, sincere responses.

2.3 The Sample

As has already been stated, developmental psychology today favors the study of people in normal life conditions, with the objective of comprehending the complexity of and factors that play a part in developmental paths. This choice of methodology has theoretical motivations, in particular to avoid an orientation centered on psychopathology, difficulty, or pathological outcomes instead focussing on optimal development and positive outcomes. This has led to a

different focus not only on risk factors but also, more importantly, on protective factors and the promotion of well-being, both psychologically and in terms
of physical health (Antonovsky 1987). Today there is broad consensus that
only by analyzing the behavior and development paths of normal adolescents,
who are not yet heavily involved in risk behavior and not yet in the care of
health and social services, is it possible to understand the functions of risk
behavior in this developmental period. The functions of risk behavior, as will
become clear over the course of this volume, are different depending on the
degree of involvement in this kind of behavior. Furthermore, by studying normative samples, we are able to comprehend not only which factors can increase
the risk of involvement but also which protective factors can counteract these
risk factors. Only by studying the interrelationship of these two factors is it
possible to comprehend why some adolescents limit their involvement in risk
behavior while others become more seriously involved and stay involved for
longer periods of time. An analysis of the latter group, while it may be able to
provide insight into risk factors, is not able to shed light on protective factors
or their diverse and complex interrelationships with risk factors. While the
absence of some factors figures as a risk and their presence as protective (as
is the case, for example, of parental supervision), others are only risk factors
(such as spending free time in nonproductive activities), and their absence
does not signify protection.

For these reasons, the study examined a normative sample composed of
adolescents (roughly 2,300) attending different types of secondary schools in
different areas of Piemonte and Aosta Valley, two regions in the northwest of
Italy. These were boys and girls who, despite difficulties and failures, were able
to face the requirements that society places upon them, primarily that of
attending secondary school. It should be noted that in the northwest of Italy,
98% of boys and girls continue their studies after middle school, at least for the
two years of secondary school. We will now take a closer look at some of the
particular characteristics of the sample based on responses to the questions in
the first part of the questionnaire, which investigates these aspects.

The sample consisted of 2,273 adolescents of both genders (46% male and 54%
female) between the ages of 14 and 19 years (38% aged 14-15, 36% aged 16-17, 26%
aged 18-19). The majority of the adolescents interviewed were born in Piemonte
(58%) followed by Aosta Valley (27%); 9% were born in other northern Italian
regions while a slightly higher percentage were born in the south (4%) than in central Italian regions (1%). Only 1% were born in foreign countries.

All adolescents in the sample resided in towns of varied dimensions in
Piemonte and Aosta Valley; more specifically, half of the subjects lived in medium-sized towns, 34% in large towns, and 16% in small towns. They attended
different types of secondary schools: 38% attended technical schools, 29%
humanities or science lyceums, 18% vocational schools, and 15% teacher's
lyceums. The sample was fairly balanced for year in school: 23% attended the
first year, 20% the second year, 19% the third year, 20% the fourth year, and 18%
the fifth year. These schools are located in towns of varied dimensions: 18% are

located in large towns (about 1,000,000 inhabitants), 42% in medium-sized towns (70,000-100,000 inhabitants), and 40% in small towns (up to about 37,000 inhabitants).

In terms of religion, the majority of the adolescents claimed to be Catholic (81%), 15% to have no religious affiliation, and 4% to belong to other religions.

As for family, there was a strong predominance of intact family units (88%) while 5% of parents were separated, 4% divorced, and 3% widowed. The average size of the family unit was four people, 68% of the adolescents had brothers or sisters, and 25% lived with other adults (mostly aunts, uncles, or grandparents) in addition to their parents. As for the education levels of the parents, which were similar for mothers and fathers, 19% earned a certificate of completion of primary school, 30% a certificate of completion of middle school, 28% a secondary school diploma, roughly 10% a university degree, and about 10% a diploma from a professional training course. In terms of occupation, the majority of adolescents' mothers had stable employment while about one third did not work outside the home. Mothers' occupations, identified from the professional categories specified by the National Institute of Statistics (ISTAT 2001b) in Italy, were as follows: white-collar jobs (22%), sales (21%), intellectual professions (20%), and a significant number were technical professions (13%) and craftswomen (12%); 9% had nonqualified professions, and 3% were in the managerial or entrepreneurial category. Of the fathers, 89% had stable employment; a large percentage was employed as craftsmen or in agriculture (33%), 17% in white-collar jobs, 13% in sales, 13% in technical professions, 11% in managerial, and 8% in intellectual professions. In terms of parents' places of birth, frequency distributions were essentially similar for fathers and mothers. The degree of mobility was fairly high, with 56% of mothers from Piemonte or Aosta Valley and 24% from southern Italy, Sicily, or Sardinia. Similar statistics existed for fathers as well.

2.4 Presentation of Results and Statistical Analysis

For reasons of space and clarity, this volume does not report all the results of the research but rather focuses on an analysis of the functions of risk behavior; many other results obtained from the study and analyses carried out have not been included. First of all, a selection was made of the descriptive results that did not constitute the goal of the study. Analyses of highly specific subsamples or of particular themes were, for the most part, also omitted. For a more in-depth examination, readers can refer to the various contributions cited throughout the text and reported in the bibliography. In adherence to the aims of the research, the following chapters are the response to the demands of a challenging two-part objective. The first part was to display the results along with the indication of the statistical analyses performed and the empiric foundation of the interpretations in order to allow other scholars working in this field to evaluate the findings. The second part was to make the book easy to read and comprehend, even for nonspecialists and, in particular, for those who work with adolescents as teachers, educators, psychologists, and in health services. In the attempt to meet this challenging goal, we chose not to display the data in the fashion typical of scientific publications but in the form of figures and tables that synthesize the results of the numerous rigorous statistical analyses performed. For some of the results, we opted to insert the results directly into the text instead of displaying them graphically. For each figure, the type of statistical analysis performed is specified while the significance value and other specific statistical indexes have been omitted. All the results reported in the figures are statistically significant with $p<0.05$, meaning that there is a negligible probability (equal to or less than 5%) that the result is due to chance. In other words, the differences found (for example, between the frequencies or means) and the relationships identified (for example, in the case of correlation, variance, and regression analyses) are very likely to be caused by some systematic reason. The decision was made not to differentiate the significance values in the figures where $p<0.05$ (which are the least frequent) from those where $p<0.01$ and $p<0.001$, always with the aim of making the volume easy to read. Not significant yet conceptually relevant relationships are identified by the abbreviation n.s. (not significant) and by a broken line.

The reader will also find summaries in which results are represented in a conceptual synthesis. Although always based on analyses of the data, these syntheses cannot be traced directly to a specific statistic.

As for the statistics used, the reliability and dimensionality of the scales were controlled respectively with Cronbach's alpha (α) and principal component analysis. In the first part of each chapter, mainly preliminary techniques were used, such as frequency, chi-squared test, and correlation analysis (Cohen and Cohen 1983). The authors also used the most powerful and well-known statistic models (ANOVA, MANOVA, regression, logistic, and discriminant analysis). The majority of these models belong to the family of the Generalized Linear Models (Nelder and Wedderburn 1972; McCullagh and Nelder 1983; Dogson 1990). As already mentioned, the present study is based on empirical cross-sectional data; the results are interpreted in the light of the complex theoretical framework, which is presented in Chap. 1. The longitudinal continuation of this study, which is currently taking place, could give further suggestions to and eventually strengthen the validity of the relationships that constitute the core of this theory. We hope, however, that even in its current form it will be able to expand the horizons of readers, providing them with new prospectives and knowledge.

CHAPTER 3

Psychoactive Substance Use

> I smoke joints because I like to… but only when I'm with my
> friends, just to have a few laughs… smoking alone is sad…
> smoking pot is something you should do with friends.
>
> *[Boy, science lyceum, first year]*

3.1 Psychoactive Substance Use: Tobacco, Alcohol, and Marijuana

Psychoactive substances are defined as any substance, natural or synthetic, that is capable of affecting the nervous system and altering its biochemical order, thus provoking changes in mood, perception, mental activity, and behavior. Among these substances we find tobacco, alcohol, and marijuana. These three substances in particular are first used by many children during adolescence, and over the years of adolescence, changes can be witnessed in their attitudes toward the substances and the style and context in which they use them.

Although all three fall under the category of psychoactive substances, there are profound differences in tobacco, alcohol, and marijuana in terms of their effects on the nervous system, the way they are considered by society, and the meanings attached to them. As far as their effect on the nervous system is concerned, tobacco has a stimulating, exciting effect, alcohol depresses psychological activity, and marijuana has a sedative, euphoric, psychedelic effect (Julien 2005). But the effects of these different substances do not depend solely on their different chemical structures or on their action mechanisms on a cerebral level; these effects are actually closely associated to objective and subjective parameters as well. Objective factors include the method of administration, the quality and quantity of the substance used, the frequency - occasional or systematic - of use, and the physical characteristics of the substance user (gender, age, weight, etc.), while subjective factors include the personal characteristics of the substance user and the circumstances in which the substance is consumed. The knowledge possessed by subjects, their expectations, and the meaning they place on the use of a particular substance influence and modify their reactions and the way they perceive themselves and the world around them: euphoria, well-being, inner tranquillity, and disinhibition are just a few of the sensations that may be experienced. It follows that the subjective experience that results from the use of the same substance can either be relatively similar or can, in different subjects or at different times, be entirely different. The circumstances of use, as the subject perceives it, also assume a great deal of importance. In fact, the physical and social characteristics of the environment in which the substance is consumed (for example, the familiarity or strangeness, or the pleasantness or hostility of the context) influence the subjective perception of the experience and the function that is attributed to it.

A second aspect analyzed here that differentiates the three substances is the way they are considered by society and, most importantly, their distinction as either legal or illegal. While tobacco and alcohol are legal drugs, marijuana is illegal. The legality of alcohol and tobacco facilitate their acceptance by society, their spread, and their consumption. However, the fact that these substances are legal can also lead to an underevaluation of the potential dangers associated with their use. In fact, anything that is seen as common or frequently occurring can be viewed as normal, regardless of the harmful effects it may have. Today, it is age that defines smoking and alcohol as acceptable for adults while these behavior types are disapproved of in children and adolescents. In contrast, the label of illicit drug, which has been attached to marijuana, contributes to emphasizing the risks tied to its consumption and also introduces the aspect of sanctions. Nevertheless, the very common yet highly deceptive distinction between "light drugs," such as cannabis, and "heavy drugs," such as cocaine or heroine, can lead us to associate minor risks to "light drugs," which, indirectly, leads to increased use of these substances. In reality, the distinction between light and heavy drugs is groundless; recent studies on the biochemical characteristics of various psychoactive substances and their effects on a neurophysiological level have demonstrated similarities in the way they function. In reality, specific circuits of the brain are assigned to neuron mediation and the reinforcement of pleasure, and all substances, regardless of whether they are labeled heavy or light, activate the same reinforcement systems in the brain. Furthermore, the harmfulness and toxicity levels, both in the short and long term, of various substances on the organism have been proven by numerous studies (Julien 2005).

Summary 3.1 summarizes the different factors that influence the impact that a given substance has on the subject. As is shown here, the most important role is played by the individual's cognitive mediation.

As we will see more clearly throughout the course of this chapter, the different social considerations of different substances affect the meanings that adolescents assign to use of these substances. For example, the fact that alcohol and tobacco use is extremely common, socially accepted, considered normal in adults, and permitted by law, encourages adolescents to act out this behavior, which for them is symbolic of adulthood even though it is actually only an outward appearance of adulthood. On the contrary, as marijuana is illegal, its use is more frequently associated with transgression and rebellion toward the adult world.

Summary 3.1. Main factors that contribute to how a psychoactive substance is perceived.

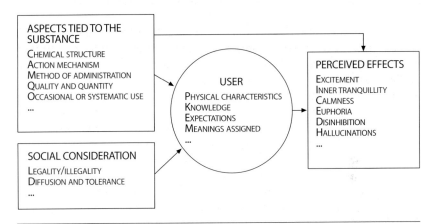

CIRCUMSTANCES OF USE

PHYSICAL AND SOCIAL CHARACTERISTICS OF THE ENVIRONMENT, FAMILIARITY OR UNFAMILIARITY OF THE CONTEXT, PLEASANTNESS OR UNPLEASANTNESS OF THE SITUATION

ASPECTS TIED TO THE SUBSTANCE
CHEMICAL STRUCTURE
ACTION MECHANISM
METHOD OF ADMINISTRATION
QUALITY AND QUANTITY
OCCASIONAL OR SYSTEMATIC USE
...

USER
PHYSICAL CHARACTERISTICS
KNOWLEDGE
EXPECTATIONS
MEANINGS ASSIGNED
...

PERCEIVED EFFECTS
EXCITEMENT
INNER TRANQUILLITY
CALMNESS
EUPHORIA
DISINHIBITION
HALLUCINATIONS
...

SOCIAL CONSIDERATION
LEGALITY/ILLEGALITY
DIFFUSION AND TOLERANCE
...

3.1.1 Cigarette Smoking

Smoking, due to the widespread nature of its use not only among adolescents but also among adults, is often considered the least serious of the different types of risk behavior. It is not associated with psychopathological or deviant processes, it does not provoke any sort of immediate danger (as with dangerous driving or alcohol abuse), and it is socially tolerated (unlike antisocial behavior, for example). Nevertheless, it has been proven that smoking is not simply a behavior that *can* be harmful to one's health, smoking *is* harmful to the health both in the short and long term. Nicotine is comparable to other psychoactive substances, as it affects the central nervous system, partially altering its biochemical equilibrium and affecting the brain's reinforcement centers (Julien 2005). But above all, smoking is strongly correlated to cardiovascular and pulmonary diseases and has been shown to increase the risk of developing certain forms of cancer.

Despite its harmfulness, cigarette smoking is very common. Among the adolescents in our sample, 70% had smoked at least one cigarette although only 14% had actually smoked only once[1]. In reality however, the number of actual smokers is much lower, as those who tried smoking only once cannot be considered smokers.

In order to obtain a more precise index of involvement, two questions were intersected, one related to the frequency with which subjects have smoked in their

---

[1] In the "Appendix," the questions and scales from the questionnaire have been included along with their related answers and main psychometric characteristics.

lifetimes ("Have you ever smoked a cigarette"?) and one related to the quantity of cigarettes smoked daily during the past month. In this way, five groups were created:
-    Nonsmokers: have never smoked, or smoked only one cigarette in their lifetime
-    Ex-smokers: have smoked several times in their life but have not smoked in the last month
-    Occasional smokers: have smoked a few or several times in their life
-    Moderate smokers: smoke habitually and in the past month smoked from one to ten cigarettes a day (a maximum of half a pack)
-    Heavy smokers: smoke habitually and in the last month smoked from half a pack to more than a pack of cigarettes a day.

The results (Fig. 3.1) show a large degree of differentiation in use, with 17% of adolescents who can already be considered ex-smokers, 15% who are occasional smokers, and one fourth who are habitual smokers (either moderate or heavy).

These results are in line with the national average. ISTAT data for the year 2000 (reported in 2002) reveals that one fourth (25%) of the Italian population between the ages of fifteen and twenty-four smoke habitually. Unlike almost all other behavior analyzed in this volume, no differences exist in levels of involvement by boys and girls, a sign of standardization in the behavior of the two genders. Involvement[2] (Fig. 3.2), however, is higher in older ages.

There are also significant differences in involvement by students of different types of secondary schools, with the greatest involvement by students of vocational secondary schools (Fig. 3.3).

Thus, as adolescents "grow up," they tend to smoke more and more. Similarly, adolescents who attend schools that, at least in theory, prepare them for

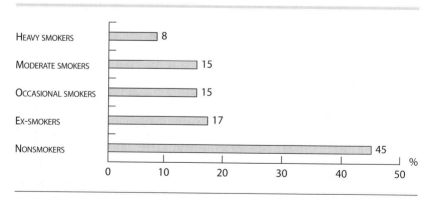

Fig. 3.1. Typology of adolescents who smoke cigarettes (percentages).

---

[2] Note that all the results reported in the figures are statistically significant, with $p<0.05$. In Chap. 2, Sect. 2.4, Presentation of Results and Statistical Analyses, the criteria for the presentation of results and for the use of statistics are explained.

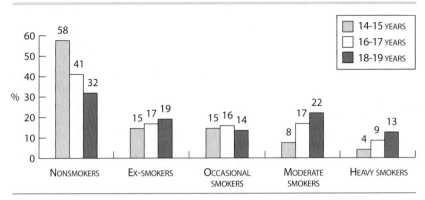

Fig. 3.2. Typology by age group of adolescents who smoke cigarettes (chi-squared).

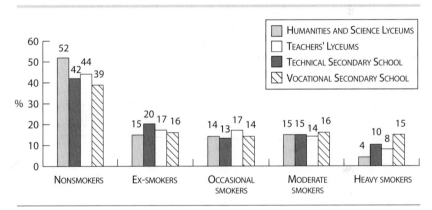

Fig. 3.3. Typology of adolescents who smoke cigarettes for type of school (chi-squared).

early entrance into the workforce also smoke more. Nevertheless, the differences in involvement between types of schools are not yet significant in the first year of secondary school (Cattelino and Bonino 2000). This finding clearly shows that greater involvement by adolescents who attend certain types of schools cannot simply be traced back to the family background or to typical socioeconomic variables, which would determine access by adolescents to different types of schools (cigarette smoking is, in fact, more common in the lower-middle social classes). An explanation of the differences between the various types of schools should be looked for within the schools themselves and, more precisely, in the different types of orientation toward adulthood they involve, the different opportunities they provide for adolescents to manifest adulthood, the different group cultures that are constructed over time, and the different levels of satisfaction adolescents find in school (Bonino and Cattelino 2002; Borca et al. 2002).

3.1.2 Alcohol Consumption

Alcohol consumption differs from use of other psychoactive substances such as tobacco and marijuana, as the harm it can cause to the health is closely connected to the quantity of the substance ingested. In fact, low consumption of alcohol is not only not harmful but can even have positive effects on the health, as it can reduce the risk of coronary arteriopathy primarily by increasing levels of the "good cholesterol" [high-density lipoprotein (HDL) cholesterol] (Julien 2005). However, although small quantities of alcohol can have positive effects, the same cannot be said of larger quantities (roughly 60 grams for females and 70-75 for males), which can compromise an individual's health and well-being on a number of levels - from the digestive tract, to the cardiovascular system, to the central nervous system.

In Italy, consumption of alcohol, especially wine, is a long-standing tradition and is deeply rooted in the national culture and economy. In recent years, however, in southern European countries (Italy and France, in particular), total alcohol consumption, along with the problems linked to it, have been gradually decreasing (Gual and Colom 1997). This decrease relates mainly to consumption of wine (according to findings by Eurostat, in Italy per capita wine consumption decreased from 33.3 liters in 1989 to 25.3 liters in 1992) while consumption of nonalcoholic beverages and beer, which contains less alcohol than wine, has increased (in Italy, per capita consumption of nonalcoholic beverages and beer has increased from 38.8 liters in 1989 to 40 liters in 1992). In recent years, consumption of hard liquor has also increased. It appears that in Italy, the typically "Mediterranean" habit of drinking wine at meals and social gatherings is slowly being replaced by a more "Nordic" style characterized by the consumption of large quantities of beer and hard liquor.

Almost all adolescents (92%) in our sample had drunk at least one glass of wine, beer, or hard liquor in their life, and 79% claim to have drunk at least once in the last six months. The most frequently consumed alcoholic beverage was beer[3], consumed by 70% of the adolescents in our survey in the last six months, followed by hard liquor (46%) and wine (42%). Boys, older adolescents, and those living in small- to midsized towns preferred wine. Therefore, it appears that wine is most often consumed by young adults living in more stable, close-knit communities. Beer, on the other hand, appears to be a more inexpensive, modern beverage that better symbolizes youth culture and is a common denominator between youth from different countries and backgrounds. The fact that beer has a lower alcohol content also makes its consumption by young people more socially accepted than consumption of beverages with higher alcohol content.

---

[3] As there is a strong correlation between the styles of consumption for beer and for other alcoholic substances, data reported in this chapter are related to beer consumption only. The data can be generalized to wine and hard liquor consumption.

Not only in Italian culture is alcohol consumption a typical phenomenon, and the international literature has emphasized that for adolescents, it is more normative to drink than to be a nondrinker (Moffit 1993; Johnstone et al. 1994). Furthermore, this data is not alarming in and of itself, as the majority of the Italian adolescents in our sample drank in moderation (two or three drinks per occasion) either habitually or occasionally (Fig. 3.4);[4] however, we cannot overlook the fact that a significant percentage of adolescents were heavy drinkers (four to six glasses of beer or more). Note that the literature considers the consumption of five to six glasses of alcohol to be a critical threshold for the health (Jessor et al. 1991; Bourgault and Demers 1997). This threshold was exceeded more than once a week in the last six months by 26% of heavy drinkers. For moderate drinkers, on the other hand, about half had never exceeded this threshold (49%), and 37% had exceeded it a maximum of five times in the last six months.

Unlike our findings on cigarette smoking, significant gender differences were found with respect to alcohol consumption: more boys drink alcohol than girls do; they also drink more frequently and in larger quantities (Fig. 3.5). Greater involvement by boys is also evidenced by the fact that boys reported having drunk more than five glasses of alcohol on an average of four to five occasions in the last six months compared with on one to two occasions for girls.

Major differences were also found between adolescents in different age groups: from 14 to 19 years old, the number of nondrinkers decreases (Fig. 3.6) while the number of moderate drinker increases.

The differences between different types of schools are also significant: larger proportions of heavy drinkers are students of technical and vocational secondary schools (Fig. 3.7). Furthermore, roughly one fourth of these students reported to have drunk more than five glasses of alcohol more than once a month in the last six months.

In considering the number of times they have been drunk in the past six

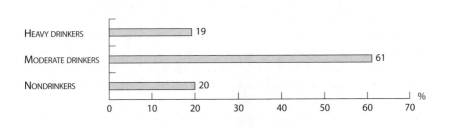

Fig. 3.4. Typology of adolescents who drink beer (percentages).

---

[4] Occasional drinkers and habitual drinkers are not distinguished in the graphs, as no significant differences were found between the two groups. The quantity consumed is what distinguishes adolescents with different styles of consumption.

months, more than half of the sample said they had not been drunk at all (53%) while 38% said they had been drunk only on special occasions. In this case as well, boys are more involved: 41% got drunk on special occasions (compared with 35% of girls), and 12% reported that they got drunk frequently (as opposed to 6% of girls). The number of times adolescents get drunk is higher at 18-19 years, but it is above all the heavy drinkers (25% of whom get drunk often or very often) who reported getting drunk frequently.

Despite the fact that alcohol consumption is high for certain adolescents and in certain situations, only a small number of adolescents from our sample claimed to have had problems tied to excessive alcohol consumption. As shown in Fig. 3.8, the most frequent problems are health-related followed by social problems (with partner, friends, or parents). Only a very small number of adolescents reported having had problems involving the authorities.

Boys reported a higher number of problems than girls of their same age, but the greatest differences are tied to the style of consumption (Fig. 3.9).

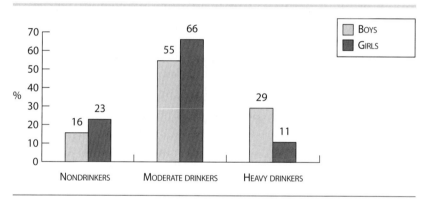

Fig. 3.5. Typology of adolescents who drink beer for gender (chi-squared).

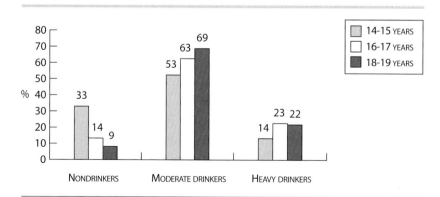

Fig. 3.6. Typology of adolescents who drink beer for age group (chi-squared).

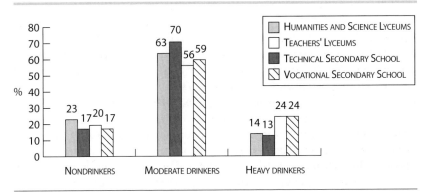

Fig. 3.7. Typology of adolescents who drink beer for type of school (chi-squared).

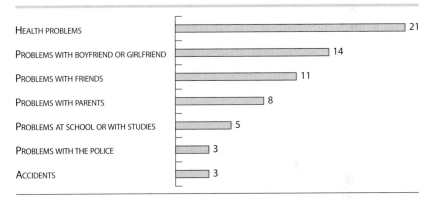

Fig. 3.8. Percentages of involvement in different kinds of problems caused by alcohol consumption.

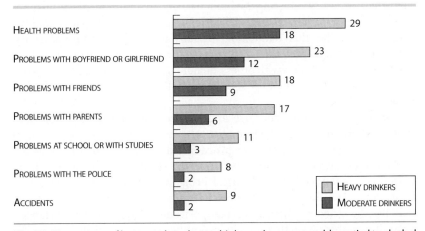

Fig. 3.9. Percentages of heavy and moderate drinkers who report problems tied to alcohol (chi-squared).

3.1.3 Marijuana Smoking

The use of illegal drugs during adolescence has become, in recent decades, such a common phenomenon that it has been categorized as one of the typical problems of this period of development. Smoking marijuana, in particular, appears to be a typically adolescent behavior not only because it generally occurs for the first time during adolescence but also because it is often abandoned upon entering adulthood.

The label of illegality placed on marijuana reflects the negative consideration and high degree of danger associated with it. However, within the realm of illicit drugs, marijuana is considered less harmful and is defined a *light* drug as opposed to a *heavy* drug, such as heroine, cocaine, or LSD. The inaccurate connotation of "light drug," as discussed previously in section 3.1, tends to diminish the perception of the risks tied to marijuana use even though, as it is now well known, all drugs have similar action mechanisms that affect the central nervous system in a similar way and, therefore, must all be considered toxic and harmful (Julien 2005).

From a pharmacological point of view, THC, the active principle contained in marijuana, has a fairly weak effect on the brain's reinforcement centers while on a cognitive level, the immediate effects of this substance, even following small doses, mainly involve the inability to carry out complex tasks requiring attention and coordination.

In considering involvement in marijuana use by a normative sample of adolescents attending secondary school, such as the one we studied, it was found that 28% have smoked marijuana at least once. Much less common were those who had, at least once in their life, consumed other types of illegal drugs (Fig. 3.10). Of the other drugs consumed, the most common were pills (stimulants or tranquilizers) and hallucinogens (LSD and ecstasy). However, only a small minority of the adolescents in our sample had used these drugs. Hallucinogenic drugs are capable of qualitatively altering one's relationship with reality, inducing the induction of hallucinations, illusions, phenomena of depersonalization, and disorientation in terms of space and time. It seems that rather than hallucinogenic substances, which induce passivity, adolescents tend to prefer activating substances, such as marijuana, which stimulate communication with others, do not induce a strong sense of dependence, and are more compatible with a normal lifestyle and acceptable psychosocial adjustment.

Involvement in substance use, and here we will consider marijuana, in particular, cannot be described simplistically in terms of use or nonuse. There are various phases that define the process of drug use and that regulate the relationship between user and substance: the preparation or approach, the initiation, and the stabilization of use. During the approach phase, which generally takes place through interactions with significant people in the individual's life, the individual forms a certain position on psychoactive substances. Thus, it is in this phase that the adolescent begins to see substance use as a more or less acceptable possibility. Next is the initiation phase, in which the adolescent tries the substance and decides whether or not to repeat the experience. The successive phase, in which substance use becomes stabilized, only occurs for some; this phase can vary greatly, ranging from occasional to habitual use or addiction.

Based on these various phases, we have constructed a typology of adolescents who smoke marijuana. The following four groups have been identified:

- Nonsmokers: have never smoked marijuana in their life or have smoked only once
- Ex-smokers: have not smoked marijuana in the last six months
- Occasional smokers: have smoked marijuana between one and six times in the last six months
- Habitual smokers: have smoked marijuana from two to three times in the last month to everyday for the last six months.

The results displayed in Fig. 3.11 show the wide variation in use, with 72% of the sample in the nonsmoker group, 6% who suspended use, and 11% who smoked marijuana occasionally or habitually.

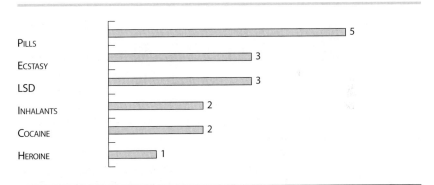

Fig. 3.10. Percentages of use of other drugs and substances.

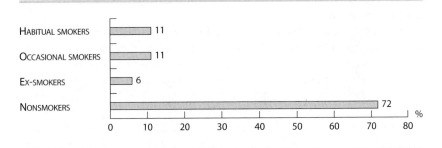

Fig. 3.11. Typology of adolescents who smoke marijuana (percentages).

Girls (82% of whom had never smoked marijuana or had suspended use, as opposed to 74% of boys) and younger adolescents are much less involved in marijuana use, especially in habitual use. Among those over 18 years of age, just under half claimed to have smoked marijuana at least once in their lives. Among them, we saw high percentages of both occasional and habitual users and boys and girls who had suspended use (Fig. 3.12).

This seems to indicate the existence of two distinct groups: the first is characterized by persistence and possibly an increase in use, and the second is characterized by the discontinuity of marijuana use (see Fig. 5.1).

Use also varies in the different types of schools and is significantly higher with regard to habitual use in vocational secondary schools (Fig. 3.13).

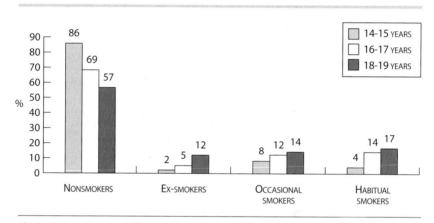

Fig. 3.12. Typology of adolescents who smoke marijuana for age group (chi-squared).

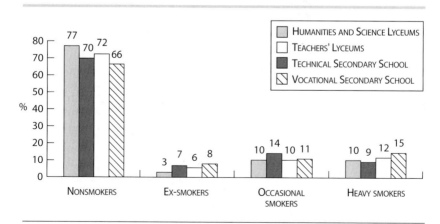

Fig. 3.13. Typology of adolescents who smoke marijuana for type of school (chi-squared).

Table 3.1 summarizes the sociodemographic characteristics of the adolescents most heavily involved in the use of the three psychoactive substances considered here.

Table 3.1. Main sociodemographic characteristics of the adolescents most heavily involved in the use of the three different substances (chi-squared).

Alcohol consumption	Cigarette smoking	Marijuana smoking
Adolescents most heavily involved are primarily: • Between the ages of 16 and 19 • Vocational and technical secondary school students No differences were found in terms of gender	Adolescents most heavily involved are primarily: • Boys • Between the ages of 16 and 19 • Vocational and technical secondary school students	Adolescents most heavily involved are primarily: • Boys • Between the ages of 16 and 19 • Vocational and technical secondary school students

3.1.4 The Use of Different Substances

Use of various psychoactive substances decreases when passing from legal to illegal substances (Fig. 3.14). It is often asked whether there is continuity in the consumption of various psychoactive substances and, more precisely, if there is a progression between smoking cigarettes and smoking marijuana and from smoking marijuana to the use of other drugs.

As a matter of fact, there are strong positive correlations between the use of certain psychoactive substances (Fig. 3.15).

This finding is not surprising as, for some time now, the literature has referred not to individual types of risk behavior but rather to "syndromes" or

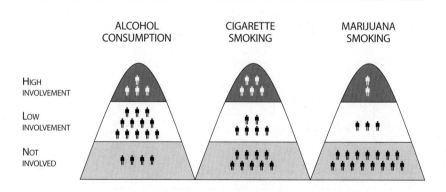

Fig. 3.14. Representation of the proportions of subjects who consume alcohol, cigarettes and marijuana (each "little person" represents roughly 5% of the total sample).

"constellations" of behavior types that have similar functions, are tied to similar psychological problems (Jessor et al. 1991), and involve the same reinforcement centers. The strong correlation between marijuana use and other types of risk behavior, such as antisocial behavior and risky driving, is also evidence of the existence of these constellations (Fig. 3.16).

This means that marijuana users are more involved in the use of other substances as well as other more action-centered types of risk behavior that share some of the same functions as substance use; for example, seeking excitement, transgression, acceptance by a group, and escape from reality.

The strong positive correlation with cigarette smoking seems to indicate that heavy smokers are at greater risk to be involved in marijuana use as well. These findings show that a progression can be seen from use of easily accessible, legal psychoactive substances, such as cigarettes or alcohol, to illegal psychoactive substances (Kandel 1978). Similarly, there can also be a progression from "light" to "heavy" drugs. It should be noted, however, that a large percentage of adolescents who have smoked cigarettes do not move on to marijuana smoking, just as the majority of those who have smoked marijuana either do not go beyond the experimentation phase of marijuana use or aban-

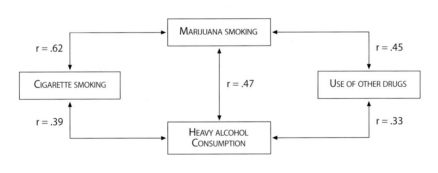

Fig. 3.15. Correlation between the use of different psychoactive substances.

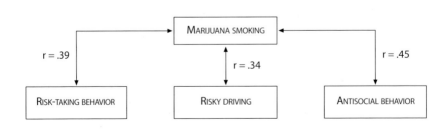

Fig. 3.16. Correlation with other types of risk behavior.

don use altogether. Only a small percentage of adolescents become habitual marijuana users, and only this group is at risk for progression to use of other stronger, more harmful illegal substances.

Figure 3.17 displays the proportion of regular marijuana smokers that are also cigarette smokers and the proportion of users of other drugs that are also marijuana smokers. As we can see, adolescents who consume illegal drugs generally consume legal drugs as well (a finding that provides further evidence of the hypothesis of the continuity and progression in the use of different substances).

Nevertheless, the involvement both in legal and illegal drugs seems to involve only a small percentage of adolescents (38% of habitual smokers are also marijuana users, and 42% of marijuana users also use other drugs), a sign that in a normative sample, progression could be just one of the possible paths that adolescents can take.

HABITUAL MARIJUANA SMOKERS

Ex CIGARETTE
SMOKERS

NONSMOKERS
OF CIGARETTES

OCCASIONAL
CIGARETTE SMOKERS

HABITUAL
CIGARETTE SMOKERS

HABITUAL MARIJUANA SMOKERS ARE, IN MOST
CASES, ALSO HABITUAL CIGARETTE SMOKERS

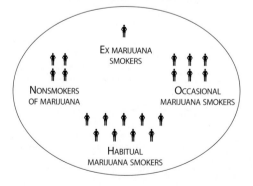

USERS OF OTHER DRUGS

Ex MARIJUANA
SMOKERS

NONSMOKERS
OF MARIJUANA

OCCASIONAL
MARIJUANA SMOKERS

HABITUAL
MARIJUANA SMOKERS

USERS OF OTHER DRUGS ARE, IN MOST CASES,
ALSO MARIJUANA SMOKERS

Fig. 3.17. Habitual marijuana smokers and users of other drugs.

3.2 Age and Context of Initiation

The approach to cigarette smoking appears to be especially strong between the ages of 13 and 15; more than half of the adolescents in our sample claimed to have tried smoking at this age while very few smoked their first cigarette after the age of 16. The habit, on the other hand, takes about one year to develop; for the majority, smoking becomes a habitual behavior between the ages of 14 and 16 (Fig. 3.18).

Boys smoke their first cigarette (average age 13 years) roughly six months earlier than girls (average age 14 years) although no gender differences were found in terms of the age when the behavior stabilized.

For the majority of Italian adolescents, the period of first approach to substance use coincides with the passage from middle school to secondary school. This transition is often experienced as and interpreted by society as an indicator of "growing up," and it is no coincidence that it is precisely at this age that adolescents, for the first time, begin to act out behavior types that are common, accepted, and considered "normal" in adults, such as cigarette smoking and alcohol consumption.

The average age of initial approach to alcohol consumption occurs earlier - around 12-13 years of age - when adolescents are still at middle school. It should be noted that 22% of the adolescents in our sample drank for the first time before the age of 10 (as we will see, however, the early age of initiation to alcohol consumption does not constitute a risk factor). In our sample, finally, the average age of first-time marijuana use occurs later than the first cigarette - around 15 years old. Thus, there are different critical ages for the initiation of different psychoactive substances and for the stabilization of their use (Fig. 3.19).

In general, legal substances are tried earlier than illegal ones, and the passage from one school to the next (from middle school to secondary school or from the second to the third year of middle school) represents a time of greater risk. Transitional periods, which bring about changes in the lives and identities of subjects, require adolescents to undergo a kind of restructuring in order to adjust to the new situation. It is precisely because of the need to confront this change that some adolescents are at greater risk for an approach to illegal actions and sub-

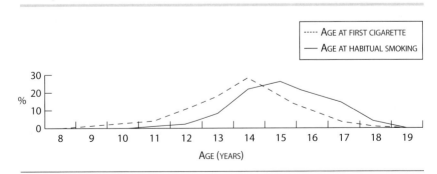

Fig. 3.18. Age of initiation and stabilization of cigarette smoking.

stances. For some, substance use is only experimental, while for others drug use can become a part of their new identity, leading to habitual substance use.

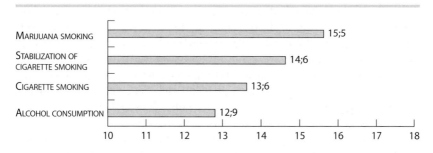

Fig. 3.19. Average age of initiation for use of different psychoactive substances (years;months).

3.2.1 Precociousness, Contexts of Use, and Risk

As far as cigarette and marijuana smoking are concerned, the precociousness of initiation seems to be a risk factor for stabilization and increase of use. The age at first cigarette or marijuana use is negatively correlated with the frequency and quantity of consumption of psychoactive substances. The relationship between precociousness and risk is also easily deducible when we look at groups differentiated by level of involvement: heavy smokers began smoking when they were around 13 years old, and the behavior became a habit before the age of 15. On the other hand, occasional smokers smoked their first cigarette at about age 14 and smoked occasionally since the age of 16. Moderate habitual smokers fall just between these two groups.

The same relationship between precociousness and style of consumption can be found for marijuana smoking. As is shown in Fig. 3.20, the younger the age of initiation, the more habitual the use. To contrast, those who discover the substance later give it up more easily.

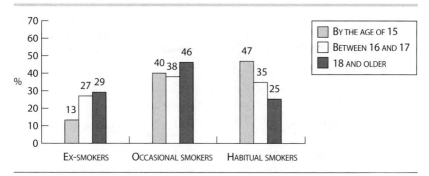

Fig. 3.20. Age of initiation in relation to typology of adolescents who smoke marijuana (chi-squared).

For alcohol consumption, however, although the age of first approach is quite young, precociousness of initiation seems to have no effect on the degree of use during adolescence. No significant relationship was found between the age of initiation and the intensity of use; in other words, moderate and heavy drinkers cannot be distinguished by the age of first approach to alcohol. In this case, the potential risks tied to the early age of initiation could not only be reduced but even eliminated by the context in which alcohol is consumed for the first and successive times. The first experience with alcohol consumption occurs within a social setting; 43% drank for the first time with their family, 55% with friends, and only 2% alone. A relationship was found between the age of first alcohol consumption and the people who were present on that occasion: almost all (85%) of those who drank for the first time before the age of 10 years old did so in the company of their family during a celebration or special occasion of some sort, as is traditional in Italy. However, the inverse was found when considering those who drank for the first time between the ages of 16 and 17; of these adolescents, only a small percentage (12%) drank for the first time with their family while almost all (87%) were in the company of friends. The remaining 1% were alone.

The context of initiation can also have an effect on the style of alcohol consumption adopted during adolescence; initiation in the company of family, even at an early age, generally leads to the most positive outcomes. Among moderate drinkers, a greater percentage of adolescents drank for the first time with their family while among heavy drinkers, a higher percentage initiated with friends (Fig. 3.21). In short, in Italy, it is not the age of initiation that seems to influence the seriousness of alcohol consumption in adolescence but rather the conditions under which this initiation occurs.

In adolescence, successive alcohol consumption also occurs in social contexts and not alone. Adolescents, unlike adults, do not drink alone. While the use of other psychoactive substances and the carrying out of other types of risk behavior generally occurs in the company of peers, alcohol is often consumed in the company of adults as well and therefore among people of different generations. More precisely, 75% claimed to have drunk alcohol at least occa-

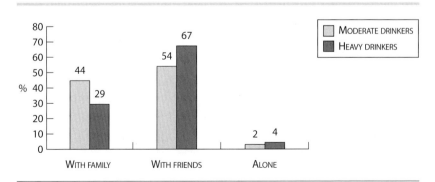

Fig. 3.21. Relational context in which first consumption of alcohol occurs (chi-squared).

sionally with their family, and 87% claimed to have drunk at least every once in a while with friends. In this case as well, the style of consumption is related to the relational context in which it occurs. Moderate drinkers drink with their families more frequently than heavy drinkers, who tend to drink more often in the company of friends.

From these data, adults seem to take on a very important instructive role that directly effects how the behavior is acted out. Adults act as models and controls through the rules and limits they impose but also as vehicles to transmit the cultural values tied to alcohol consumption. In other words, adults offer the context in which drinking occurs (for example, a holiday or special occasion) while at the same time communicating the meanings that have been assigned to drinking by the cultural environment that the adolescent is a part of; in Italian culture, drinking is tied mainly to conviviality, shared happiness, and physical and emotional relaxation.

3.3 Homogeneity Within Peer Groups

It has been shown that psychoactive substance use in adolescence is not a solitary activity and that the group has an important influence on the way substance use occurs: cigarette smokers, drinkers, and marijuana users spend many hours a week with their peers and reported having many friends who are also involved in the use of psychoactive substances, so much so that friend models and hours spent with friends are good predictors of use (Fig. 3.22).

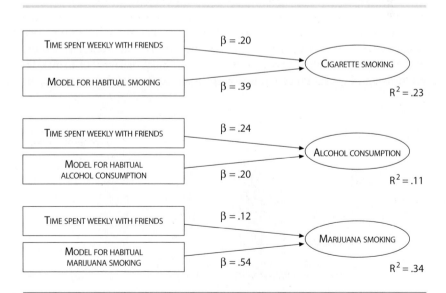

Fig. 3.22. Variables related to friends (multiple regression).

As shown by regression analyses, in passing from legal to illegal substances, friend models, especially for marijuana use, become more important. Friends facilitate an approach to the drug because they appear as credible, reassuring models, nothing like the terrifying commonly held image of a drug addict. Thus, initiation occurs within the protective and captivating context of the group (Kandel 1986). Thanks to their peers, adolescents also have an easier time obtaining marijuana. Although this substance is highly accessible to the majority of adolescents, it is even more so when one has peers who are marijuana users (Fig. 3.23).

The data presented here are consistent with the findings presented in most of the literature on risk behavior in adolescence, which affirms that the peer group, with the behavior models it offers, can represent an element of risk for the adolescent (Jessor and Jessor 1977; Jessor et al. 1991; Plant and Plant 1992). There is a great deal of uniformity in the behavior of adolescent friends; however, there is also a tendency by those who carry out a behavior to overevaluate the number of friends involved in the same behavior. This mechanism, termed *false consensus*, induces individuals to overestimate the number of people who behave in the same way that they do; this is caused by a need to feel normal, which is in turn connected to the positive affirmation of their identity (Savadori and Rumiati 1996)

To explain the similarity between the behavior of adolescents and their friends, and thus the homogeneity of behavior within groups, various mechanisms were hypothesized, the first of which was the imitation of the behavior of others. The processes of peer influence are generally defined as active in the case of explicit pressure applied to act out a certain behavior and passive if there is a model but no explicit request to act out the behavior (Graham et al. 1991; Aloise et al. 1994). Both of these types of pressure have a substantial influence (Magnusson et al. 1986), as the opinions and models of the people affectively closest make up the relational context in which substance use occurs and, at the same time, offer reasons to either act out a behavior or to avoid it (Oetting and Beavais 1986). On this point, it should be noted that the major-

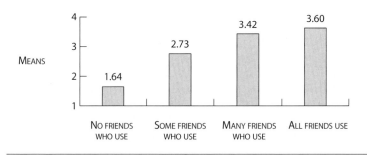

Fig. 3.23. Accessibility of marijuana in relation to friends' use (ANOVA).

ity of adolescents who use psychoactive substances reported that their friends use these substances as well and that these friends have tolerant attitudes toward or explicitly approve of the use of these substances.

The most simplistic and reductive aspects of the imitation and influence hypothesis have found fertile ground outside the realm of scientific psychology, so much so that we commonly hear the reprehensible behavior of an adolescent blamed on the influence of the "wrong crowd," or in other words, on the same reprehensible behavior acted out by the adolescent's peers. Psychology today has clarified that imitation is not a passive process that removes responsibility from the individual. Imitation occurs primarily in the initial phase of the approach to a particular substance, yet from the very beginning, it is accompanied by more complex psychological processes, most importantly the active construction of identity through the sharing of the values and behavior of the group. From this standpoint, friends offer behavior models that adolescents adopt not so much - or not only - because they are imitating these models but because personal advantages are obtained and a self-image is constructed through identifying with others.

Recently, the direction of causality between adolescents' behavior and the behavior of their peers has also been put up for discussion, contrasting the theory of influence with that of social selection (Ennett and Bauman 1994; Engels et al. 1997; Engels 1998) and postulating therefore a sort of attraction between those who behave in the same way (Eiser et al. 1991). According to this model, the selection of friends who drink or smoke is the consequence and not the cause of substance use (Bauman and Ennett 1996). In other words, the existence of similarities in behavior and attitudes leads adolescents to prefer the company of certain boys and girls and to seek them out as friends.

In reality, both the hypothesis of influence and that of selection play an important role in comprehending the behavior of adolescents. While the hypothesis of social influence seems useful in explaining experimentation and occasional use of substances, the selection hypothesis appears more appropriate in explaining habitual use.

3.4 Parents: Models and Attitudes

Can the models and attitudes of family members have an influence on the adolescent's involvement in the use of psychoactive substances? As far as alcohol consumption is concerned, we have already seen that drinking with the family provides adolescents with models of moderation, an external control over the quantity of the substance consumed at a time, and, above all, a chance to understand the cultural values of alcohol consumption.

If we consider cigarette smoking, parental models have a protective function. In fact, as we can see in Fig. 3.24, adolescents who are nonsmokers have a significantly lower number of parents who are smokers while those who smoke habitually have a significantly higher number of parents who are both smokers. This result is consistent with other studies (den Exter Blokland et al. 2004; Harakeh et al. 2004).

Parental smoking may also play an indirect role by affecting youths' susceptibility to peer influences and friendship selection. For instance, in a study of Engels and colleagues (Engels et al. 2004), parental smoking seemed to affect the selection of new friends: in particular, adolescents with smoking parents were most likely to become affiliated with smoking friends.

Within the family, the models offered by siblings - older brothers in particular - are also important (Lloyd and Lucas 1998). Girls especially are more likely to smoke when they have brothers who smoke (Fig. 3.25): older sibling could be perceived as credible models to imitate and could encourage more strongly the processes of identification, being more similar to the adolescent than are the parents.

We can hypothesize that the older sibling model is an important factor

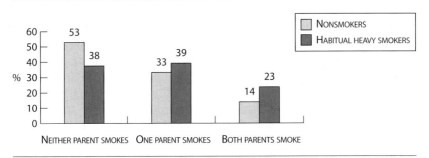

Fig. 3.24. Parental model for cigarette smoking (chi-squared).

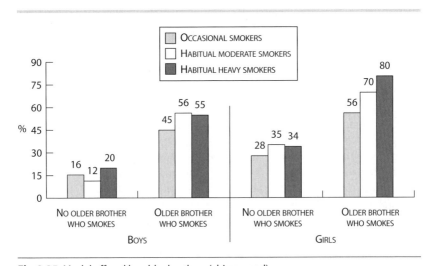

Fig. 3.25. Model offered by older brothers (chi-squared).

linked to the concept of social images of smokers and drinkers. In other studies, positive relations were observed between smoker and drinker prototypes and adolescents' intention and willingness to smoke and drink in the future (Spijkerman et al. 2004).

Even more important than parental behavior models is the parents' explicit disapproval of adolescents' smoking, which was found to be significantly less in boys and girls who are seriously addicted smokers (Fig. 3.26).

Even the fact that parents' know their sons or daughters smoked was found to be an important aspect: parental knowledge is correlated to greater involvement in smoking by the adolescent (Fig. 3.27).

The importance of this aspect can be explained not only by the fact that, when smoking becomes a daily habit, adolescents have a difficult time hiding it from their parents but also by the fact that a parent's knowledge that their child smokes can be interpreted as indirect, implicit approval.

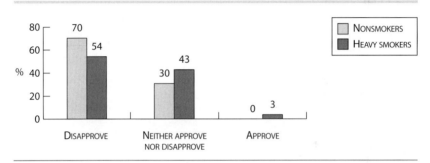

Fig. 3.26. Attitudes of parents toward cigarette smoking (chi-squared).

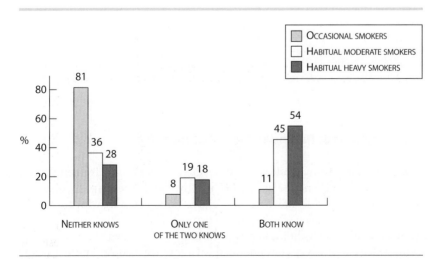

Fig. 3.27. Parental knowledge of children's smoking (chi-squared).

The findings with regard to parental models and attitudes seem to indicate that both these aspects are important in influencing smoking by adolescents (Fig. 3.28). The most important role, however, is carried out by parental knowledge of adolescent behavior, which suggests that the family, through its attitudes, can play an important protective role even when the model presented is one of risk.

A disapproving attitude by parents constitutes an important protective factor even where illegal substances are concerned. In this case, however, the most related factors are the models provided by friends and the accessibility of the substance (Fig. 3.29).

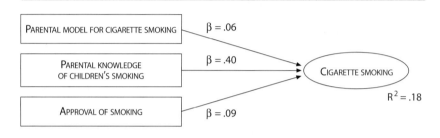

Fig. 3.28. Parental behavior and attitudes (multiple regression).

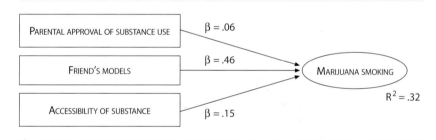

Fig. 3.29. Various variables related to parents and friends (multiple regression).

3.5 Functions of Psychoactive Substance Use

While there are many studies that describe adolescent involvement in risk behavior in general and the use of psychoactive substances in particular, very few are able to provide information useful to understanding why, despite the obvious risks associated with smoking cigarettes and marijuana and drinking large quantities of alcohol, adolescents initiate and prolong use of these substances. Based on a very common medical approach, people put their health at risk by carrying out inappropriate behavior and consuming harmful substances because they are unaware of the risks involved with these behavior types. As we will see in Chap. 8, this model, according to which healthy actions are the necessary consequence of accurate information, is groundless. As far as the possible outcomes tied to the consumption of substances are concerned, the majority of young people have accurate knowledge, but this awareness is not a sufficient deterrent. Our data also reveal that adolescents are aware that tobacco, alcohol, and marijuana can cause serious health problems (Fig. 3.30), but in spite of this knowledge, as we have seen, experimentation with these substances occurs in a large number of subjects. Alcohol, which in small doses can actually be beneficial, is considered by adolescents to be the substance that, if consumed daily, can create the most health problems. This belief is probably tied to the greater experience young people have with the effects of alcohol abuse compared with the effects of other substances. The perception of risk is significantly lower among adolescents who are most heavily involved in psychoactive substance use (Fig. 3.31).

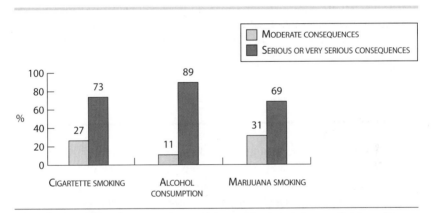

Fig. 3.30. Perception of risk tied to the use of psychoactive substances (chi-squared).

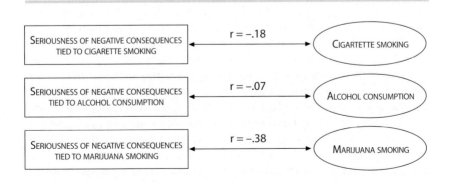

Fig. 3.31. Correlation between perception of risk and use.

This relationship between variables can be attributed to the influence of a reduced awareness of the risks involved with substance use and the more likely cause, the effect that experience with a substance has on modifying the user's attitude toward it. It has been demonstrated that cognitive dissonance, created by the discrepancy between knowledge (knowing that a behavior is harmful) and action (acting out the behavior in spite of this knowledge), can lead to modifications of attitudes in order to regain a degree of coherence between thought and behavior.

But if the perception of risk is high even among those involved in substance use, why do some adolescents, at a certain point of their lives, decide to become smokers or drinkers? And why do some adolescents, at a certain point, give up using these substances while other persist in or even increase their use? In order to respond to these questions, it is necessary to reflect on the functions that different behavior types, including risky or clearly harmful ones, can serve in the eyes of the adolescents who are acting them out. The use of psychoactive substances during adolescence can perform a number of functions that are closely tied to the main developmental tasks that adolescents find themselves faced with and to the various contexts of experience. Here we analyze the main functions involved, which can be traced back to adulthood, experimentation, the ritual function, transgression, and the need for control and escape.

3.5.1 All Grown Up

Becoming an adult is one of the crucial tasks of adolescence, which concludes in the acquisition of this new social status. And yet, in modern Western society, the awkward condition of being "suspended" between two worlds - that of children and that of adults - is increasingly prolonged. The use of psychoactive substances, especially cigarettes and alcohol, can serve the function of allowing adolescents to precociously affirm their adulthood. This affirmation occurs in the absence of obligations, responsibilities, challenges, or other essential aspects of adulthood that cannot yet be achieved by the adolescent, and it constitutes a simple, immediate, and also extremely superficial way to feel grown up.

The adulthood function facilitated by substance use is clearly suggested by the relationship between this behavior and other typically adult behavior, such as being involved in affective relationships with someone of the opposite sex, having sexual intercourse, having a job, or valuing independence in making decisions (Fig. 3.32). Although cigarette smoking and alcohol consumption as well as marijuana smoking can be used by adolescents to make them feel or appear grown up, the type of adulthood achieved is different, depending on the type of substance used. Cigarette smoking and alcohol consumption are common behavior types considered normative in adults; acting out these types of behavior, therefore, allows adolescents to feel like adults by doing what adults do. The same cannot be said for marijuana smoking, which is characteristic of certain groups of young people but not of adults. It follows that such behavior has a more transgressive connotation: growing up in opposition to or in spite of adults.

In smoking cigarettes, adulthood is in a certain way anticipated, but only for younger adolescents and girls does affirming oneself as "grown up" take on

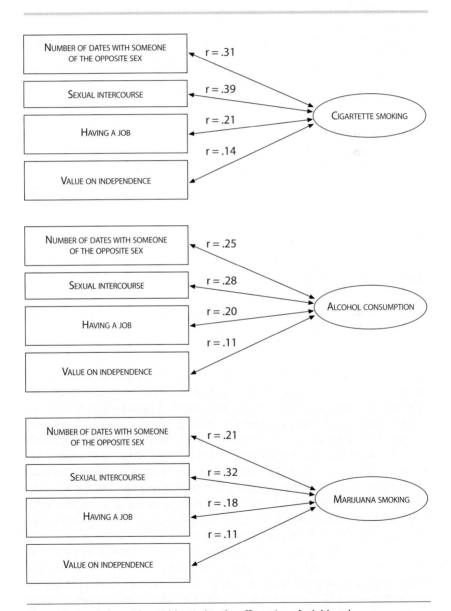

Fig. 3.32. Correlation with variables tied to the affirmation of adulthood.

a transgressive meaning: as adolescents get older, involvement in smoking rises, becomes socially acceptable, and serves different functions. Still, different processes come into play in alcohol consumption. As drinking occurs both in the company of peers and adults and is common among both, it probably allows the adolescent to identify with both adults and peers, forming continuity between past, present, and future and between the family and friend context.

The precocious need to appear as adults is, in our culture, also tied to a strong push by the means of mass communication toward consumption of adult consumer goods. This push is created by strong economic interests that seek out new areas of the market to target among the young and very young. Nevertheless, some groups are more oriented toward a precocious achievement of adulthood than others. Among these we find, for example, young adolescents who use highly visible, ostentatious behavior to distinguish themselves from the world of children, a world which is still very close at hand and which they are still often included in. Then there are the students of technical and vocational secondary schools, in other words, schools that should prepare adolescents for an early entrance into the workforce although this aim appears to be more theoretical than realistic. These students may feel more impelled to grow up quickly while lyceum (humanities, science, and education) students, for example, having many more years of school ahead of them and a later entrance into the workforce, have an easier acceptance of the "suspended" adolescent condition and show less orientation toward adulthood (Bonino and Cattelino 2000).

3.5.2 Cigarettes, Marijuana, and Transgression

Complementary to the function of anticipated adulthood, substance use can also serve a transgressive function that, in the case of cigarette smoking and alcohol consumption, consists of acting out adult behavior when not yet actually an adult. This kind of transgression is aimed primarily at affirming a social status that is not yet recognized by society. It is for this reason, for example, that the adolescents in our sample tended to hide their cigarette smoking. The transgressive function connected to early achievement of adult status is found mainly in cigarette smoking and is more relevant for girls and younger adolescents. Moving on to consider alcohol, transgression is not achieved through moderate drinking. As we have seen, many adolescents initiate drinking in a family context under the guidance and control of their parents. Furthermore, alcohol is an integral part of adult culture, and therefore, transgression is not achieved through drinking alone but rather by passing socially accepted limits. Smoking marijuana, which involves the consumption of an illegal substance, appears to be even more transgressive (Adalbjarnardottir and Rafnsson 2002). Having made these distinctions, transgression is nevertheless involved in all three substances considered, and the use of these substances is correlated with other behavior having similar values, such as anti-social and risk-taking behavior and risky driving (Fig. 3.33).

The transgressive function is felt most strongly by boys, which can be traced back to their greater involvement. Boys feel a stronger desire to increasingly expand their freedom and independence and are therefore more inclined to transgress and seek ways to affirm themselves through illegal or barely legal actions. However, the transgressive function is felt most strongly by those who do not identify with the values of the community, who do not find personal gratification in the school setting, and who have a weak internal locus of control. In fact, all of these variables are related to the degree of involvement in the use of psychoactive substances (Figs. 3.34, 3.35, 3.36).

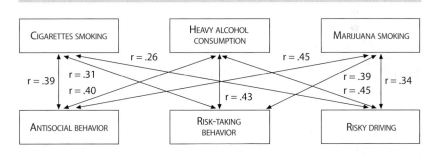

Fig. 3.33. Correlation with other types of risk behavior.

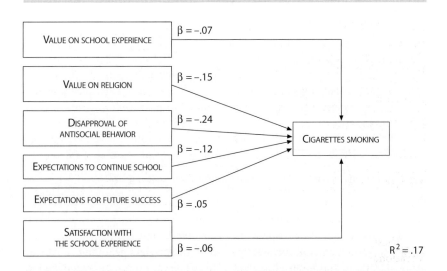

Fig. 3.34. Personal variables and cigarette smoking (multiple regression).

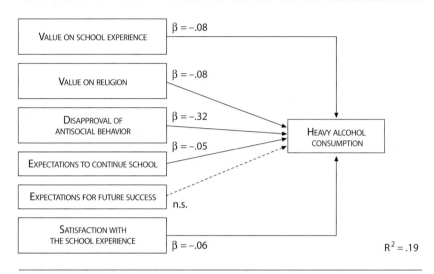

Fig. 3.35. Personal variables and heavy alcohol consumption (multiple regression).

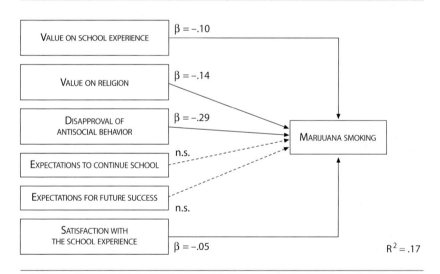

Fig. 3.36. Personal variables and marijuana smoking (multiple regression).

These characteristics are present to a greater degree in students who attend vocational and technical secondary schools and are less prevalent in lyceum students (Bonino and Cattelino 2002). This observation can be traced back to greater involvement in substance use by the former than the latter.

Another risk element is tied to the low presence of models for conventional behavior among friends, accompanied by a greater orientation toward friends when making important decisions and a low compatibility (that is to say, a low degree of agreement) between friends and parents.

In Fig. 3.37, some of these relationships have been reported. In reality, these adolescents seem to be only superficially anticonventional and do not lack elements of conventionality and conformity; they are actually more easily influenced by consumer and hedonistic values (Carlson and Edwards 1990) that are shared by their peer group, members of which are habitual consumers of psychoactive substances.

The transgressive function that, as we have said, is characteristic of high levels of alcohol consumption is not carried out by moderate consumption

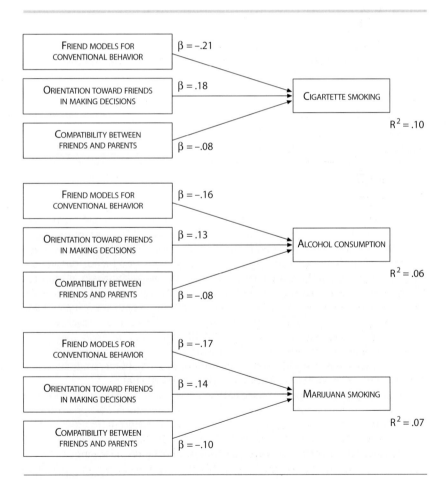

Fig. 3.37. Variables related to peers (multiple regression).

of alcoholic substances. Moderate drinkers, due to their style of consumption and the fact that this style is considered acceptable by society, have characteristics that differentiate them both from heavy drinkers and non-drinkers (Box 3.1).

Box 3.1. Moderate Drinkers

Unlike other psychoactive substances, alcohol, when consumed in moderate quantities, is not harmful to the health. It seems that in small doses, alcohol can even act as an important protective factor against coronary heart disease. Also, from a psychological and social standpoint, moderate alcohol consumption takes on an important role during the years of adolescence. As we have seen, the majority of adolescent drinkers are moderate drinkers. These boys and girls are, on the whole, well adjusted: they identify with the values of the community, they have a strong internal locus of control, and they are involved in family and school activities. For these young people, alcohol consumption, precisely because it is moderate, is neither a source of problems nor a strategy for escaping from difficulties. For this reason, there is a clear difference between moderate drinkers, and heavy drinkers for whom alcohol consumption is accompanied by serious problems. But moderate drinkers also differ from nondrinkers. The two groups have in common their involvement in daily activities and their attitudes of acceptance and identification with the rules of society. However, moderate drinkers appear to be more involved in their communities, more open to social relationships, and more willing to try out new roles and new tasks.

Based on all of our analyses, moderate drinkers appear to be more active participants in the life of the community; they spend more time with their families as well as with other adults, and many of them are involved in church groups or do volunteer work. These adolescents also have active social lives: they are at ease with their teachers and with their classmates, spend time with friends outside the school context, and are often involved in an affective relationship or reported having numerous dates with people of the opposite sex. As far as free time activities are concerned, again, moderate drinkers differ from both heavy drinkers and nondrinkers. Heavy drinkers generally use their free time unproductively, without any clear plan or activity; nondrinkers, on the other hand, generally spend their free time at home; moderate drinkers seem to be better able to coordinate their obligations at home with their obligations outside the home, study time, and community life, and to rest with social and sports activities.

This ability by moderate drinkers to have varied experiences, to make plans for their lives and for their futures, and to build broad and varied social networks made up of both peers and adults, leads these adolescents to report having greater confidence in themselves, their abilities, and their futures and to be less affected by negative sentiments such as alienation, stress, and depressed feelings.

3.5.3 What Is It Like? Experimentation

Another function that can be carried out by using psychoactive substances consists in experimenting with new sensations and the effects that various substances can have on the individual. Similar to the adulthood function, the experimentation function is also tied to the development and consolidation of a new identity, which is achieved through testing limits and exploring possibilities (Kandel and Logan 1984; Bishop et al. 1997). This experimentation function, which translates as a search for new, unusual, and extreme sensations, including altered states of consciousness, comes into play mainly with heavy alcohol consumption and marijuana smoking and is stronger in those adolescents whose aim in using these substances is to get drunk or high. This function is common to excessive alcohol consumption and marijuana use as well as other risk behavior, such a risky driving and risk-taking behavior, acted out in order to experience strong sensations (Fig. 3.38).

The experimentation function, which by definition relates to experiences, is felt primarily by adolescents who have only brief forays into risk behavior, by those who give up use early on, and by those who are first coming into contact with substances - generally the youngest adolescents. This function is also more relevant for boys than for girls. In fact, the development of a male identity follows paths that are tightly linked to experimentation while female identity develops mainly through making commitments (Palmonari 1997).

Other personal and social characteristics are also able to increase involvement in heavy drinking and marijuana use aimed at experiencing new sensations and testing limits. These types of behavior occur more frequently in those who have greater difficulties in testing their limits and experimenting in other areas, such as the school context, for example, or in more mature ways, such as reading, reflection, and free-time spent in constructive, organized activities (Fig. 3.39).

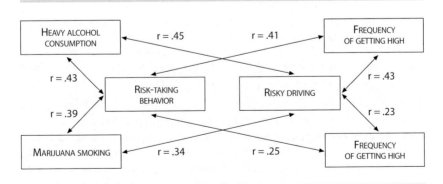

Fig. 3.38. Correlation with other types of risk behavior.

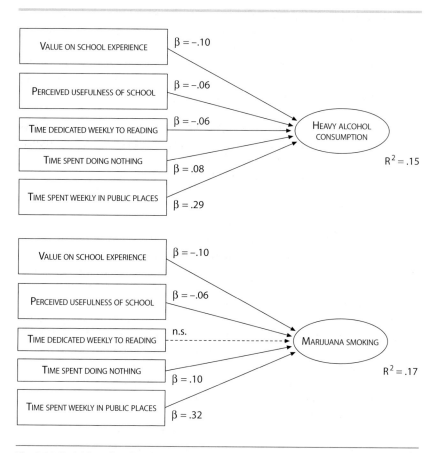

Fig. 3.39. Variables related to the experimentation function (multiple regression).

3.5.4 The Ritual Function

Throughout the course of adolescence, boys and girls invest a great deal of time and energy in friendships. As adolescents seek to gain autonomy from parental figures, close friends become an important source for defining their identities. As a result, belonging to a peer group, with its rituals and behavior requirements, becomes a highly significant experience both for the development of identity and the subjective well-being of the youngest adolescents (Cattelino 2000). The ritual function played by the use of psychoactive substances is closely tied to adolescents' need to define themselves and to begin to maintain relationships with others, especially with their peers. The ritual function was also stressed by adolescents themselves in individual interviews (Giannotta et al. 2004).

The actions involved in drinking and smoking contain a series of ritual behavior types that range from, in the case of smoking, lighting one another's cigarette or joint; passing around the lighter; holding, inhaling, and putting out the cigarette or joint; and so forth. In the case of drinking, helping oneself to a drink, sipping, exchanging glasses, and, of course, raising a glass to drink a toast are all ritual-type behavior marked by the characteristics of simplification, exaggeration, and repetition.

Consuming alcohol and smoking with peers often emerge as rites of passage, rites of initiation, or bond-forming rituals. As was discussed previously, both cigarette smoking and alcohol consumption are common, socially accepted behavior among adults; thus, in the eyes of adolescents, carrying out these types of behavior often signals a passage from childhood to the adult world. This aspect appears to be more relevant for girls and younger adolescents, who have a greater need to communicate and greater difficulties in communicating their independence and adulthood in a visible way. Instead of representing a passage from childhood to adulthood, smoking marijuana, as it is illegal, could act more as an initiation rite or rite of passage into a group of young people - a group that differs greatly both from the world of children and the world of adults. Furthermore, smoking cigarettes or marijuana, much like drinking certain alcoholic beverages, is often more or less explicitly requested, if not actually required, by certain groups in order to be accepted, making these types of behavior actual rites of initiation and belonging.

But even more than rites of passage, smoking and drinking appear to be bonding rituals or ritualized ways to create relationships within the group, to bring the group's members together and to create a shared emotion. This need to share actions and emotions is also tied to the great similarity in the behavior of adolescents within a group. In the case of alcohol consumption, the bonding ritual brings together groups of adolescents, but it also unites adolescents with adults and elderly people. Drinking is often a ritual that creates a sense of joy when it occurs in the context of a celebration, and in other situations, it can transform a neutral situation into a festive, joyful occasion.

Adolescents do not drink alcohol to quench their thirst or to bring out the taste of certain foods, nor do they drink to deal with the difficulties of daily life: they drink when they are with friends, during their free time, or on weekend nights. One of the fundamental aims of drinking alcohol is, thus, to create a feeling of joy, facilitated by the moderate disinhibition that occurs as a result of moderate alcohol consumption. This need to be part of a group, to come together, and to relate with others also applies to adolescents who use other psychoactive substances; in fact, these adolescents spend a great deal of time with their peers, have quality relationships with them, and receive support from them (Fig. 3.40).

It should also be noted that the ritualistic nature of these types of behavior can also help adolescents face certain critical moments, for example, when they find themselves alone, meet someone for the first time, or are faced with a person they do not know well. Perhaps it is also for this reason that adoles-

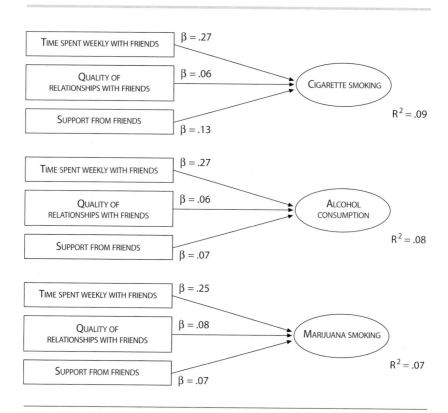

Fig. 3.40. Variables related to relationships with peers (multiple regression).

cents who drink reported having less difficulties in asking someone of the opposite sex out for a date even when they are not in a stable relationship with that person (Fig. 3.41).

The need to create a bond through consuming psychoactive substances together is felt more strongly by boys who, compared with girls of the same age, tend to have larger groups of friends whose ties are based on the sharing of behavior. Girls' social relationships, on the other hand, are more individualized, often consisting in friendships with one other person (Camerana et al. 1990; Cattelino 2000).

The ritual formation of bonds through the use of substances is also characteristic of other adolescents who, either because of immaturity tied to age or to lacking cognitive and relational capacities, are unable to find more mature ways of feeling like part of a group, have difficulties in planning shared actions based on other activities, and are unable to create bonds through deeper forms

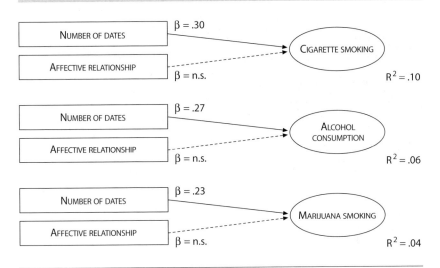

Fig. 3.41. Variables related to affective relationships (multiple regression).

of sharing. These adolescents spend their free time in nonproductive, unplanned activities (mostly sitting around not doing anything or in public places) and generally do not use dialogue and communication to deal with problems. In light of this, formal groups, and church groups in particular, act as protective factors, as they generally have specific aims and organized activities that transcend simply spending time together. In these groups, bonds are generally formed through the sharing of ideals, and the activities are more or less rigidly planned. Thus, there is no need to drink or smoke together in order to feel like a group or to do something while waiting for someone to come up with an idea that everyone can agree on, as often occurs in informal groups where activities are generally improvised and where there is a constant need to be recognized as a group by the sharing and continuous repetition of behavior.

3.5.5 Marijuana Use as an Escape

In habitual marijuana smokers, much like those who consume large quantities of alcohol in order to get drunk, substance use can no longer be interpreted in terms of experimentation or temporary transgression. In these adolescents, who repeatedly get high or drunk, substance use seems to be a means of escape from a present situation that is unfulfilling and marked by conflicts - with friends or parents - that they do not know how to resolve or perhaps even to express (Summary 3.2).

Summary 3.2. Main characteristics of heavy drinkers and heavy marijuana users.

- Prevalently boys in the older age groups (16-17 and 18-19 years)
- Most attend vocational schools
- Low self-esteem and lack of confidence in coping skills
- Pessimistic expectations for the future
- Reported high levels of alienation
- Have had several academic failures, and school for them is not a place where they find personal fulfillment
- Strongly oriented toward the peer group
- Have little dialogue with and receive minimal support from their parents
- Spend free time in nonproductive, nonorganized activities
- Spend a great deal of time outside the home and many hours in public places and video arcades
- Involved in a number of risk activities

Box 3.2. High-risk Adolescents

When analyzing the various types of risk behavior, whether tied to the use of psychoactive substances or externalized actions such as antisocial behavior, risky driving, or other risk-taking behavior dictated by a need to feel strong sensations, there is always a minority of adolescents who are heavily involved in risk; depending on the specific behavior considered, this group ranges from 8-12%. These adolescents have particular characteristics that differentiate them from their peers who are either uninvolved in risk behavior or involved at low levels.

First and foremost, the majority of these heavily involved adolescents are boys between the ages of 16 and 19, most of whom attend vocational secondary schools followed by technical secondary schools. As for their personal characteristics, these adolescents generally have lower self-esteem than their peers, have less confidence in their academic abilities, feel less able to confront the difficulties of daily life, and have more pessimistic expectations for future success. They also perceive themselves to be more insecure and reported high levels of alienation, stress, and depressed feelings. They feel their conception of life is neither similar to that of their parents nor to that of their friends although they appear to be more oriented toward their friends in making important decisions.

High-risk adolescents also differ from their peers in the way they use their free time and in their perception of their context (Piko and Vazsonyi 2004). They are implicated in multiple types of risk behavior (these adolescents are often heavy smokers, habitual marijuana smokers, heavy drinkers, sexually promiscuous, and implicated in antisocial behavior and risky driving), and they spend most of their free time outside the home in informal groups and in nonproductive, unplanned activities (like sitting around doing nothing or walking/driving around without a destination) or seeking amusement in coffee shops, video arcades or discos. They are often boys and girls who come from families where a cultural division has

For this reason, marijuana use and excessive alcohol consumption, resulting in altered consciousness, can appear to be emotional strategies for resolving difficulties (Labouvie 1986). However, these strategies are actually illusory attempts to confront problems that, in reality, are not confronted but denied or forgotten for the time being only to re-emerge just as real as ever and often aggravated by the use of the substance. As we saw in the introduction to this chapter, one of the physiological effects of psychoactive substances is the alteration of cognitive capacities, which in turn leads to greater difficulties in confronting and resolving complex tasks. For this reason, it is clear how these strategies actually become a vicious cycle in which the problems that adolescents seek to escape from by getting high or drunk become even more difficult to resolve.

Box 3.2 lists the main characteristics of adolescents at high risk for involvement. These characteristics are typical not only of heavy users of psychoactive substances but also of the adolescents most heavily involved in other types of risk behavior, such as risky driving, risk-taking behavior dictated by a desire for strong sensations, and antisocial behavior.

Box 3.2.

formed between parents and children, caused, for example, by immigration, urbanization, or rapid changes in lifestyle and values. These adolescents do not see their parents as points of reference or sources of support, and the parents themselves seem to have given up on parenting.

Not even school is experienced or perceived as a resource. High-risk adolescents have generally had to repeat more years during their school careers than other adolescents, and they often leave primary school with a negative judgment of their capabilities. They are very unsure about both their present and future and, because of this, do not view the school as useful for their future job and for their adult lives but rather as an experience that has no real point. Within the school context, these adolescents do not have satisfying relationships with their teachers and classmates, which is intensified by a sense of uneasiness that is tied to a lack of confidence in their scholastic capabilities, a lack of importance attributed to the school experience, and low expectations to continue school. These adolescents dedicate a very small amount of time to study, and they have strong intentions to drop out of school; in many cases, they have already stopped attending school for periods of time.

From this description, we can clearly see the serious difficulties for high-risk adolescents. Although it should be kept in mind that this group represents a minority of adolescents, it cannot be ignored or overlooked. For these young people, use of psychoactive substances and heavy involvement in other risk behavior function mainly as escape methods - ways of avoiding difficulties and responsibility. Pessimism about a future that they cannot imagine and that they have difficulties working toward combined with a lack of self-esteem and dissatisfaction with their present lives and contexts leads these young people to opt for actions and sensations - such as getting drunk or high - that let them escape their problems and their inability to confront these problems in a more well-adjusted way.

Summary 3.3 provides an overview of the main functions carried out by the use of the three psychoactive substances considered.

Summary 3.3. Main functions carried out by psychoactive substance use.

Alcohol consumption	Cigarette smoking	Marijuana smoking
• Anticipation of ADULTHOOD, by drinking to act like an adult	• Anticipation of ADULTHOOD, by imitating adult behavior (mainly students of technical and vocational secondary schools)	• Anticipation of ADULTHOOD, by acting in opposition to or in spite of adults
• TRANSGRESSION, tied to alcohol abuse (primarily in boys who drink excessively)	• TRANSGRESSION, tied to anticipation of a typically adult behavior (especially in the youngest adolescents and girls)	• TRANSGRESSION, tied to the illegality of the substance (mainly students of technical and vocational secondary schools)
• TESTING oneself and one's reactions; tied to heavy consumption and getting drunk (especially in occasional drinkers)		• EXPERIMENTATION with the effects that the substance can have on the individual by getting high (especially in those trying the substance for the first time and in the youngest adolescents)
• RITE OF PASSAGE (mostly for younger adolescents, girls, and those approaching alcohol for the first time)	• RITE OF PASSAGE (mostly for younger adolescents, girls, and those approaching cigarettes for the first time).	• RITE OF INITIATION (especially for 16- to 17-year-olds)
• RITUAL OF JOYFULNESS AND BONDING, between different generations	• BONDING RITUAL, to form a connection with other young people (especially for boys and the youngest adolescents)	• BONDING RITUAL, to connect with other young people (especially for boys)
• ESCAPE from difficulties and confrontation of problems through getting drunk frequently		• ESCAPE from difficulties and confrontations through repeatedly getting high

3.6 **Protective Factors**

Protective factors are the combination of variables and personal and contextual characteristics that are able to limit adolescents' involvement in risk behavior. For a long time, these factors were overlooked by an approach that was more focussed on identifying risk factors, and only recently have protective factors begun to be considered in order to better comprehend the different paths that involvement in various types of risk behavior can take and, based on this information, develop effective prevention strategies (Jackson et al. 1997; Deković 1999).

In recent years, it has been found that protective factors act both by promoting personal abilities useful in overcoming the various developmental tasks and by promoting greater well-being through the reduction, balancing, neutralization, or compensation of risk factors. Therefore, it is clear that there is a dynamic interaction between risk factors and protective factors (Stattin and Magnusson 1996). As Rutter pointed out (1987, 1993), these factors should not be considered as static qualities of an individual but rather as resources that the individual can turn to in times of need. From this perspective, protective and risk factors interact over time, competing to influence not so much developmental outcomes as developmental paths. Furthermore, in a developmental, constructivistic, interactionistic perspective - like the one we have assumed - a protective factor is not necessarily so at all ages or for all adolescents. For instance, there are different antecedents and outcomes of marijuana use initiation during adolescence that are linked to different risk and protective factors (Ellickson et al. 2004). For this reason, we seek, in this section, to evidence the possible gender differences and differences between adolescents of different age groups in order to better understand which variables maintain their protective value throughout adolescence and which, on the other hand, are effective at different times or for different adolescents.

Protective factors can be described according to their different tendencies. For example, some can be represented along a continuum ranging from a minimum to a maximum of protection; others on a continuum where risk and protection are found at either end, (i.e. parental support); others appear as a u-shaped tendency (i.e. parental control); others still can be described by their presence or absence (i.e. participation in a church group).

As we have already seen through our analysis of the functions of psychoactive substances, the disapproval of antisocial behavior, value on the school experience and religion, satisfaction with the school experience, and expectations to continue school are important personal protective factors that are related to adolescents' choices. Those who are gratified by the school experience, who are dedicated to their studies, and who recognize the values of respect for others and the rules of society work to reach their goals of growth through strategies and across paths that are nondetrimental and not exclusively external. In this section, we will analyze other protective factors, examining in particular the role of knowledge about risks, the role of the school experience, the use of free time, and the relationships between adolescents and their parents and friends.

3.6.1 What Type of Knowledge Is Most Useful?

As we already noted (Fig. 3.31), the perception of risk and knowledge of the possible negative consequences involved in certain behavior is a protective factor. However, the relationship between knowledge and behavior has often been emphasized without discussing other relevant aspects that are related to individual decisions and the adoption of a certain lifestyle. Thus, based on a medical model that is common yet ineffective, it is believed that being aware of the risks involved in a given behavior is the strongest deterrent to keep us from carrying out that behavior. As we have mentioned, this approach, which is the basis of a number of advertising slogans used even recently in prevention campaigns, is more or less ineffective. In reality, human action is not based exclusively on cognitive evaluations but is tightly linked to emotional, affective, relational, and social factors.

While our study results show that awareness of the physical and psychological risks involved in the use of psychoactive substances is, in fact, a protective factor (Fig. 3.42), it also emerged that this knowledge alone is not sufficient to prevent involvement in various types of behavior (the values of R^2 are actually quite low). The figure shows how awareness of risks is more protective in the case of marijuana smoking while for alcohol consumption, it has practically no influence.

When examining the specific knowledge of the potential negative consequences tied to substance use, a rich and complex picture emerges. As far as cigarette smoking is concerned, adolescents pointed out physical risks

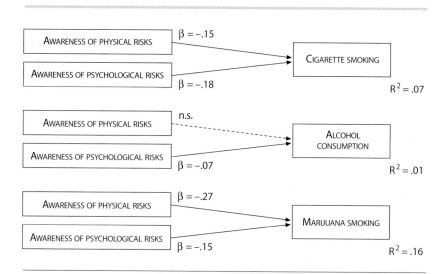

Fig. 3.42. Awareness of risks on use of psychoactive substances (multiple regression).

ranging from respiratory problems and the possibility of developing cancer to shortness of breath, coughing, impotence, and heart disease. They also pointed to risks with psychological implications ranging from addiction to aesthetic drawbacks (such as yellow fingers and teeth) to smelling bad and being irritable.

Also, in the case of heavy alcohol consumption, the awareness of risks is articulated in terms of symptoms such as headache and nausea, liver-related problems, and gastrointestinal and cardiovascular problems. In addition to these potential consequences, subjects also mentioned problems related to alcoholism, cognitive problems, personality and mood disturbances, compromising behavior, and damage to social relationships.

Finally, as far as marijuana use is concerned, the most frequently cited consequences were dependence, deficit in cognitive performance, damage to the central nervous system, the possibility of progressing to other types of drugs, and the jeopardizing of certain social relationships.

Further exploratory analyses conducted showed that not all knowledge has the same effect in protecting adolescents from serious and lasting involvement in substance use. For example, medical consequences, even when related to serious, but not immediate, health problems, do not appear to be good deterrents. However, knowledge related to the negative repercussions that a behavior could have in the here and now appears to be an important protective factor. So, for example, the idea of having yellow teeth and smelling bad after smoking a cigarette or a joint or of having bad breath after drinking too much alcohol seems to be more protective than being aware of the risk of developing cancer as an adult.

Other types of knowledge that serve as protective factors are closely tied to the developmental tasks typical of adolescence, such as becoming increasingly independent, consolidating relationships with friends, and defining one's personal identity. So, for example, knowledge of the risk of addiction or damage to the central nervous system that substance use can cause assumes a protective value. For adolescents on the path to achieving greater independence, the risk of having to depend on someone or something represents a serious threat. In the same way, damage to the central nervous system or to cognitive abilities can affect the entire redefinition of the self, which also occurs through ideas and reasoning. For this reason, damage to the brain, and to the cognitive capabilities connected to it, represent a threat to the entire identity more so than the consequences connected to damage of any other organ.

These findings are evidence that it is not the knowledge related to more serious consequences that is the most effective and that scare tactics are clearly not the appropriate approach to prevention for adolescents. On the one hand, the awareness of the potential risks - which could compromise the present lives of young people, their relationships, their appearance, and their deepest identity - is, on the other hand, a good protective factor. Summary 3.4 lists the types of knowledge that have the strongest protective value.

Summary 3.4. Overview of the most useful types of knowledge.

In the prevention of psychoactive substance use, some types of information are more useful than others. The most useful information is related to:

- Potential negative repercussions on one's present life or near future
- Potential immediate advantages of noninvolvement
- The possibility of compromising the achievement of developmental tasks (definition of the self and identity, independence, and social relationships)

3.6.2 The School Experience

School represents an important life context beginning from early childhood and plays a key role in the years of adolescence, so much so that adjustment to school is an important developmental obligation and failure in the adjustment process often translates into a deep sense of discomfort (Fonzi 2002).

Precisely because the school experience today plays such an essential role in helping adolescents to construct a sense of their personal identity and in defining their relationships with social institutions (Palmonari and Rubini 1998), it can play an important protective role for various types of risk behavior. Figures 3.43, 3.44, and 3.45 display the results of a multiple regression analysis where variables related to school success, perception of self as a student, and relationships with teachers and classmates were the predictors of use for different psychoactive substances.

From these analyses, it emerges that there are numerous variables connected to the school experience that play a protective role. In particular, not

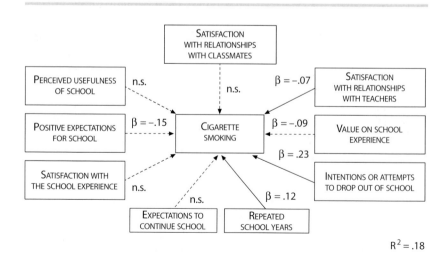

Fig. 3.43. School-related variables and cigarette smoking (multiple regression).

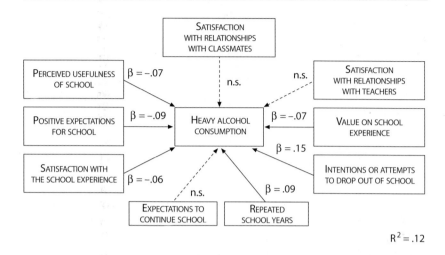

Fig. 3.44. School related variables and heavy alcohol consumption (multiple regression).

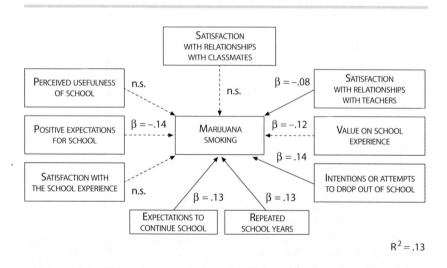

Fig. 3.45. School related variables and marijuana smoking (multiple regression).

wanting to drop out of school, a low number of repeated school years, and high expectations for school were protective factors for use of all three substances considered. Other variables act as protective factors only for some substances: value on school experience and satisfying relationships with teachers contribute to reducing involvement in cigarette and marijuana smoking; a perception of the school as useful to one's present and future protects against alcohol abuse.

Table 3.2 summarizes the variables tied to the school experience. To extract these data, a multiple regression analysis was conducted on the sample stratified by gender and age group. What emerges is that adolescents who value the school experience, who reported satisfactory relationships with their teachers, who are successful in the educational context, and, above all, who have high expectations for school are less involved in habitual or heavy use of psychoactive substances. These adolescents are probably successful in creating a strong personal identity through dedication and commitment to the academic institution and do not feel the need to seek out alternative or superficial ways of affirming adulthood or feeling successful. On the contrary, students who are not gratified in the school experience, who have experienced serious failures such as failed school years, and who have considered dropping out, have a greater tendency to use psychoactive substances and the effects they produce as emotional escape strategies and to seek out transgressive, highly visible, yet purely superficial ways of affirming their personal identity.

Table 3.2. Factors tied to school experience based on gender and age (multiple regression).

Protective factors		
Cigarette smoking	**Heavy alcohol consumption**	**Marijuana smoking**
Protective factors are: • Good relationships with teachers • High positive expectations for school • Value on the school experience Quality relationships with teachers are protective mainly for girls and adolescents aged 16-17 The other two aspects are more protective for boys and adolescents 16-17 years old	Protective factors are: • Perceived usefulness of the school • Satisfaction with the school experience • Value on the school experience • High positive expectations for the school Valuing the school experience is more protective for girls, while perceived usefulness of school is more important for boys. High expectations for the school experience are a very good protective factor for all adolescents	Protective factors are: • Value on the school experience • Good relationships with teachers • High positive expectations for school Good relationships with teachers are mostly protective for girls and adolescents aged 16-17; the other two aspects are protective for all the adolescents considered
Factors that increase the probability of involvement		
Cigarette smoking	**Heavy alcohol consumption**	**Marijuana smoking**
The factors that increase the probability of involvement are: • Repeated school years • Intentions or attempts to drop out of school These factors increase risk for boys and are most prevalent in adolescents from 16-17 years old	The factors that increase the probability of involvement are: • Repeated school years • Intentions or attempts to drop out of school Repeating a school year is only a risk factor for boys and the youngest adolescents	The factors that increase the probability of involvement are: • Repeated school years • Intentions or attempts to drop out of school Intention to drop out of school is a risk factor both for boys and girls in all age groups

3.6.3 Use of Free Time

The contexts in which adolescents spend their free time and the activities they take part in outside the school setting can be important risk or protective factors for the use of psychoactive substances. However, the influence of contexts and, above all, the context in which free time is spent, should not be viewed with a deterministic approach; it is now clear that the individual has an active role in selecting and shaping these contexts.

Over the last decades, free time has become more and more important in the lives of adolescents. Free time often represents the only - or at least the preferred - opportunity for adolescents to make decisions independently, giving young and very young people the opportunity to give shape to their own identities and to contribute actively to the construction of their lifestyles. From our analyses, we found that the use of free time has an important role in either encouraging or limiting the use of various psychoactive substances by adolescents (Figs. 3.46, 3.47, 3.48).

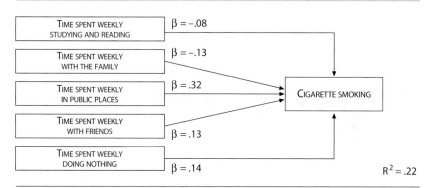

Fig. 3.46. Variables related to free time and cigarette smoking (multiple regression).

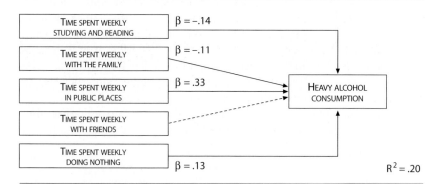

Fig. 3.47. Variables related to free time and heavy alcohol consumption (multiple regression).

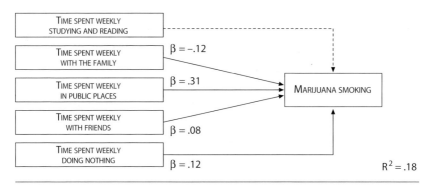

Fig. 3.48. Variables related to free time and marijuana smoking (multiple regression).

Time spent with the family and time spent studying or reading are protective factors for psychoactive substance use. While on one hand time spent with one's parents limits the opportunities for experimentation with risk behavior, on the other hand, it offers adolescents the possibility to assume adult behavior and attitudes by relating to adults as equals. Furthermore, by spending time together, a tighter bond is formed between parents and adolescent children, facilitating dialogue and narration, which is so important in the definition of one's self. Through this sharing and dialogue, adolescents can find constructive strategies for the resolution of problems.

Time dedicated to studying and reading offers adolescents a chance to reflect on themselves and the meaning of their lives and choices; it also offers them an opportunity to see other points of view and develop different reasoning strategies. All of these cognitive capabilities constitute useful life skills that probably help the adolescent to confront different situations and, thus, to avoid using substance abuse as an easy escape.

On the contrary, time spent doing nothing, and especially time spent in public places, can represent risk factors for adolescents. Those who do not dedicate time to studying and their families and who do not find other constructive ways of spending their free time are more exposed to risk and boredom and are more likely to use or abuse substances as a superficial, and also relatively ineffective, way to fill the sense of emptiness they feel with strong sensations. For these adolescents, substance use can also be a superficial way to form a bond with friends in the absence of shared ideas or plans.

Table 3.3 summarizes the variables tied to the use of free time. These finding are based on a regression analysis conducted on the sample, stratified for gender and age group.

Table 3.3. Factors tied to free time based on gender and age group (multiple regression).

Protective factors		
Cigarette smoking	**Heavy alcohol consumption**	**Marijuana smoking**
Protective factors are: • Time spent studying and reading • Time spent with the family On the whole, free time is strongly related with cigarette smoking for adolescents aged 14-15. Time dedicated to studying is protective mainly for boys and the youngest adolescents (14-15 years) while for girls, time spent with the family has a greater importance	Protective factors are: • Time spent studying and reading • Time spent with the family All in all, free time is strongly related with heavy alcohol consumption for boys and adolescents aged 16-17. Time spent with the family is more protective for girls 16-17 years old	The only protective factor is: • Time spent with the family Although it is significant for all groups, time spent with the family has a greater importance for girls
Factors that increase the probability of involvement		
Cigarette smoking	**Heavy alcohol consumption**	**Marijuana smoking**
The factors that increase the probability of involvement are: • Time spent doing nothing • Time spent in public places • Time spent with friends Time spent doing nothing, although significant in all groups, has the greatest importance on the youngest adolescents. Time spent in public places appears to be a risk factor for boys and girls of all ages	The factors that increase the probability of involvement are: • Time spent doing nothing • Time spent in public places Time spent doing nothing, while significant for all groups except for adolescents 18 and older, is a stronger risk factor for girls. Time spent in public places poses a risk for boys and girls of all ages but is especially important for boys and adolescents 18 and older	The factors that increase the probability of involvement are: • Time spent doing nothing • Time spent in public places • Time spent with friends These factors are significant for boys and girls of all ages. However, boredom is a greater predictor of implication for boys and adolescents 18 and older while spending time in public places has a greater importance on substance use by adolescents 16-17 years old

3.6.4 External Regulation, Support, and Control

The adolescents most heavily involved in the use of all three psychoactive substances considered here appear to have a weaker internal *locus of control* than their nonusing peers. In fact, as we have seen, they disapprove less of antisocial behavior and they do not identify as strongly with the values shared by society (for example, they attribute less value to religion and the school experience). These same adolescents have greater difficulties managing their activities and their free time, spending hours doing nothing, or passing time in public places.

Along with this general trend toward transgression and difficulties in self-regulation and self-control, other factors tied to relationships with friends and parents also come into play. From our data, it appears that it is neither the family structure - whole or divided - nor the parents' profession or academic background that influences adolescents; all of these factors were found to be not significant. Therefore, we can go beyond a simplistic view in which the children of divorced or separated parents are necessarily at greater risk. These parents can also play a protective role by carrying out the two main functions of the family: support, which means being readily available and open to dialogue, and control, which entails establishing and enforcing rules of behavior for inside and outside of the home (Cattelino et al. 2001).

In an analysis of the family's functioning, the influence of parents or, rather, the type of relationship that exists between parents and children, has a primary role. A balance between support and control creates the foundation not only for the construction of a positive self-perception (Jackson et al. 1998; Cattelino et al. 2001) but also for the reduction of risk of serious and persistent involvement in psychoactive substance use (Bonino and Cattelino 2000).

The results reported in Fig. 3.49 confirm the protective role played by a combination of support and control. Table 3.4 provides a summary of the protective factors tied to the family context. These results were obtained by conducting regression analyses on the sample stratified by gender and age group. The picture that emerges from these analyses shows how the effect of support and control changes for boys and girls and as adolescents get older. Therefore, parents must be able to flexibly alter their attitudes over the course of this "group effort," which having adolescent children represents for the family (Scabini 1995; Scabini et al. 2005 in press).

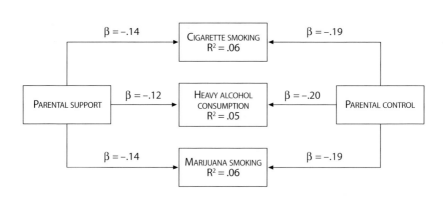

Fig. 3.49. Parental support and control and the use of different psychoactive substances (multiple regression).

Table 3.4. Protective factors related to the family context based on gender and age (multiple regression).

Cigarette smoking	Heavy alcohol consumption	Marijuana smoking
Protective factors are: • Parental support • Parental control Support and control were significant for all groups, but they appear to be most protective for adolescents aged 16-17; support appears to be more protective for the girls	Protective factors are: • Parental support • Parental control Control is more protective for boys while support has a greater protective role for adolescents aged 16-17	Protective factors are: • Parental support • Parental control While support and control have a protective function for boys and girls of all ages, they have a greater importance on girls and adolescents 16-17 years old

Through an authoritative parenting style, the family plays a protective role both by helping adolescents acquire a greater ability to self-regulate and by alleviating the adolescent's feelings of discomfort through dialogue and emotional support (Cattelino et al. 2001; Ciairano et al. 2001). In this way, families can limit the risk that their adolescent sons and daughters will turn to psychoactive substances in order to escape from reality and unpleasant feelings.

With regard to cigarette smoking in particular, an authoritative parenting style, characterized by a high degree of support and control, plays a protective role both for involvement and for giving up smoking; in other words, this parenting style can limit the behavior to the experimental phase (Fig. 3.50).

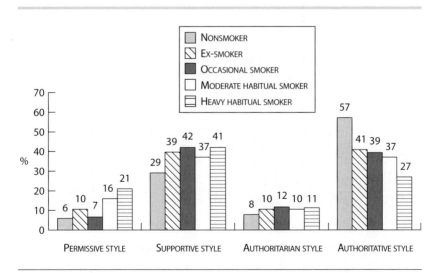

Fig. 3.50. Parenting style and adolescents' cigarette smoking (chi-squared).

A balanced union of empathetic support and strictness also appears to be decisive in adolescents' involvement in smoking, which, unlike other psychoactive substances, enjoys a fairly high degree of social acceptability. This parenting style may result in less desire to anticipate adulthood, less need for transgression, less orientation toward the group, greater acceptance of one's status as an adolescent, greater social competence, and greater ability to take on difficulties thanks to open dialogue with the family (Bonino and Cattelino 2000).

Even a supportive parenting style characterized by a high degree of support and little control can be protective, especially for the oldest adolescents and for girls. An authoritarian style, on the other hand (low support and high control), and above all a permissive style (little support and low control), are risk factors and are characteristic of the relationships between the most heavily involved adolescents and their parents.

As for marijuana smoking, the family climate of ex-smokers differs both from those of adolescents who have never felt the need to smoke marijuana and of habitual smokers (Fig. 3.51).

The adolescents who have never tried marijuana tend to come from families where there is an authoritative parenting style characterized by well-defined rules and strong emotional support. Adolescents who have given up smoking marijuana come primarily from families where there is a high degree of emotional support but very little strictness - both for behavior inside the home and outside of it (Cattelino and Bonino 1999). While the absence of control and limits can explain both the greater ease with which these adolescents became involved and their greater need to put themselves to the test, the high degree of support they receive probably plays a protective role, helping them

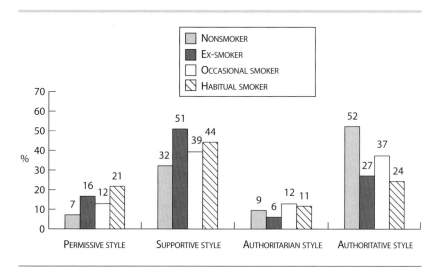

Fig. 3.51. Parenting style and adolescents' marijuana smoking (chi-squared).

to give up smoking marijuana. In the case of habitual users whose use is not limited to an initial experimental phase and who are mainly looking for a means of escape, the family appears to be nonexistent - not at all strict but also not at all supportive, even less so than in the families of occasional smokers.

Also, in the case of alcohol consumption - or more precisely, alcohol abuse - an authoritative parenting style appears to be the most protective (Fig. 3.52).

In addition to the family, friends can also play an important protective role in limiting heavy and persistent involvement in substance abuse (Figs. 3.53, 3.54, 3.55). Our findings clearly show that the most protective factor offered by friends is a model for nontransgressive lifestyles. Having friends who dedicate time to studying and organized, productive activities allows adolescents to see conventional models and identify with their peers, establishing significant relationships with them without turning to the use or abuse of psychoactive substances.

For boys, we also see the importance of self-regulatory efficacy, especially in the presence of friends whose behavior is transgressive. The ability to "be yourself" in the face of peer pressure is a strong protective factor and can have a major impact on the choices an individual makes. This result is consistent with other studies showing that self-efficacy beliefs predicted psychosocial outcomes (Caprara et al. 2004).

Another interesting aspect that emerges from our data is the role played by the perceived relationship between one's friends and parents. A greater orientation toward friends in making important decisions, low compatibility - or, rather, a low compatibility and therefore conflict between friends and parents - and transgressive friend models significantly increase the risk of involvement in substance use. In these situations, substance abuse can act as an inef-

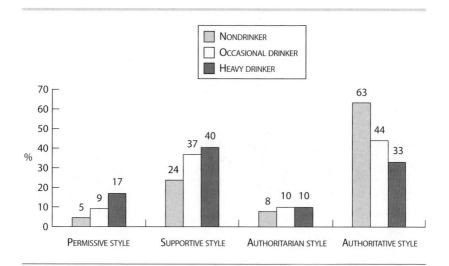

Fig. 3.52. Parenting style and adolescents' alcohol consumption (chi-squared).

fective coping strategy carried out mainly in an attempt to escape conflict and tension. This aspect of conflict between friends and parents is a good predictor of legal substance use (tobacco and alcohol), which shows that adolescents who use illegal substances have deeper, more internal difficulties and conflicts. Alternatively, it could be hypothesized that cigarette smokers and drinkers, whose transgression is more limited, are more aware of these conflicts while adolescents who smoke marijuana heavily may be less able to assign meaning to their difficulties through cognitive elaboration.

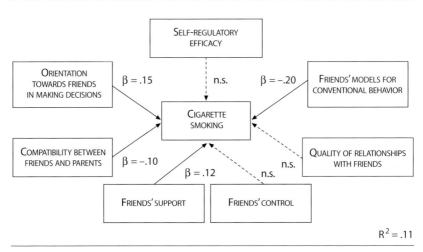

Fig. 3.53. Variables related to peers and cigarette smoking (multiple regression).

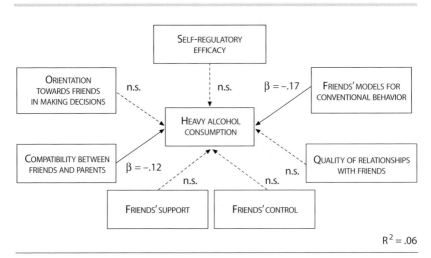

Fig. 3.54. Variables related to peers and heavy alcohol consumption (multiple regression).

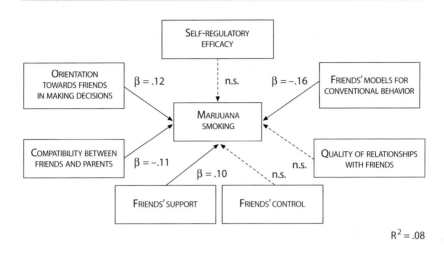

Fig. 3.55. Variables related to peers and marijuana smoking (multiple regression).

Table 3.5 summarizes the variables tied to relationships with friends. To extract these data, a multiple regression analysis was conducted on the sample, stratified by gender and age group.

Table 3.5. Factors tied to peer-related aspects (multiple regression).

	Protective factors	
Cigarette smoking	**Heavy alcohol consumption**	**Marijuana smoking**
Protective factors are:	Protective factors are:	Protective factors are:
• Self-regulatory efficacy	• Self-regulatory efficacy	• Compatibility (degree of agreement) between friends and parents
• Friends' models for conventional activities	• Compatibility (degree of agreement) between friends and parents	• Friends' models for conventional activities
• Compatibility (degree of agreement) between friends and parents	• Friends' models for conventional activities	Friends' models are protective for both genders in all age groups, and compatibility between friends and parents, while significant for both boys and girls, is particularly protective for adolescents 16-17 years old
Compatibility between friends and parents is protective for adolescents 16-17 years old and older while friends' models for conventional activities are protective for all age groups and both genders. For boys self-regulatory efficacy is also protective	• Friends' control Self-regulatory efficacy is protective for boys only while control by friends is only protective for adolescents 18 and older. Both of the other aspects are protective for both genders and for all age groups	

cont. ▸▸

Table 3.5. *Cont.*

Factors that increase the probability of involvement		
Cigarette smoking	**Heavy alcohol consumption**	**Marijuana smoking**
The factors that increase the probability of involvement are: • Friends' support • Orientation toward friends in making decisions Substantial friends' support is accompanied by greater involvement in cigarette smoking by adolescents 18 and older while a greater orientation toward friends in making decisions is significant only in adolescents younger than 18	The factors that increase the probability of involvement are: • Quality of relationships with peers • Orientation toward friends in making decisions An orientation toward friends in making decisions appears to be a risk factor for girls and adolescents aged 16-17. Having quality relationships with friends is only significant for adolescents 18 and older while a high degree of support from friends is significant for boys only	The factors that increase the probability of involvement are: • Friends' support • Orientation toward friends in making decisions Orientation toward friends in making decisions is significant for all groups except for those 18 and older. Support has a greater importance for boys and is not significant for the youngest adolescents (14-15 years old)

Summary 3.5 offers a theoretical overview of the main protective factors tied to the family, school, friends, and free-time contexts. These protective factors have been linked to the different functions that the use of various psychoactive substances can perform for adolescents.

Summary 3.5. Main protective factors related to family, school, friends, and free-time contexts in relation to the functions of psychoactive substance use.

Protective factors	Related functions
FAMILY • Parental models • Older sibling models • Attitudes of explicit disapproval • Alcohol consumption in the family context • Parental support • Parental control	Parental models for nonsmoking and moderate alcohol consumption encourage: • IDENTIFICATION with adults • Imitation and adoption of a healthy style of consumption and healthy lifestyle Sibling models (especially older siblings) for nonsmoking encourage: • IDENTIFICATION with young people • Imitation and adoption of a healthy style of consumption and healthy lifestyle The explicit disapproval of substance use: • Favors control and monitoring • Communicates information on the harmfulness of cigarette smoking, marijuana use, and heavy alcohol consumption Alcohol consumption in the family context favors: • IDENTIFICATION • Adoption of a moderate style of consumption • A BOND between generations • A SENSE OF BELONGING to the adult world and to the community • The sharing of CULTURAL VALUES tied to moderate alcohol consumption (as opposed to ESCAPE or abuse) • BONDING and JOYFULNESS RITUAL

cont. ▶▶

Protective factors	Related functions
	A balanced combination of support and control encourages: • The use of dialogue and exchange as methods of AFFIRMING oneself and one's ADULTHOOD • SELF-ENHANCEMENT, through the sharing of ideas, feelings, expectations, plans, etc. • AUTONOMY, through establishing equal relationships • Use of COPING STRATEGIES, based on verbalization and comparison • Internalization of rules and values vs OPPOSITION to them • Processes of EXTERNAL REGULATION and SELF-REGULATION
SCHOOL EXPERIENCE • Value on academic achievement • Satisfaction with the school experience • Good relationships with teachers • Perceived usefulness • Expectations to continue school • High positive expectations for future success	Viewing school as a meaningful, satisfying experience encourages: • SELF-AFFIRMATION • STRENGTHENING OF A POSITIVE IDENTITY • Involvement in society's institutions and the adult world instead of TRANSGRESSION and OPPOSITION • ASSUMING RESPONSIBILITIES and obligations as opposed to ESCAPE from them
PEERS • Models for noninvolvement in cigarette and marijuana smoking and moderate alcohol consumption • Models for nontransgressive behavior or conventional behavior • Compatibility between friends and parents	Friends' models encourage: • IDENTIFICATION and adoption of healthy patterns • Fewer occasions for consumption • Reduced availability of substances The perception of friends as nontransgressive, involved in conventional activities, and having values similar to those held by one's parents favors: • The creation of a BOND based on the sharing of ideas and organized, constructive, activities as opposed to nonproductive or oppositional activities • The perception of SOCIAL ACCEPTANCE unrelated to the use of psychoactive substances • EXPERIMENTATION with roles and socially accepted, nondangerous actions • The perception of continuity with the values of the adult world and with society as opposed to TRANSGRESSION, OPPOSITION, and ESCAPE
FREE TIME • Time spent studying and reading • Time spent with the family • Belonging to a religious group	Time spent per week reading and studying, time spent with the family, and belonging to a religious group encourage: • SELF-AFFIRMATION and the CONSTRUCTION OF IDENTITY, through reflection, ideas, comparison, and prosocial behavior • The reinforcement of a SENSE OF BELONGING to the community • Reflection on the meaning of one's existence and of the meaning of one's actions, both for oneself and others • PLANNING SKILLS and COMMITMENT • Use of effective COPING STRATEGIES • Internalization of values as opposed to opposition to them • SOCIAL VISIBILITY, through participation in constructive activities

CHAPTER 4

Risk-Taking Behavior and Risky Driving

> For me drinking with friends on a Saturday night or smoking a cigarette isn't about breaking the rules anymore, they're just things I normally do... for me, now, breaking the rules means going 250 km an hour in my car... in four or five years even that won't be about breaking the rules... breaking the rules is only tied to driving now because we're 18 and it's something new for us...
>
> *[Boy, science lyceum, fifth year]*

4.1 Risk-Taking Behavior

Risk-taking behavior is behavior that endangers the personal safety of those that carry it out and, in some cases, the safety of others. This type of behavior is enacted in order to provoke excitement and strong sensations and is extremely common in adolescents. At this point in their development, not only are boys and girls constantly faced with new possibilities and alternatives, but they also feel the need to make new commitments and reinforce those made previously (Bosma and Jackson 1990) and to experiment with roles and behavior different from those that are characteristic of childhood. In this kind of experimentation, inherent in the process of personal growth and maturation, adolescents often find themselves acting out behavior that can put their physical, psychological, and social well-being at risk.

Numerous studies have shown that risk-taking and experimenting with actions and sensations during adolescence can play a role in overcoming the developmental tasks tied to the achievement of autonomy (Jack 1989), adulthood, and individualization (Palmonari 1997). Pursuing new activities and taking initiative are characteristics of typical adult behavior; however, sometimes this need to take on new tasks can lead to, for more or less extended periods of time, experimentation connected to challenging personal limits and assuming, at times, even serious risks (Irwin and Millstein 1986).

While it is true that involvement in risk is very common during adolescence, it is also true that risk-taking is not limited to this period of development; many adults seek risks in a variety of different environments, first and foremost in sports but also in driving, games, the stock market, and betting and gambling. The widespread nature of this behavior has led to a belief that there are certain personality types that have a constant need for intense, unusual, new sensations - personalities that require high levels of stimulation because of their unique biological makeup. In particular, Zuckerman (1983) considered "sensation seeking," or the need to feel a variety of new, strong, complex, enthralling sensations, as a personality trait with a strong biological substrate that involves various neurotransmitters (dopamine, norepinephrine, catecholamine) and the limbic system. Associated with this trait is a need to run physical and social risks with the precise aim of provoking strong sensations, which these individuals experience as extremely exciting and pleasurable. Other personality traits often associated with experiencing sensations are impulsiveness and the need for high levels of stimulation. However, personality traits and biological components cannot, on their own, explain why involvement in dangerous behavior is more characteristic of certain periods in the course of a lifetime (such as transitional periods) and of certain social groups. Furthermore, it is also now clear that there is a circular relationship of reciprocal influence between behavior and biochemical changes.

For this reason, in order to comprehend the reasons for involvement in risk-taking behavior, it is necessary to refer to the functions that the different types of risk-taking behavior serve for those who act them out. By studying functions, we can distinguish between the different meanings that the same behavior can have when acted out by an adolescent or an adult and better understand the differences in involvement between different subjects. The deliberate assumption of risks in order to feel strong sensations and intense excitement appears to be a phenomenon with a great deal of variation in which adolescents differ, both in the extent of the risks they take and their reasons for taking them (Shapiro et al. 1998). As for the extent of risks assumed, numerous studies, ours included, have examined the different levels of risk implied in various behavior types and different patterns of involvement (Bonino and Cattelino 2000; Wiesner and Silbereisen 2003). Excitement and sensation seeking can occur in a wide variety of ways, from using psychoactive substances, to watching thrillers, playing games, gambling, playing sports, seeking danger and speed, breaking rules and acting deviantly, and having promiscuous sex. Also, while some individuals act out risky or problematic behavior habitually, others stop at the experimental phase (Levitt et al. 1991; Cattelino and Bonino 2000). The explanation for differences in levels of involvement can be found in the functions that the different types of risk-taking behavior serve. These functions are tied to the development of an adult identity and to the consolidation of relationships with adults, peers, and the broader social context. More precisely, with regard to identity, acting out risk-taking behavior can fulfill a need to challenge oneself, put oneself to the test in order to learn about one's potential and limits, reflect on oneself, and present oneself to others in a certain way. Risk taking is also encouraged by our current cultural context that offers numerous models for challenge and self-display, emphasizes extreme sports and places strong sensations and hedonistic values above all else.

Based on this description, it is evident that in order to understand the reasons and factors that facilitate or limit involvement in risk-taking behavior, it is essential that we consider the combination of interactions that form between various personal resources and contextual opportunities (Silbereisen and Todt 1994a; Chisholm and Hurrelmann 1995). This model, which examines human actions within a specific developmental and cultural context and seeks to comprehend the aim of these actions, has proven to be particularly useful in studying risk-taking behavior; these are actions that have not been carried out by chance or by mistake but have been deliberately chosen and pursued in order to provoke strong sensations and excitement in the full awareness of the risks and dangers that these actions imply.

4.1.1 Males and Risk

The types of risk-taking behavior we analyzed include acting out dangerous behavior for the pleasure it brings; practicing various activities in a risky manner because it is exciting, and risking personal safety when out at night because it is exciting[1]. Fifty-six percent of the adolescents in our study claim to have carried out at least one risk-taking behavior in the last six months even though, for most of these young people, this behavior was a form of experimentation (Fig. 4.1).

Boys are more implicated in risky actions than girls[2]: 68% of boys reported carrying out at least one risk-taking behavior in the last six months as opposed to 45% of girls (Fig. 4.2). By comparing the means for involvement on the scale of risk-taking behavior, the greater involvement of boys was confirmed (Fig. 4.3).

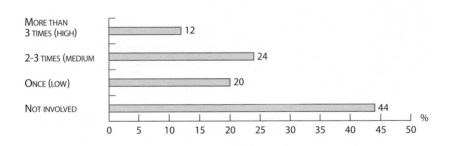

Fig. 4.1. Involvement in risk-taking behavior (percentages).

---

[1] In the "Appendix," the full questions and scales from the questionnaire have been reported, along with their related responses and main psychometric principles.
[2] Note that all the results reported in the figures are statistically significant, with $p<0.05$. In Chap. 2, Sect. 2.4, Presentation of Results and Statistical Analyses, the criteria for the presentation of results and for the use of statistics are explained.

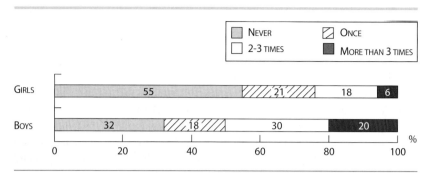

Fig. 4.2. Involvement in risk-taking behavior for gender (chi-squared).

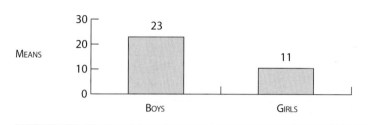

Fig. 4.3. Means for involvement in risk-taking behavior for gender (ANOVA).

Unlike the findings reported in Chap. 3 on psychoactive substance use and cigarette smoking in particular, our findings showed no sign of a gradual standardization in the behavior of boys and girls; risk-taking behavior appears to be a property of the male identity. As far as age is concerned, no statistical differences emerged in the various age groups between 14 and 19 years of age, which seems to indicate a degree of stability in this behavior over time. However, significant differences were found between subjects on different educational tracks, with higher levels of involvement found in students of technical secondary schools (Fig. 4.4).

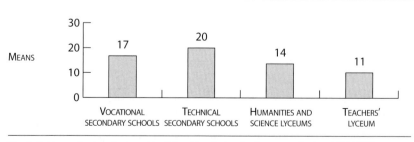

Fig. 4.4. Means for involvement in risk-taking behavior for type of school (ANOVA).

But why are boys and students who attend technical secondary schools more willing to risk their personal safety, and why do they find so much excitement in carrying out risky actions? The reasons behind boys' greater involvement in risk-taking behavior can be traced back to cultural, media, and consumer models that emphasize the role of risk and challenge as methods of self-affirmation for boys in particular. Other reasons are tied to males' and females' different processes of personal identity construction and the different opportunities available to boys and girls. Recent literature has shown how, for boys, experimentation is a central part of the process of constructing a positive identity whereas for girls, taking on commitments is more important in this process (Palmonari 1997).

Our data also confirm this interpretation: boys were found to be more involved than girls in all types of risk behavior that involve outward, highly visible behavior such as risky driving and antisocial behavior. At the same time, boys were also found to be less involved than girls in activities and groups that require a stable commitment (Figs. 4.5 and 4.6).

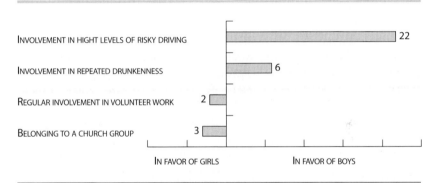

Fig. 4.5. Comparison between the percentages of involvement of boys and girls in various types of activities.

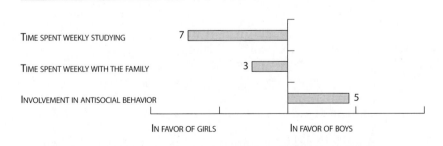

Fig. 4.6. Comparison between the proportional means for boys and girls for involvement in various types of activities.

This experimentation with actions and sensations that is typical of boys and students of technical secondary schools can also be explained by the greater vulnerability of these individuals to consumer models and their greater tolerance for experimentation, even when risky.

Another element to be considered is the increased difficulties in entering the workforce in recent decades, a difficulty which, in Italy, presumably clashes even more strongly with the expectations of technical secondary school students. Although very different, the educational paths undertaken by their peers who attend lyceums or vocational secondary schools have in common a greater sense of clarity with regard to the future: those who attend lyceums are more oriented toward continuing their education after obtaining a diploma and have long-term plans for their personal success and entrance into the adult world. Identifying oneself as a student or, more specifically, as a successful student, is typical of the lyceum student (especially humanities and science lyceums) and appears to give these adolescents a strong sense of positive identity. On the other hand, those who attend vocational secondary schools are oriented toward early entrance into the workforce. Many of them are not even certain that they will finish school and obtain a diploma (Fig. 4.7). While the world of work clearly does not hold great opportunities for these students, at least they have the security of knowing that they want to and have to look for work.

Technical secondary school students, however, are uncertain about whether or not they will carry on their educations after obtaining a diploma, and they are uncertain about entering the workforce. Many of them enrolled in this type of school because they did not particularly excel in school and they wanted to obtain a diploma that would be useful at the end of the five years of sec-

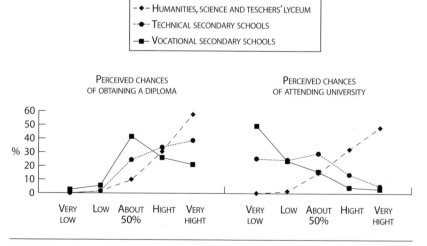

Fig. 4.7. Percentages of expectations for academic achievement (chi-squared).

ondary school. However, as the years go by, a decreasing number of Italian students intend to terminate their studies after completing secondary school, and a growing number report plans to attend specialization courses or to enroll in university. Most likely this uncertainty about whether or not to remain a student and about either entering the adult world early but with great uncertainty or remaining in the educational system - in short, this "in-between" social status - results in a greater need to experiment with new roles and activities, some of which are risky.

Adolescents who enroll in different types of secondary schools also differ from one another in terms of the personal resources they possess, such as their temporal perspective, greater or lesser vulnerability to consumer and risk models, perception of self as a student (Bonino and Cattelino 2002), and others. Table 4.1, summarizes some of these differences, evaluated through variance analyses, of the personal characteristics of students attending different types of schools.

Table 4.1. Means for personal characteristics of adolescents attending different types of schools (MANOVA).

	Humanities, science, and teachers' lyceums	Technical secondary schools	Vocational secondary schools
Expectations for future success	++[a]	+++	+
Overall satisfaction with self	++	+++	+
Self-confidence in coping	+++	++	+
Positive perception of own academic abilities	+++	++	+
Self-regulatory efficacy	+++	++	+
Sense of alienation	++	+	+++
Depressive feelings	++	+	+++

[a] A greater number of plus signs (+) corresponds to a higher mean

These characteristics, during the years of school attendance, interact with the opportunities that the various types of schools offer their students in terms of self-image, development of adequate coping skills, and possibilities for experimentation and confrontation (Bonino and Cattelino 2002). Thus, the greater involvement of technical and vocational school students in risk-taking activities can also be attributed to the lack of opportunities offered by these schools.

As far as the greater involvement of boys is concerned, the aspects considered previously, tied to the affirmation of a strong, well-defined masculine identity, also interact with a cultural context in which there continue to be major differences in educational styles, types of control, and role expectations in the socialization processes of boys and girls, especially in Italy and in the south of Europe (Claes et al. 2003). Adolescent males are generally given more freedom (Fig. 4.8) than are females, and there is a certain degree of tolerance for their transgressive or risk-taking behavior. These factors can lead boys to identify the assumption of risk as a means of demonstrating their courage, virility, and strong will. The fact that girls are less involved in behavior types that are dictated by a desire for strong sensations can be explained by their greater involvement in family and school life, greater participation in organized groups, the greater control they are subjected to, and above all, the greater pressure placed on them by adults to conform to the conventional expectations of society.

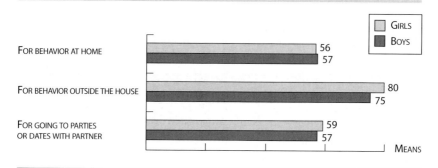

Fig. 4.8. Proportional means for perceived parental control (MANOVA).

Summary 4.1 provides an overview of the main characteristics of the adolescents who are most implicated in risk-taking behavior dictated by a desire to feel strong sensations.

Summary 4.1. Main characteristics of the adolescents most involved in risk-taking behavior.

Sociodemographic characteristics

The most heavily involved adolescents are generally:
• Boys
• Students of technical or vocational secondary schools

Other characteristics linked to sociodemographic characteristics

The most heavily involved adolescents are:
• More sensitive to media and consumer models
• More oriented toward experimentation
• More involved in other risk behavior
• More uncertain about their future
• Less involved in constructive activities and regular engagements
• Less subject to parental control for behavior outside home

4.2 Functions of Risk-Taking Behavior

First of all, the dangerous actions considered here are acted out with the express purpose of provoking strong sensations, or in other words, because of the intrinsic excitement involved in acting out these types of behavior. As we have said, the pursuit of new, enthralling sensations, which leads to the assumption of physical and social risks, is a very common phenomenon, although for most people this kind of behavior is limited to adolescence; only for some does it precede, accompany, and follow this phase of development. The hedonistic quest for excitement is often linked to certain personality traits (Zuckerman 1983) and involves more or less conscious decision-making processes. The choice to carry out risk-taking behavior derives from a combination of perceptions and evaluations (Moore and Gullone 1996; Parsons et al. 1997), tied as much to the costs as to the benefits recognized in a certain action within a given physical and social context and at a given time.

Consistent with the literature (Jessor et al. 1991), our analyses of the psychosocial concomitants point to the presence of a syndrome of risk-taking behavior. A strong positive correlation exists between dangerous actions and psychotropic substance use, antisocial behavior, risky driving, and sexually promiscuous behavior (Fig. 4.9).

The correlation coefficients, calculated for the sample stratified by gender and age, are quite high in all cases, but there are some differences: the association between risk-taking behavior dictated by a need for strong sensations and other types of risk behavior is stronger for girls than for boys (except for the strong correlation with risky driving). This finding suggests that, for girls, all risk behavior assumes an experimental function aimed at trying out new behavior types and feeling new sensations. Differences were also found in the strength of the associations between adolescents in different age groups: with age, the strength of the correlations between risk-taking behavior and cigarette smoking and between risk-taking behavior and risky driving decreases;

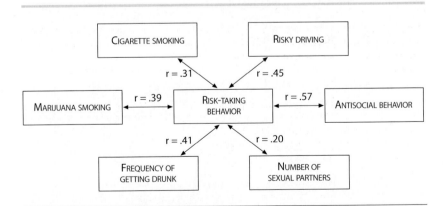

Fig. 4.9. Correlation with other types of risk behavior.

at age 16-17, there is a peak in the strength of the correlations between risk-taking behavior and marijuana smoking and between risk-taking and antisocial behavior. These findings could indicate that, with age, smoking cigarettes and driving gradually lose their connection with sensation seeking and become part of the normal lifestyle of certain adolescents. At the same time, the strong correlations found in adolescents 16-17 years old show how, at this age, many types of risk behavior, particularly transgressive, illegal behavior such as smoking marijuana and antisocial behavior, are acted out in order to feel strong sensations.

Thus, these high correlations indicate that all types of adolescent risk behavior analyzed in this book can be considered means by which to experience new sensations and strong excitement, particularly in the forms that involve the highest number of adolescents. At the same time, they also indicate that different types of behavior can perform similar functions. However, the risk-taking behavior types examined here have at least two functions that should be taken into consideration: For some adolescents, the pursuit of risk and excitement is a way to test themselves, to reinforce their sense of identity, and to gain greater social acceptance. In contrast, for other adolescents, these same behavior types are just illusory means of escape.

4.2.1 Self-Affirmation and Experimentation

The challenge component along with the need to put oneself to the test in order to discover one's potential and limits are both important aspects of risk-taking behavior. The challenge aspect is particularly important for those who identify less strongly with the values shared by society, attributing little importance to health, religion, and the school experience while at the same time having a strong desire for independence and a low disapproval of antisocial behavior (Fig. 4.10).

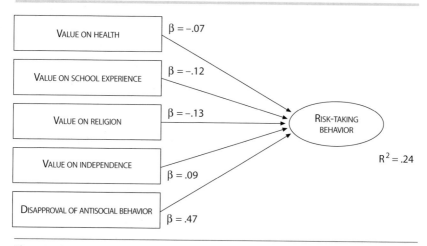

Fig. 4.10. Personal variables (multiple regression).

These characteristics are present to varying degrees in boys and girls and in adolescents of different ages. In girls and in the youngest adolescents, the variables more related to involvement in risk-taking behavior are a high value on independence in decision-making, a low value on religion, and a low disapproval of antisocial behavior. For boys and older adolescents, on the other hand, predictors of high involvement, in addition to low disapproval of antisocial behavior, are low value on the school experience and low value on health. These results point to the fact that for all adolescents, self-affirmation carried out through risk-taking behavior takes on a transgressive meaning; for girls and younger adolescents, this is tied mainly to a desire for independence, while for boys and older adolescents it is linked to a clear opposition to the establishment.

The need to put oneself to the test is also connected to a positive self-perception, a high confidence in one's ability to confront difficulties, and a weak internal locus of control for health (Fig. 4.11). Therefore, aspects connected to a high level of self-control - although this sense of control is often only an illusion - combine with other aspects such as a fatalistic view of life and health. It is for this reason that challenging fate and danger can be a strategy for affirming oneself and one's ability to control events and avert danger.

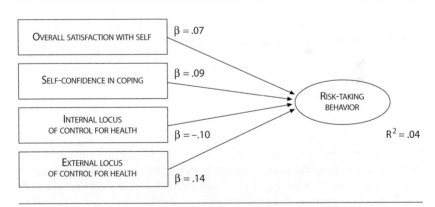

Fig. 4.11. Variables related to self-perception (multiple regression).

Different aspects of self-perception are relevant adolescents of different ages in different ways. In the youngest adolescents (14-15 years old), greater involvement in risk-taking behavior is tied to a positive self-perception characterized by high levels of personal satisfaction and high confidence in the ability to face problems. In older age groups, the perception of having little control over one's health and well-being assumes greater importance.

The need to know one's potential and to exert control over events during periods of profound change, such as adolescence, is quite common; however, buys and girls manifest this need in different ways. In boys, self-affirmation is achieved through highly visible behavior, and control is exerted mainly upon the surrounding environment; girls on the other hand, as we will discuss in Chap. 7, tend to exert control over themselves, their physical appearance, and food.

The need for highly visible self-affirmation and constant challenges to one's limits in the pursuit of excitement is felt most strongly by those who, for various reasons, perceive a greater deal of uncertainty in their present condition. It follows that those who frequently use these acts to strengthen their sense of identity generally find little gratification in school experience, view school experience as not particularly useful to their personal achievement, and have low expectations to continue school (Fig. 4.12). Dangerous conduct becomes a glaring way to be seen, to demonstrate courage and strength to oneself and to others, and to succeed in overcoming fears and limits, demonstrating in this way one's ability to succeed in life.

4.2.2 Identification and Social Acceptance

The function of strengthening personal identity that risk behavior performs is tightly linked to social acceptance and desirability within the peer group. Our data show that the adolescents who are most involved in risk conduct have a secure place within a group of peers; they reported spending the majority of their free time in the company of friends, having numerous dates with someone of the opposite of sex, and being attractive (Fig. 4.13).

The data can be interpreted based on studies of ritual behavior. The acting out of risk-taking behavior can represent a rite of passage, a bonding ritual, or even a courtship ritual: exaggerated actions, the repetition of these actions, and a high emotional charge can signal the passage from childhood to adulthood, facilitate (if not regulate) access to certain groups, and solidify the bond between those who take part in these rituals.

However, it was also found that certain young people, boys in particular, have a difficult time resisting pressure by their peers to perform transgressive or dangerous actions (Fig. 4.14). Therefore, it would appear that, at times, involvement in risk, more than being a way to experience excitement, is the consequence of a lack of self-regulatory efficacy.

4.2.3 Escape Through Action and Excitement

While for some adolescents risk-taking behavior dictated by a desire for excitement is a way, however dangerous, to reinforce a sense of their personal identity, to test their abilities, and to feel like part of the group, for other adolescents where these types of behavior persist, these same actions appear to be escape methods used to avoid confronting difficulties and developmental tasks.

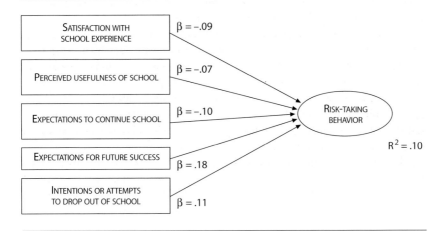

Fig. 4.12. Variables related to the school experience (multiple regression).

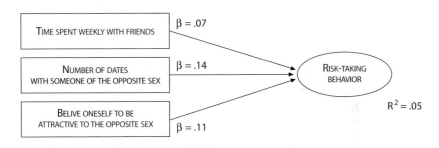

Fig. 4.13. Variables related to relationships with peers (multiple regression).

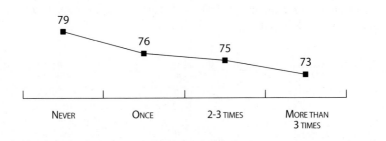

Fig. 4.14. Proportional means for the perception of ability to resist peer pressure (self-regulatory efficacy) in boys with different levels of involvement in risk-taking behavior (ANOVA).

This function is felt more strongly by adolescents with characteristics similar to those of the high-risk group described in Box 3.2.

Our data, which are consistent with other studies on risk and high susceptibility to boredom (Levitt et al. 1991), reveal greater involvement in risk-taking behavior by adolescents who have difficulties in organizing their free time constructively and who spend long hours in public places (coffee shops, discotheques, video arcades) or sitting around doing nothing (Fig. 4.15). Apart from being a way to avoid boredom, the pursuit of excitement through risk appears to be a means by which to escape a present reality that offers little fulfillment and little opportunity for achievement.

For this reason, the young people who are uninterested in school, have a difficult time seeing the point in what they are doing, intend to drop out of school, have unsatisfactory relationships with their parents, do not use dialogue to deal with their difficulties, and are very oriented toward their friends - friends who offer weak models for conventional behavior - are the ones most involved in risk-taking behavior (Fig. 4.16).

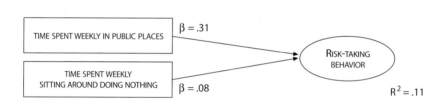

Fig. 4.15. Variables related to use of free time (multiple regression).

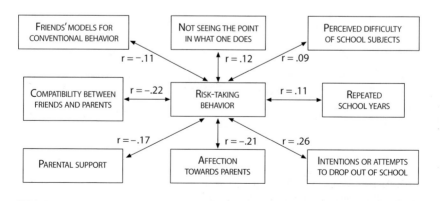

4.16. Correlations between variables tied to the escape function.

In reality, this escape from difficulties through action and excitement is actually inadequate and illusory: persistent involvement in risk-taking behavior acted out in order to feel strong sensations does not succeed in placating feelings of unease but is actually associated with an increase in such feelings (Fig. 4.17).

Summary 4.2 outlines the main functions of risk-taking behavior.

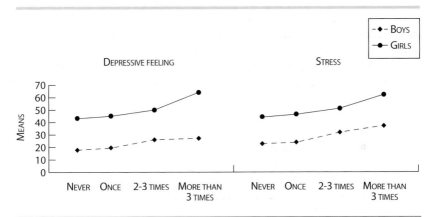

Fig. 4.17. Means proportion for depressive feelings and stress in adolescents with different levels of involvement in risk-taking behavior (MANOVA).

Summary 4.2. Main functions performed by risk-taking behavior.

Risk-taking behavior
• EXPERIMENTATION and SENSATION SEEKING
• SELF-AFFIRMATION, through showing off and attempting to control situations
• CHALLENGE and AUTONOMY, through experimentation (especially for girls and the youngest adolescents) or through opposition (especially in adolescents aged 16-17 years old)
• CHALLENGE and TRANSGRESSION (in all groups but particularly for boys)
• COPING STRATEGY, tied to self-affirmation and conflict resolution (for the youngest adolescents)
• SOCIAL ACCEPTANCE and VISIBILITY, through showing off and the sharing of behavior
• RITE OF PASSAGE, through tests of courage (especially for the youngest adolescents and the group characterized by the lowest level of involvement)
• BONDING and BELONGING RITUAL, through the sharing of behavior and the emotions related to the behavior
• COURTSHIP RITUAL, through showing off (especially for boys)
• ESCAPE (especially for adolescents most heavily and persistently involved)

4.3 Driving in Adolescence: A Step Toward Independence

One of the main developmental tasks during adolescence is the achievement of increasing autonomy from parental figures. This need for greater autonomy is felt both by young people and by society, which requires that adolescents become increasingly independent and take on responsibilities within the community. In Italy today, the process of gaining emancipation in terms of behavior, emotions, and values, culminating in the achievement of independence from one's family of origin, is long and gradual. It appears that this process has come to rely heavily on relationships with the peer group - a context in which adolescents can develop new affective relationships; come into contact with new values, ideas and opinions; and make decisions about various aspects of their daily lives (such as how to spend their free time, how to dress and so on).

In light of this, the ability to move from one place to another - to and from school, out with friends, and anywhere one wants to go - becomes extremely important. Having or being able to drive a car or other motor vehicle allows adolescents to move freely from one place to another and facilitates the acquisition of greater autonomy. Moving from one place to the next becomes easier and faster; one can travel farther from home and come home more quickly whenever one wants. For this reason, gaining access to a motor vehicle can be an important event in the development of an adolescent and can lead to a number of changes in lifestyle (Williams 1998). Being able to drive a car or scooter allows boys and girls a greater freedom of movement and autonomy from their parents on a practical level, but it can also facilitate the process of separation from one's parents and the achievement of psychological autonomy. This process is certainly not linear; on the contrary, it is complex and tortuous, often involving ambivalent or contradictory behavior characterized by leaps forward and frequent steps backward. For this reason, the act of distancing themselves and then returning to their home territories and their families with their own car or scooter acquires both a practical and affective meaning. Driving can encourage the process of emancipation by allowing for a separation from the environment and the relationships of the adolescent's childhood, both in a physical-spatial sense and a psychological sense. Adolescents are aware of the functions carried out by driving on another, less practical level as well. As shown in recent studies, the car, beyond its pragmatic value, is conceived by most adolescents as a vehicle for freedom and independence, or even for personal affirmation.

4.3.1. Adolescents at the Wheel

Sixty-two percent of the adolescents in our sample had driven an automobile, motorcycle, or scooter in the past six months, and 40% possessed their own means of transportation. There were a significantly greater number of male drivers than females (Fig. 4.18), which is consistent with the findings of other studies (Vavrik 1997). The highest percentages of drivers of different forms of transport were found among boys (Fig. 4.19),[3] but the most common were motorcycles (125-cc engine or higher) and scooters.

The greater frequency of driving by boys and the fact that they more frequently possess their own vehicle is in part connected to the greater freedom and independence that male adolescents enjoy compared with their female counterparts, who are subject to greater control (Scabini 1995; Cattelino et al. 2001).

Differences were also found between age groups, with the number of drivers increasing with age (Fig. 4.20).

It was also found that 40% of adolescents between the ages of 14 and 17, or in other words, under the legal age to drive a car in Italy[4], had actually driven a car (Fig. 4.21)[5]. Underage driving is not a phenomenon typical of Italy or Europe, and it is a particular risky behavior much neglected (Lam 2003).

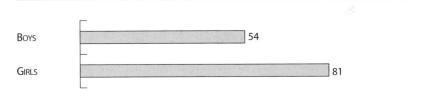

Fig. 4.18. Percentages of involvement in driving for gender (chi-squared).

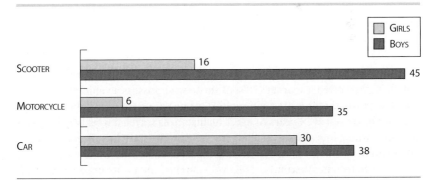

Fig. 4.19. Percentages for different vehicles driven for gender (chi-squared).

---

[3] The sum of the percentages is greater than 100 because many adolescents had driven more than one means of transportation.

[4] By Italian laws, at the moment of data collecting, adolescents were allowed to drive a scooter (lower than 125-cc engine) from the age of 14 without a specific driving license, while in 2004 a specific driving license was introduced. A motorcycle (125-cc engine or higher) can be driven from the age of 16 with a specific driving license (type A). Only from the legal age of 18 it is possible to obtain the learner's permit and after that a car driving license (type B).

[5] The sum of the percentages is greater than 100 because many adolescents had driven more than one means of transportation.

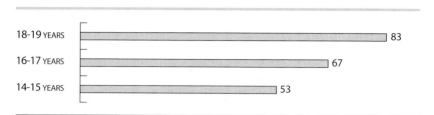

Fig. 4.20. Percentages for involvement in driving for age group (chi-squared).

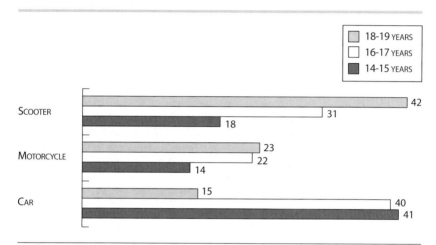

Fig. 4.21. Percentages for vehicles driven for age group (chi-squared).

The majority of young drivers have their own means of transportation, which is most often a scooter (78% of those who possess a vehicle), a form of transportation that is quite fashionable among young Italian adolescents and that can be driven at 14 years of age. The distances traveled weekly vary greatly: those who generally travel the greatest distances are boys (an average of 30-50 km driven in an ordinary week compared with 10-30 km for girls), older adolescents, technical secondary schools students, and those who live in small- to medium-sized towns. The fact that adolescents who live in small towns drive more can be explained by contingent needs related to the fact that the schools they attend are often not located in the towns where they live or that they have to travel greater distances in order to meet friends or take part in recreational activities. Furthermore, small- and medium-sized towns are generally not as well served by public transport as larger cities. Also, people in small- and medium-sized towns perceive driving as less risky because traffic is less intense. But in addition to these practical reasons for the greater involvement in driving by adolescents from small towns, there are other reasons of a more psychological nature. Adolescents who live in small towns must travel farther away from home in order to feel autonomous and free from the watchful eyes of people who know them. This need is felt to a much lesser degree by those who live in larger cities where often, even next-door neighbors do not know each other and where it is not necessary to travel great distances in order to feel free and anonymous.

Returning to gender differences in driving involvement, it was found that boys not only drive more than girls but they also drive more at night: 70% of boys reported to have driven after 8 o'clock in the evening at least occasionally in the last six months compared with 45% of girls. As we will see in the following section, driving at night is a risk factor for motor vehicle accidents.

4.4 Risky Driving

While driving allows adolescents to reach objectives that have a strong positive impact on their development, it is counted as a risk behavior because it is potentially more dangerous to the health and safety of adolescents than other behavior types that do not enjoy the same level of tolerance and social acceptance. In comparison to many other types of risk behavior, in Western culture, risky driving constitutes to be one of the most frequent and most accepted ways of carrying out risky actions. However, it is also one of the most dangerous, at times leading to extremely serious or even deadly outcomes. Despite the intense emotion stirred by adolescent suicide or deaths provoked by substance abuse, in Italy as well as in other European Union countries, motor vehicle accidents are the leading cause of death for adolescents and young people between the ages of 15 and 24. According to data published by ISTAT (1998, 2001a, 2001b, 2004), since the 1990s, there has been a constant increase in road accidents: from 161,782 registered in 1990, to 190,031 in 1997, to 211,941 in 2000. These accidents caused the deaths of 6,410 people while another 301,559 people were injured to varying degrees seriousness.

Parallel to the increase in the number of vehicles in circulation over the last ten years, the number of accidents and injuries, while there has been some fluctuation, has also tended to increase. However, the number of deaths has decreased constantly due to technological improvements in automobile safety (air bags, lateral reinforcement bars, headrests in the back seats), more effective medical care, and new laws on safety (helmets and safety belts made mandatory). The mortality rate (number of deaths per one hundred accidents) decreased from 4% in 1991 to 3% in 2000. However, contrary to the trend in recent years in the overall youth mortality rate, the mortality rate for car accidents involving young people shows no sign of decreasing. While the number of deaths of young people between the ages of 15 and 34 dropped from 11,284 in 1997 to 9,902 in 1999, the percentage of deaths caused by motor vehicle accidents rose from 27% (3,037 deaths) in 1997 to 31% (3,048 deaths) in 1999.

Fifteen percent of the adolescents in our sample reported having had accidents caused by their own negligence. More of these accidents involved boys

(17% compared with 12% girls), consistent with the data furnished by ISTAT that show higher involvement by young boys in road accidents and in fatal accidents; 83% of adolescents aged 15-17 and 87% of those 18-20 who died in 2000 following road accidents were boys.

As our data show that in the first years of adolescence, the vehicle used most frequently was the scooter (cars were also driven in the last six months by many adolescents but only on occasion). These vehicles also appear to be the most dangerous: a much lower percentage of car drivers have had accidents than drivers of two-wheeled vehicles (Fig. 4.22).

These results are consistent with the national data for Italy. Based on the ISTAT in cooperation with the Automobile Club of Italy (ACI) data (2001), of the boys and girls aged 15-17 who died driving in the year 2000, 85% were driving scooters and 4% motorcycles. Among the drivers who were injured, 91% were driving scooters. Twenty-one percent of those who died as passengers were on scooters or motorcycles, as were 27% of those who were injured. As adolescents get older, car use becomes more common. Between the ages of 18 and 20, the percentage of those who died at the wheel of a car reached 59% and for injuries, 49%.

Most of the road accidents that occur in the evening hours of the weekend involve adolescents and young adults. Our data also show a positive correlation between the frequency of nighttime driving and accidents. In Italy, "the Saturday-night disasters" is a term used often by the media to refer to the high number of accidents caused by young people that occur on Saturday night, or more precisely, in the early hours of Sunday morning, often after leaving discotheques. This phenomenon, which began in the 1980s, has become even more substantial in recent years; the number of Saturday-night accidents reported by ISTAT rose from 3,215 in 1980 to 8,450 in 2000. In the last ten years, Friday nights have also seen a growing number of accidents. In 2000, between the hours of 10 o'clock on Friday night and 6 o'clock on Saturday morning (Friday-night accidents) and 10 o'clock on Saturday night and 6 o'clock on Sunday morning (Saturday-night accidents), 15,326 accidents occurred, with 917 deaths. Friday- and Saturday-night accidents account for 44%

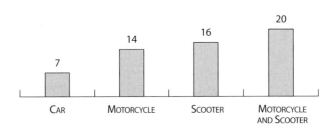

Fig. 4.22. Percentages of accidents for vehicles driven (chi-squared).

of all nighttime road accidents, and the deaths and injuries caused by these accidents account for 48% and 46%, respectively, of the deaths and injuries in nighttime road accidents. Thus, a high level of danger is the main characteristic of this type of accident: the average number of deaths in one hundred Friday- and Saturday-night accidents is six while the annual average for all accidents is three deaths per one hundred.

In many cases, the cause of these accidents can be attributed to the drivers' precarious psychological and physical conditions, which negatively influence their driving ability. Fatigue, physical exhaustion, and the assumption of psychotropic substances reduce attention level, slow reflexes, and decrease the perception of risk. At night, driving becomes particularly demanding: low visibility makes driving more difficult, and the absence of traffic, instead of making the task easier, is often a risk factor, leading to higher speeds. During the nighttime hours, drivers are also more vulnerable to drowsiness, which is a determining factor in many accidents. Drowsiness increases reaction times, causes lapses in attention, and reduces the ability to identify important stimuli (Horne and Reiner 1995). These elements can negatively impact driving performance, reducing the ability to perceive danger and to react immediately (Lucidi et al. 1998).

Our data also reveal strong relationships between driving under the influence of psychoactive substances (alcohol and marijuana) and traffic-code offenses on the one hand and road accidents on the other (Fig. 4.23).

As mentioned previously, young drivers (60% under the age of 30), and boys in particular (90%), are most often responsible for the accidents occurring during the nighttime hours of the weekend (ISTAT 1997). The fact that these individuals drive more frequently at night is not the only explanation. According to many authors, young drivers' lack of experience in managing their drowsiness is an important element (Summala and Mikkola 1994). These studies found that adolescents often believe they can remain attentive through the force of their will, even when they have a strong physical need for sleep. In reality, when the need for sleep is high, the will to stay awake and attentive is not enough to allow the driver to avoid the negative influence of drowsiness

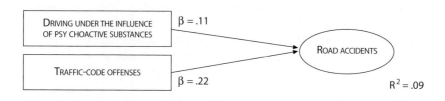

Fig. 4.23. Different offenses (multiple regression).

on driving ability. The behavior and activities young people take part in on weekends can also have a negative influence on their attention level. A study conducted on a sample of adolescents found that not only were attention levels lower at night than in the day, but attention levels decreased even further for boys and girls who had consumed alcohol and was lower for those who had been in discotheques than for those who had been in pubs or at parties (Lucidi et al. 1998). Possible explanations for these findings include physical tiredness, the fact that music at very high volumes can decrease sensitivity to certain stimuli, and the possible use of drugs that can be easily obtained in discos.

In our sample as well, the interaction of hours spent in discotheques with driving after having consumed alcohol or smoked marijuana was strongly related to involvement in road accidents; so much so that when this variable was introduced into a multiple regression analysis, it eliminated the effects of nighttime driving (Fig. 4.24).

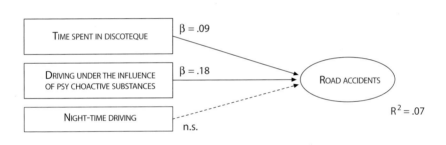

Fig. 4.24. Multiple regression.

4.4.1 Offenses, Risks, and Accidents

Based on our data, the risks and offenses committed by adolescents behind the wheel are many and varied, ranging from driving without a license and adequate attention to safety (evidenced by not wearing a safety belt or helmet), to traffic-code offenses and driving under the influence of alcohol or drugs. As far as driving without a license is concerned, our study revealed a significant percentage of adolescents who claim to have driven illegally in the last six months (Fig. 4.25). As we have already mentioned in this chapter, it is mostly the youngest adolescents who have driven a car despite not being of legal age to do so.

As for driving safety, adolescents reported infrequent use of safety belts and helmets when alone (19% reported never using these devices while only 9% reported using them regularly). However, these safety devices are used more frequently by adolescents when they are not driving and are passengers (13% never and 22% always), which confirms that actively assuming risks as a driver is often linked to an underevaluation of danger and greater perception of control. Our analyses of helmet and safety belt use also revealed the importance of both friend and adult models for the use of these devices (Fig. 4.26). The model offered by the best friend, followed by the father's model, is the best predictors of safety belt or helmet use. The maternal model does not have an influence (not even in the sample stratified by gender) despite the fact that in modern society people of both genders drive. This greater sensitivity to the paternal model seems to confirm that adolescents tend to associate driving with the male identity.

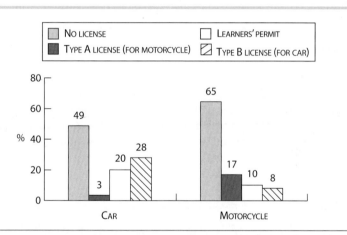

Fig. 4.25. Percentages for the vehicles driven in relation to type of driver's license.

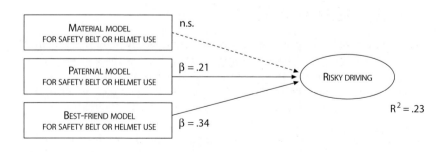

Fig. 4.26. Models for safety belt or helmet use (multiple regression).

Scarce attention to safety, which involves not only adolescents but their parents as well, is accompanied by a general lack of attention, which is confirmed by a high number of traffic-code offenses of various types, especially those related to speed limits, safe braking distance, and giving the right of way (Fig. 4.27).

Boys have a more risky driving style than girls, with a mean of 17 on the scale of traffic-code offenses compared with a mean of 13 for girls. Not only do boys have a higher mean on the general scale, they are also more involved in all the offenses considered here. In terms of age and school attendance, 16- to 17-year-olds (average age = 16) and technical secondary school students (average age = 17) are the most involved in risky driving.

Other differences are tied to the vehicles driven: the highest levels of involvement were found in those who, in the past six months, drove more than one type of vehicle (car, motorcycle, scooter), followed by motorcycle drivers. Car drivers were found to be the most respectful of traffic codes (Fig. 4.28). Figure 4.28 reports the means for four types of traffic offenses: exceeding the speed limit by at least 30 kilometers per hour, driving at high speeds in the vicinity of a school, racing at high speeds), failure to give the right of way (failure to stop at a stop sign, running a red light, cutting in), dangerous driving style (defying chance in traffic, taking risks in order to make driving more exciting), failing to respect safe braking distances, and entering no-traffic zones.

Failure to respect traffic codes is one of the main causes of road accidents (Fig. 4.29). In confirmation of this statement, our data clearly indicate that accidents do not occur in relation to the number of kilometers driven in an ordinary week: it is not those who drive the most who have the highest probability of having an accident but, rather, those who have a dangerous driving style.

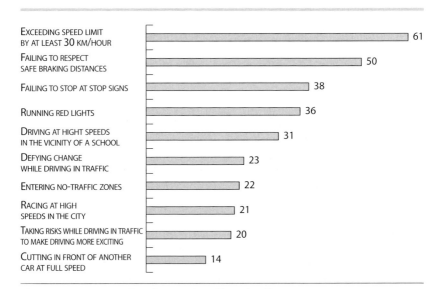

Fig. 4.27. Percentages of involvement in traffic-code offenses.

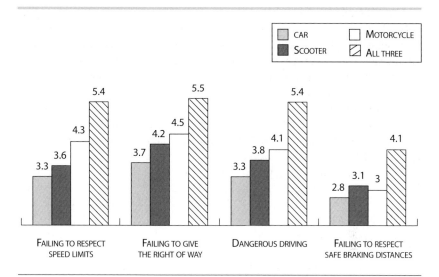

Fig. 4.28. Means for traffic-code offenses in relation to vehicle driven (MANOVA).

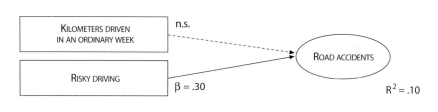

Fig. 4.29. Multiple regression.

Considering different groups of adolescents divided by gender, age group, and vehicle used, the types of offenses that were related to involvement in road accidents changed (Summary 4.3).

In fact, multiple regression analyses revealed that, for boys, the best predictors of involvement in accidents were failure to give the right of way, and speeding, while for girls, the best predictors were the failure to respect safe braking distances and failure to give the right of way. When analyzing the sample stratified for age group, the regression model revealed no significant findings for the youngest age group, while for 16- to 17-year-olds, failure to give the right of way was found to be a predictor of involvement in accidents, as was speeding for adolescents 18 and older. Failure to respect safe braking distances was also found to be a predictor for both of these age groups.

Our data also reveal that the variable most related to accidents by car drivers is the failure to respect safe braking distances while for scooter drivers it is the failure to give the right of way. Accidents by motorcycle drivers are associated mainly with dangerous driving practices carried out with the aim of making driving more exciting.

Summary 4.3. Main causes of road accidents (ANOVA).

Failure to respect safe braking distances:

• Especially for girls

• For adolescents aged 16 or older

• For car and scooter drivers

Excessive speed:

• Especially for boys

• For adolescents 18 and older

Failure to give the right of way:

• For adolescents of both genders

• For young people 16-17 years old

• For scooter drivers

Dangerous driving:

• Especially for motorcycle drivers

Data related to the widespread nature of traffic offenses and to the causes of accidents are consistent with the findings reported by ISTAT/ACI (2001). These findings show that the large majority of accidents (77%) reported in 2000 by public safety authorities were caused by driver negligence: distraction and indecisive driving were the most frequent circumstances (20%), followed by speeding (12%) and failure to respect safe braking distances (11%). Also, according to national reports, driver error is the determining factor in the greatest number of deaths (68%) and injuries (78%). On the national level, the most dangerous offenses are driving against traffic, which produces the highest mortality rate (seven deaths per one hundred accidents), followed by excessive speed, which in Italy in the year 2000 was the cause of 25,180 accidents with 1,275 deaths and 36,982 injuries. Although driving against traffic may seem like a rare event, it is actually much more frequent than one might think. The second type of violation, speeding, is, on the other hand, extremely common, widely tolerated by society, and grossly underestimated in terms of its dangerousness.

Along with the emphasis on speed that long characterized automobile companies' advertising campaigns - campaigns that have only recently shifted some of their focus to the theme of safety as a promotional feature - our culture has adopted an attitude that considers traffic offenses as acceptable or even necessary in certain situations in order to proceed expeditiously. This attraction to speed is accompanied by a behavioral style, which is increasingly common in our society, based on competition, hurry, and the need to stand out from the crowd. Confirming this fact, the individuals who adopt this type of behavior commit a greater number of speed limit violations (West et al. 1993).

In addition, as we will see later in this chapter, it must also be noted that, compared to other traffic offenses, serious sanctions are rarely imposed for speed limit violations, and the punishment for these offenses is generally a fine.

4.4.2 Driving Under the Influence of Psychoactive Substances

Numerous adolescents involved in our study reported having driven under the influence of alcohol or after having smoked marijuana (Fig. 4.30). Boys are more involved than girls only for driving after consuming alcohol while there are no statistically significant differences for driving after having smoked marijuana or taking passive risks - in other words, being the passenger in a vehicle driven by someone who has used psychoactive substances.

As shown in Fig. 4.23, driving under the influence of psychoactive substances is related to involvement in road accidents although much less so than other traffic-code offenses that do not involve the use of psychoactive substances (non-substance-related offenses contribute to twice as many accidents as those related to driving under the influence of substances). Despite this fact, the use of psychotropic substances, narcotics, and alcohol is usually identified in the media as the primary cause of many fatal accidents - both on Saturday night and otherwise - involving adolescents and young people on their way home from discotheques. The attention directed to these episodes by the media and the emotional interest they provoke, given their dramatic consequences, has contributed to making the Saturday-night accident the prototype of accidents involving young people and substance use their prototypical cause (Box 4.1).

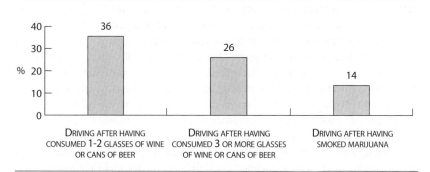

Fig. 4.30. Percentages for driving under the influence of psychoactive substances.

Box 4.1. Road Accidents and Heuristic Reasoning

The use of psychoactive substances is often believed to be the prototypical cause of accidents involving adolescents and young people. This belief, in virtue of heuristic reasoning - which leads us to believe that the most probable events are the ones that are most representative of a particular category (the representativeness heuristic) or that we can recall most easily (the availability heuristic) - causes us to overestimate the relationship between the consumption of alcohol or drugs and road accidents, which, based on statistical findings, actually appear to be relatively infrequent. As shown by national statistical data, only a small percentage of the accidents that occurred in 2000 were caused by drivers whose psychophysical state had been altered by the consumption of alcohol (1.5% of accidents) or drugs (0.1% of accidents); the causes of the vast majority of accidents were linked to errors made by the driver.

The emphasis placed on accidents caused by driving under the influence serves a self-protective function for most adults and for adolescents who either do not use psychoactive substances or do not combine alcohol consumption and drug use with driving. The belief that accidents are caused by drivers that are drunk or high allows those who do not drink and do not use drugs to feel safe, removed from all danger and clearly differentiated from the high-risk group. These cognitive processes also lead to self-exonerating strategies for other offenses, which, when compared to driving under the influence, appear less serious in the eyes of those who commit them. This advantageous comparison allows us to overlook the risks that we expose ourselves to, forgetting that the majority of accidents are caused by errors and a dangerous driving style characterized by systematic violations of the traffic code.

National data show that, although less numerous, accidents tied to alcohol or drug abuse have a high danger level for those involved in them. This category of accidents has one of the highest mortality rates: 7% as opposed to 3% for accidents caused by driver errors. A risk this high is tied to the changes in the driver's psychophysical state induced by the substances consumed, which can seriously compromise performance and the ability to judge one's limits and the limits of the vehicle. Psychoactive substances affect the central nervous system, altering perception, increasing the amount of time that passes between the perception of a stimulus and the response, and altering behavioral reactions (Julien 2005). According a report by ISTAT/ACI (2001), in accidents caused by an altered psychophysical state, the driver loses almost all control of the vehicle, unable to reduce the effects of the impact by braking or turning, often with very serious consequences. In Box 4.2, the influence of psychoactive substance use on adolescents' driving ability and driving style has been examined in greater detail.

Box 4.2. **Driving Ability, Driving Style, and the Consumption of Psychoactive Substances in Adolescence**

Several authors (Elander et al. 1993; Deery and Love 1996a) have identified two different variables related to motor vehicle driving: first, there is *driving ability*, which includes specific driving tasks and can be improved with practice; second, there is *driving style*, which refers to decision making when driving both in terms of how one decides to drive and the habits acquired over time. Both aspects can be influenced negatively by alcohol consumption, even in moderate doses. For example, it was found that even low quantities of alcohol increase times of perception (Deery and Love 1996b) and reaction to danger (West et al. 1993), aspects that are tied to driving ability. It was also found that, again, after consuming only low quantities of alcohol, drivers' responses to dangerous situations became more abrupt, an aspect tied to driving style (Deery and Love 1996b). The effects of substances on the nervous system increase in relation to the quantity of the substance ingested, and those who drink large doses of alcohol run greater risks than those who drink in moderate quantities (Gruenewald et al. 1996).

Adolescents at greatest risk are those who habitually consume psychotropic substances. It was found that an increase in consumption of beer and hard liquor leads to a corresponding increase in road accidents, as does the passage from occasional to habitual use of marijuana. Hard liquor consumption in particular, given the high alcohol content, coincides with broader involvement in serious accidents; this involvement is further reinforced by frequent consumption.

It should be added that driving while intoxicated is even more dangerous for young drivers than for adults. In fact, adolescents who have accidents after drinking alcohol have lower blood-alcohol levels than adults, and when blood-alcohol levels are the same, the risk of being involved in a serious accident is greater for young drivers. This can be explained first of all by adolescents' lack of experience in drinking combined with risk factors such as inexperience in driving and frequent nighttime driving to and from places such as bars, discos, or parties where alcohol is consumed. Thus, alcohol seems to reinforce the risk of road accidents that already exists for adolescents due to other factors.

Furthermore, adolescents who have consumed alcohol are generally unable to offer an accurate judgment of their own state of drunkenness (Turrisi et al. 1993): they feel they are capable of controlling a vehicle just as they can when they are sober, and they underestimate the dangers tied to driving under the influence of psychoactive substances. Some authors have found that the greater the frequency of driving after drinking, the more inaccurate the evaluation of the risks involved in this behavior (Deery and Love 1996b).

To explain this finding, it must be noted that, despite the positive relationship between involvement in road accidents and frequency of driving while intoxicated (Williams et al. 1986), this conduct often has no negative consequences either in terms of accidents or fines and trouble with the police (Farrow 1985; 1987). Driving numerous times after having drunk alcohol or riding with drivers that have been drinking without ever meeting with problems leads adolescents to underestimate the dangerousness of their behavior (Finken et al. 1998). The more previous experiences one has had with episodes involving driving under the influence of alcohol or drugs that have not led to negative outcomes, the lower one's perception of the risks involved in this activity. Along the same lines, a group of authors has found that the individuals most involved in risky behavior judge these actions to be less risky than do those who have never experienced them (Benthim et al. 1993). Successfully overcoming a situation that involves risks also inspires confidence in one's ability to control events, leading to an underestimation of potential risks and negative consequences (Johan 1990); this is caused by an error in perception tied to the mistaken generalization of previous experiences, which leads individuals to believe that, through their actions, they can completely control the outcomes of situations that, in reality, can have serious consequences.

For these reasons, adolescents, unlike adults, underestimate the relationship between road accidents and the consumption of psychoactive substances. They can recall numerous examples of situations, experienced firsthand or by friends, where driving under the influence of alcohol or drugs did not lead to adverse outcomes. Thus, they do not consider Saturday-night accidents to be prototypical but, rather, exceptions, and they defensively attribute these accidents to the errors or inability of others (McKenna 1993). In this case as well, it is due to heuristic reasoning that adolescents attribute less risk to driving while intoxicated. This flawed judgment leads adolescents to carry out this behavior more frequently (Lavery and Siegel 1993; Moore and Gullone 1996), consequently increasing the risks to their safety.

4.4.3 Fines

Despite the large number and great variety of offenses committed and risks assumed, only 10% of the adolescents in our study reported having been fined in the last six months (the same period considered for offenses). In terms of the main sociodemographic characteristics, boys reported receiving more fines than girls (14% compared with 5%) while there were no significant differences between age groups, students who attended different types of school, and those who lived in towns of different sizes. There were, however, differences in the distribution of the fines depending on the type of vehicle used; those who in the past six months drove a number of different types of vehicles (automobiles, motorcycles, and scooters) and motorcycle drivers reported receiving fines more frequently (Fig. 4.31).

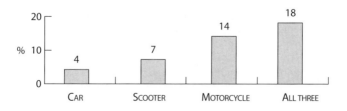

Fig. 4.31. Percentages of fines in relation to vehicle driven (chi-squared).

Risky or reckless driving, speeding, and - to a lesser extent - the number of kilometers traveled per week, were found to be related to fines (Fig. 4.32). Driving at night, failure to wear a safety belt or helmet, failure to give the right of way, and failure to respect safe braking distances do not appear to influence fines despite the fact that these offenses were found to be extremely common and strongly associated with road accidents.

The fact that there is no relationship between fines and the failure to wear a safety belt or helmet clearly shows the tolerance that exists for this type of offense. Previously, we saw that numerous adolescents either do not use or only occasionally use these safety devices. The same can be said for other offenses as well, including failure to respect safe braking distances, which are considered less important and which the police tend to overlook. The low number of fines is a clear signal that, unlike other forms of antisocial behavior, such as aggression, theft, or vandalism, risky driving enjoys a high degree of social tolerance.

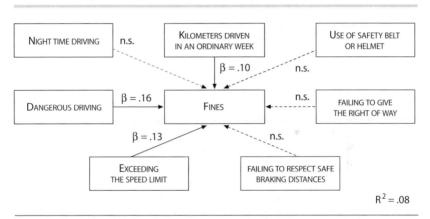

Fig. 4.32. Variables related to driving (multiple regression).

4.5 Functions of Risky Driving

As we have seen, adolescents, and adolescent males in particular, are a risk category for risky driving. This can be explained in part by a lack of experience and reduced capacity to recognize and respond appropriately to unexpected situations. In addition to these factors, as shown by our data and confirmed by the literature (Williams 1998; Begg and Langley 2004), this group has a driving style characterized by high speed, underestimation of safe braking distances, dangerous passing, and failure to give the right of way to other vehicles and pedestrians. Inexperience can account for part of the offenses and accidents involving adolescents, both boys and girls, but this explanation on its own is insufficient to provide an understanding of adolescent's implication in this risk behavior. Risky driving styles are not caused by inexperience alone but by other factors also directly related to age. Among these, there is the deliberate will to experience strong sensations (Jonah et al. 2001; Iversen 2004) and the thrill of risk (note that there is a strong positive correlation between risky driving and risk-taking behavior dictated by a desire to experience strong sensations), as well as a low capacity to perceive and cognitively elaborate the presence of risk (Mayew and Simpson 1990). As boys tend to drive more in general and to be more implicated in risky driving, the functions carried out by this type of behavior appear to be more closely tied to male identity.

In the following paragraphs, we will seek to analyze the main functions that risky driving serves for adolescents and to identify, based on these functions, the risk and protective factors for this type of behavior.

4.5.1 Adulthood, Self-Affirmation, and Experimentation

Driving a vehicle offers the opportunity to achieve a great deal of independence and helps young people to feel like adults. Furthermore, in Italy, the type of vehicle driven is closely related to age[6]: from age 14, boys and girls are allowed to drive scooters with engines smaller than 125-cc; from age 16, adolescents can take the type-A license, which allows them to drive motorcycles with 125-cc engines or larger; and at 18 years of age, adolescents - now legally adults - can take the type-B license, which permits them to drive a car. It follows, therefore, that the type of vehicle driven can also be used to signal one's age and to show that one is "growing up." Driving vehicles with increasingly powerful engines can truly be seen as a rite of passage to adulthood. The desire for independence combined with the desire to put oneself to the test and to show that one is grown up is so strong that many adolescents, as we have already seen, drive motor vehicles without having the legal permission to do so and also presumably without having the knowledge and ability that driving requires.

This same function, linked to the anticipation of adulthood through the assumption of typical adult behavior, is also carried out by dangerous driving. Young people who have risky lifestyles reported involvement in many types of behavior that signal adult status. In particular, they more often reported having a job, they smoke and drink more, and they have more sexual intercourses (Fig. 4.33).

---

[6] By Italian laws, at the moment of data collection, adolescents were allowed to drive a scooter (lower than 125-cc engine) from the age of 14 without a specific driving license, while in 2004 a specific driving license was introduced. Motorcycle (125-cc engine or higher) can be driven from the age of 16 with a specific driving license (type A). Only from the legal age of 18 it is possible to obtain the learner's permit and, after that, the car driving license (type B).

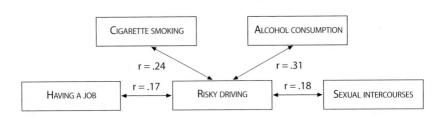

Fig. 4.33. Correlation with types of behavior tied to the anticipation of adulthood.

Risky driving, besides being a way to display an adult identity, if only superficially, allows some adolescents, younger boys in particular, to affirm themselves in a highly visible way, and to show that they are secure, fearless, and fully able to control themselves and the situation. Our findings show that for adolescents aged 14-15, the perception of always being able to make important decisions for their lives is tied to a greater number of traffic-code offenses; for adolescents aged 16-17, overall satisfaction with oneself is a predictor of traffic-code offenses. Similar to the case of affirmation of adulthood, this self-image is often only an appearance and is not actually accompanied by confidence in oneself and abilities. These characteristics, which are tied to superficial forms of self-affirmation, are found more frequently in boys and those who attend technical and vocational secondary schools. These adolescents appear to be more influenced by hedonistic and consumer values, values that the schools they attend provide little opportunity to reflect upon critically.

It should also be kept in mind that in Italy, risky driving conduct is boosted by the production of ever faster and ever-more powerful cars and motorcycles and by many adults who offer negative models in terms of respect for traffic code. The automobile industry in Italy, despite recent economic crises, has in recent years appealed to the youngest consumers by offering them increasingly powerful models, with aerodynamic lines and characteristics similar to the cars and motorcycles that race in Formula One, Motorcross, and rallies (just consider the lines, accessories, and colors of the products produced to appeal to young people). Boys and technical secondary school students are likely the groups that are most influenced by these consumer models and by the bad example of certain adults, both of which are models that contribute to the social acceptance and spread of driving styles characterized by risk-taking and high speed.

Once again, it should be noted that self-affirmation often occurs through exhibiting not only one's own qualities but also one's possessions and abilities. In Western society, young people and adults often use their means of transportation to communicate something about themselves (for example, their strength, their power, their wealth, or their agility) and as a way to increase their sex appeal. A positive relationship between risky driving and perception of self as attractive to the opposite sex was found in boys, young adolescents (14- to 17-year-olds), and technical secondary school students while this relationship was not significant for other groups. Once again, it appears to be the most immature adolescents (the youngest) and the least active participants in the school experience (boys) who seek superficial forms of self-affirmation.

Also tied to the strengthening of identity is the need to put oneself to the test in order to know, experience, and confirm one's abilities, potential, and limits. This need, which is felt more strongly by those who have a greater sense of their lack of a well-defined role in society, is often associated with anti-conventional traits and transgressive attitudes, which in our sample were expressed by a low disapproval of antisocial behavior and a low recognition of values such as the importance of religion, the school experience, and one's own health (Fig. 4.34).

The transgressive function of risky driving has some unusual characteristics and is not as strong for this type of behavior as it is for some of the behavior types analyzed in other chapters (substance use, antisocial behavior, precocious sexual intercourse). While it is true that traffic-code offenses represent a violation of established rules, it is also true that these offenses are common, socially accepted, and rarely sanctioned. The widespread acceptance of risky driving is evidenced both by a lack of control as well as its institutionalization in sports such as Formula One, rally races, and motorcross. This fact can explain, at least in part, the greater implication of technical secondary school students. Lyceum students find more internal, less blatant forms of self-affirmation and are therefore less involved in all types of risk behavior. On the other hand, vocational school students frequently feel the need to affirm themselves through extreme, often illegal, behavior. Dangerous driving, as it is a more moderate and socially accepted form of transgression, is unable to express to the same degree as other types of risk-taking behavior the pro-

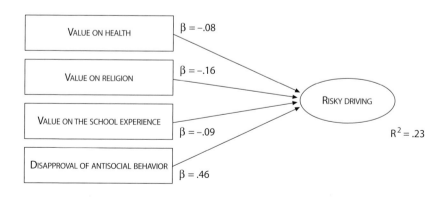

Fig. 4.34. Personal variables (multiple regression).

found difficulties of these adolescents. However, it does respond to the more moderate need for transgression and experimentation felt by technical secondary school students.

4.5.2 Identification and Peer Emulation

Risky driving, like other types of risk behavior, is tied to identification, social desirability, and peer acceptance. High levels of involvement in this type of behavior are therefore linked to the perception of being attractive to people of the opposite sex and to spending a great deal of time in the company of friends (Fig. 4.35).

But risky driving can also serve important functions tied to social confrontation, the need to differentiate oneself, to surpass one another, and to be seen and respected by one's peer group. The need for differentiation from peers is evidenced by the fact that a greater proportion of adolescents who are most involved in this behavior (15% compared with 7% of the low-involvement group) reported that their view on life is not similar to anyone else's and especially not that of their parents or friends. This need for differentiation from one's peers could translate into competition, high-speed racing, driving without hands, or other risky activities. These needs are felt more strongly by those who practice sports and who find sports teams a context in which they can express themselves (Fig. 4.36). These types of groups, based on competition and challenging limits, institutionalize confrontation and the comparison of individuals' performances.

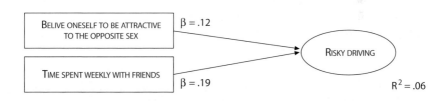

Fig. 4.35. Variables related to relationships with peers (multiple regression).

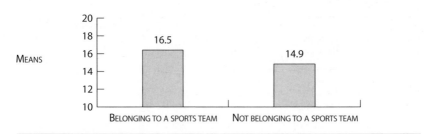

Fig. 4.36. Means for risky driving (ANOVA).

The surpassing of limits and experimentation with danger and high speed are also, like other risk behavior types, experiences judged as exciting and as having a strong component of pleasure. It should be noted that there is a strong positive correlation between risky driving and other risk-taking behavior dictated by the desire to feel strong sensations. Thus, risky driving also carries out the function of allowing the individual to experience strong emotions and sensations. This pursuit of sensations, as we will illustrate more clearly in the following section, occurs especially when accompanied by cognitive difficulties in foreseeing the possible outcomes of one's actions, by the illusion of control, and, as our data reveal, a focus on the present and scarce ability to plan one's time and activities (Zimbardo et al. 1997).

4.5.3 Adolescent Escape

The literature has repeatedly emphasized the fact that young drivers generally believe - although in reality it is rarely true - that they have full control over their own behavior and the vehicle when driving. The analyses we conducted also in part confirm this data. In reality, adolescents who commit more traffic offenses also reported a higher degree of self-confidence in coping (Fig. 4.37). These adolescents, however, also reported less certainty about their expectations to continue school, perceive a greater degree of conflict between the ideas and values of their parents and those held by their friends (Fig. 4.37), and have a weak internal locus of control for health and well-being, which they usually attribute to external causes.

From this description, we can see how risky driving can be a means, although generally illusory and ineffective, of trying to control certain aspects, relationships, and situations that cannot be controlled and are therefore perceived

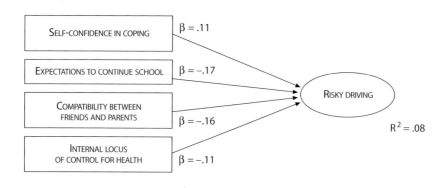

Fig. 4.37. Variables tied to the escape function (multiple regression).

as something that is forced upon them that they feel powerless to control.

Finally, driving, as we mentioned in the "Introduction," can be a way to deal with difficulties. The temporary physical and mental distance from problems can help us to see these problems with a greater degree of detachment and can therefore be useful in the resolution of those problems. Sometimes, though, this act of distancing oneself from conflicts and difficulties can last, making it more a means of avoidance or escape than of detachment. For this reason, risky driving can constitute an easy escape through actions and sensations when one lacks adequate ways of resolving problems.

This function is prevalent in adolescents who are heavily involved in risky behavior and whose characteristics are similar to those discussed in the description of high-risk adolescents in Box 3.2. These adolescents have limited personal resources, in particular, the ability to plan and organize their time, which they generally spend doing nothing or in public places, neglecting their studies and relationships with their families (Fig. 4.38). Our recent analyses of the relationships between driving style and use of free time confirm that the adolescents most involved in risky driving spend most of their free time in nonorganized activities. We also found that time spent weekly in nonorganized activities is associated with both poor planning abilities and difficulties in identifying with established roles and activities, leading to low expectations for conventional achievement and a greater need for escape (Cattelino et al. 2000).

At the same time, these adolescents tend to have a limiting, pessimistic view of their context. They do not see the school experience as a source of personal satisfaction nor do they see it as useful for their lives and future achievements; they spend little time studying and, although they continue to attend, they would like to drop out (Fig. 4.39).

These adolescents also perceive their families as distant and disinterested (Fig. 4.40) and, as we have seen, they dedicate very little time to them.

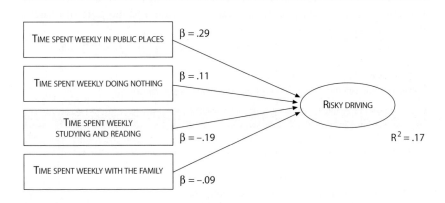

Fig. 4.38. Variables related to use of free time (multiple regression).

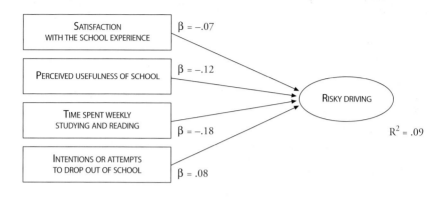

Fig. 4.39. Variables related to the school experience (multiple regression).

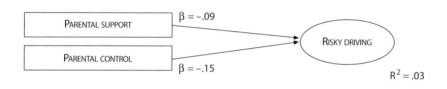

Fig. 4.40. Variables related to parenting style (multiple regression).

Therefore, all of these findings reveal that risky driving and risk, and the excitement that is tied to them, can be ways, however ineffective and potentially harmful, for these adolescents to escape from a context that is perceived as unfulfilling both through actual physical distance and the pursuit of new, intense, exciting sensations.

The main functions of risky driving are outlined in Summary 4.4.

Summary 4.4. Main functions carried out by driving and risky driving.

Driving
• AUTONOMY, both practical and psychological, through separation and return (especially for boys, technical secondary school students, and adolescents who live in small towns)
• SEPARATION, both physical and psychological, from conflictual situations
• ADULTHOOD, through acting out an adult behavior

cont. ▸▸

Risky driving
• ADULTHOOD, through the anticipation and exaggeration of an adult behavior (especially for younger adolescents and those who drive a vehicle before attaining the legal age to do so)
• EXPERIMENTATION AND SELF-AFFIRMATION, through control of the motor vehicle (especially in boys)
• SELF-AFFIRMATION, through exhibiting one's means of transportation and showing what one can do with it (especially in adolescents under the age of 18)
• SENSATION-SEEKING and EXPERIMENTATION
• IDENTIFICATION and DIFFERENTIATION from peers
• EMULATION of and SURPASSING peers (especially for those who play sports)
• TRANSGRESSION (in all groups but particularly for technical school students, boys, and drivers of scooters and motorcycles)
• COPING STRATEGY, tied to exterior means of self-affirmation
• ESCAPE (especially in older adolescents and in those who are most heavily and persistently involved)

4.6 Protective Factors

The main protective factors are related as much to adolescents' individual resources as to the opportunities that their context offers or that they create for themselves. Our data suggest that the ability to accept the rules and values of society, a high disapproval of antisocial behavior, the ability to see the sense in one's actions and one's life, a commitment to school, having short- and long-term projects (expectations to continue school), and being able to use dialogue to share and deal with difficulties are all protective factors. These individual characteristics then interact with the family, peer relationships, and the school experience.

The family plays both a direct and indirect role in influencing the driving practices of adolescents. As discussed previously, the paternal model for use of the safety belt is directly related to the same behavior in adolescent children. As the analyses conducted show a strong positive relationship between use of the safety belt or helmet and a prudent driving style (Fig. 4.41), it can be hypothesized that the parental model also has an influence on other aspects of driving.

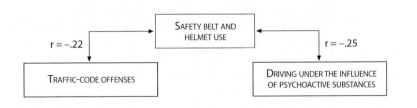

Fig. 4.41. Correlations.

The family also exerts an important indirect role closely tied to the functions of dangerous driving. Like the other types of risk behavior examined, this role is carried out through support and control. The protective role of control was found to be particularly crucial to the behavior of adolescent children. Requiring adolescents to respect curfews and give information about where they will be and with whom reduces both involvement in traffic-code offenses and driving under the influence of psychoactive substances. Particularly in terms of driving after having drunk alcohol or smoked marijuana, the influence of control and parental support has an importance, acquiring a stronger protective value (Fig. 4.42).

The multiple regression analyses conducted on the sample, stratified for gender and age group, shows that for boys and the youngest group of adolescents, control is more important (for adolescents aged 14-15, it is actually the only significant characteristic), while for girls and adolescents aged 16-17, the greatest protective comes from the interaction of parental control and support.

As for the role of friends, their behavior models can either increase or decrease involvement in risky driving practices. As we saw earlier, for example, the model offered by the best friend for using a safety belt or helmet is an excellent predictor of the adolescent's behavior. In addition, having friends who drive under the influence of psychoactive substances increases the risk both of emulation and the probability of risking one's personal safety by riding with these friends. Friends also play an indirect role in influencing the driving conduct of adolescents (Fig. 4.43); greater lengths of time spent in the company of peers is associated with risky driving. This is due to imitation as well as the reciprocal behavioral reinforcement that occurs in many group situations and the need to show off, to be the center of attention, and to emulate and surpass one another. The role of friends tends to become stronger when there is low compatibility between the views and beliefs of friends and

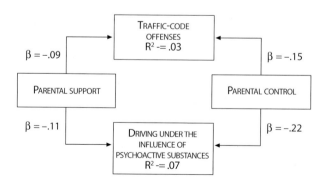

Fig. 4.42. Variables related to parenting style (multiple regression).

parents (Bina et al. 2004). The presence of conflicts in adolescents' social networks can therefore increase the risk of high levels of involvement in risky driving practices. Consistent with the literature, this occurs particularly when peers act as models for dangerous, nonconventional behavior and in adolescents who are more impulsive (West et al. 1993), who lack coping skills, and who have a low tolerance for stress and frustration (Donovan et al. 1983). However, support from and control by friends are not related.

Finally, in terms of school, being cognitively and emotionally invested in the school experience, marked by good relationships with teachers, satisfaction with the school experience, and a perception of the school as useful, is accompanied by lower involvement in risky driving (Fig. 4.44).

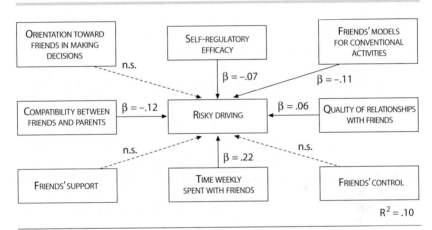

Fig. 4.43. Variables related to peer relationships (multiple regression).

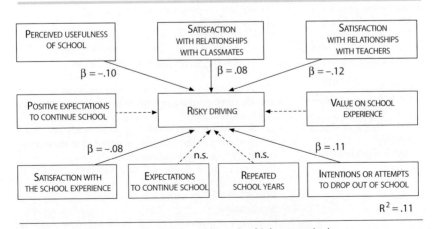

Fig. 4.44. Variables related to school experience (multiple regression).

This is due mainly to the fact that those who identify more strongly with their school and their role as students tend not to feel the need to seek out highly visible, and often transgressive, means of affirming their identities. Second, those who perceive the school experience as useful and are confident in their ability to succeed have less need to put themselves to the test and to feel capable in other contexts. Finally, dedication to studying offers a wealth of opportunities for reflection as well as functional, constructive use of free time that does not have to be filled by moving aimlessly from place to place looking for ways to overcome boredom.

A theoretical overview of the protective factors related to the family, school, friend, and free time contexts is provided in Summary 4.5. These protective factors are tied to the various functions that risky driving can have for adolescents.

Summary 4.5. Main protective factors related to the family, school, friends, and free time contexts in relation to the functions of risky driving.

Protective factors	Related functions
FAMILY • Paternal model • Control • Support	The model for safety belt and helmet use, through the processes of IDENTIFICATION, can encourage non-risky-driving behavior Control limits EXPERIMENTATION (especially for boys and the youngest adolescents) The right combination of support and control encourages: • The use of methods for SELF-AFFIRMATION that involve dialogue and confrontation • The expression of ADULTHOOD through sharing and relating with adults as equals • AUTONOMY through relating with adults as equals • The use of COPING STRATEGIES based on verbalization and confrontation as opposed to ESCAPE • Internalization of rules and values that counter the need for TRANSGRESSION
SCHOOL EXPERIENCE • Satisfaction with the school experience • Satisfaction with relationships with teachers • Perceived usefulness	Viewing the school experience as a meaningful and potentially satisfying experience encourages: • SELF-AFFIRMATION • REINFORCEMENT of a positive IDENTITY • Involvement in the institutions of the adult world as opposed to TRANSGRESSION or OPPOSITION
PEERS • Model for use of helmet and safety belt • Model for conventional behavior • High compatibility with parents	The perception of one's friends as nontransgressive people involved in ordinary daily activities with values similar to one's parents encourages: • IDENTIFICATION and DIFFERENTIATION processes based on the sharing of constructive (as opposed to destructive or oppositional) ideas and activities • The perception of having SOCIAL BONDS that are not limited by an excessive need to show off • EXPERIMENTATION with socially accepted, nonrisky roles and behavior • Perception of continuity with the values of society and the adult world instead of TRANSGRESSION and OPPOSITION

cont. ▶▶

Protective factors	Related functions
FREE TIME • Time spent studying and reading • Time spent with the family	The time spent per week reading, studying, or with the family encourage: • SELF-AFFIRMATION and IDENTITY CONSTRUCTION through reflection, comparing ideas, and prosocial behavior • The consolidation of a SENSE OF BELONGING to the community • Reflection on the sense of one's existence and on the value of one's actions for one's self and others • PLANNING and COMMITMENT • Use of effective COPING STRATEGIES • The internalization of values instead OPPOSITION to them

CHAPTER 5

Antisocial Behavior

> In my opinion, the group is just a form of security… when you do something with a group of friends you feel less responsible, it doesn't seem so serious… everyone does it, so you do it too.
>
> *[Girl, science lyceum, fifth year]*

5.1 Antisocial Behavior in Adolescence

Antisocial behavior is defined as behavior that goes against the norms, values, and principles of the community that one belongs to. The term antisocial behavior refers to a variety of different types of behavior - from aggression, to theft, to property damage, to vandalism - that are similar for the transgressive significance they hold. Only in part do these types of behavior coincide with delinquent behavior, which is characterized by more extreme illegality and the intervention of judiciary authorities and the police.

Historically, psychological research has shifted from the study of delinquency to antisocial behavior. From a methodological point of view, this has meant a move from studying official acts (criminal charges, court cases, and fines) to data supplied by the subjects themselves. In reality, as the majority of antisocial acts committed are not discovered, reported, and punished, the only way to learn of them is through the accounts of those who carried them out. Thus, the study of antisocial behavior through subjective accounts has revealed a great increase in antisocial behavior among adolescents. This increase refers to the number of adolescents implicated, the number of acts committed (de Wit and van der Veer 1991; Emler and Reicher 1995; Rutter et al. 1998), the variety of behavior types, and the seriousness of these behavior types (Born 1987; 2003; Loeber et al. 1998). Upon reaching the threshold to adulthood, after the age of 18-20 years, the widespread nature and high frequency of antisocial behavior decreases.

This trend clashes with conflicting empirical evidence. Numerous studies have pointed to the existence of strong continuity in antisocial behavior for certain individuals (Loeber and Farrington 2000; Koops and Orobio de Castro 2004). This continuity does not refer to a single behavior or behavioral category, such as physical aggression, for example (Olweus 1993; Eron et al. 1991; Smith and Sharp 1994; Frączek and Zumkley 1992) but can emerge as different types of antisocial behavior, for example, aggression at an early age followed by theft (Loeber 1990) or early disobedience followed by acts of delinquency (Farrington 1994). However, discontinuation of antisocial behavior is also common, and the majority of young people who commit acts of antisocial behavior do not go on to become career criminals; for these individuals, antisocial behavior is confined to the adolescent years (Moffit 1993; Werner 1990; Koops and Orobio de Castro 2004). The inconsistency of these results has led to the discrediting of generalized theories that traced antisocial behavior to factors that were always the same, regardless of the life-cycle period analyzed (Gottfredson and Hirshi 1990). These factors were generally ascribable to elements within the individual, such as an insufficiency of some sort or a pathology of the personality (de Wit and van der Veer 1991), or to external events, such as the role of society at large and the resulting lack of social control. These theories have given way to developmental theories on antisocial behavior that distinguish between subjects whose initiation into antisocial behavior begins early - occurring in early childhood and youth - and those, on the other hand, who begin later - during adolescence (Moffit 1993). The first group, much less numerous and consisting mainly of boys, is generally characterized by continuity; these individuals display persistent forms of antisocial behavior throughout the entire life cycle. The second group is characterized by the discontinuation of antisocial conduct; antisocial behavior in members of this group is confined to the years of adolescence (Fig. 5.1).

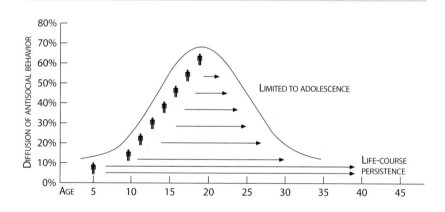

Fig. 5.1. Hypothetical illustration of the change in the diffusion of involvement in antisocial behavior over the course of the lifetime (the *continuous line* represents the well-known antisocial behavior curve for age; the *arrows* represent the duration of involvement in antisocial behavior) [Figured derived from Moffit 1993].

During adolescence, these two types of antisocial behavior coexist, but each has its own specific etiological factors and characteristics. In particular, antisocial behavior that begins precociously and unfolds over the course of one's existence until adulthood originates in childhood and is rooted in early socialization processes (Loeber 1990) and factors that, over the course of successive development, lead to the crystallization of this behavior (Frączek and Zumkey 1992; Patterson et al. 1992). This group is comprised mostly of boys, who appear to be more vulnerable to violent behavior caused by physical characteristics linked to neurological development such as hyperactivity, attention disorders, and difficult temperaments (Moffit et al. 2001). Adolescent antisocial behavior, on the other hand, is a response to the typical needs of this developmental period and cannot be understood or controlled without considering the characteristic developmental tasks of these years.

The move from generalized theories on antisocial behavior to developmental theories has led to the gradual abandonment of traditional explanatory models (Paternoster and Brame 1997), which traced antisocial and criminal conduct to genetic or biological characteristics, to poor socialization and to inadequate internalization of the norms that regulate society caused by deficiencies or personality pathologies or to deficiencies in terms of social factors (socioeconomic status, residing in degraded neighborhoods, the break-up of society and the family, loss of values, and so on). These models have been replaced by interactionistic and multicausal models that consider the contribution of a number of factors of an individual and social nature. Tracing antisocial behavior in a deterministic way to one or more antecedent causes fails to explain how, beginning from the same initial risk conditions, many outcomes are possible and these outcomes do not necessarily coincide with a career of antisocial behavior. Empirical evidence based on longitudinal studies has led us to conceive antisocial behavior more as a path or a process than the product or effect of antecedent causes and has encouraged researchers to focus on the risk mechanisms and the protective factors that have an impact on different psychosocial contexts over the course of development (Wiesner and Silbereisen 2003).

In keeping with this type of theoretical approach, the types of antisocial behavior examined in this chapter, which are considered normal during adolescence (Silbereisen and Noack 1988), are analyzed in the context of the subjects' lifestyles taking into account characteristics of the adolescent period and objectives for growth in this phase of the life cycle. Through analyzing the interactions between antisocial behavior and the main contexts of adolescent development - family, school, peer group, and so-called "fourth context" (Silbereisen and Todt 1994a) of free time - we have sought to bring to light the main functions performed by the types of antisocial behavior for the adolescents who put these behavior types into effect and, based on this, to identify the main risk and protective factors for this type of conduct.

5.2 Multiple Forms of Antisocial Behavior

As mentioned previously, antisocial behavior includes a wide variety of behavior types that defy the norms of society. This chapter examines three categories of antisocial conduct that, while not exhaustive, include the most frequent and often the only manifestations of antisocial behavior to be found in a normative sample of adolescents. These categories include physical aggression against peers[1], theft and vandalism, and violation of the norms of obedience and honesty toward parents and teachers. These three aspects represent distinct factors within a factor analysis of the main components (Fig. 5.2)

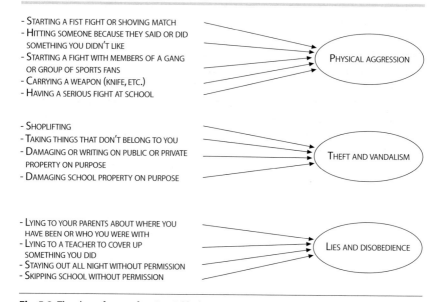

Fig. 5.2. The three forms of antisocial behavior.

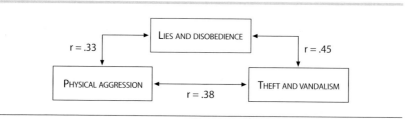

Fig. 5.3. Correlation between different forms of antisocial behavior.

---

[1] The full questions and scales from the questionnaire along with their related responses and main psychometric characteristics are reported in the "Appendix."

and are examined separately because, on the one hand, they involve different types of individuals, and on the other hand, show different tendencies over time. Thus, it is reasonable to presume that they absolve different functions. Furthermore, physical aggression differs in that it causes more serious harm and for the fact that it involves direct attack while theft, vandalism, lies, and disobedience are generally less direct and less detrimental in terms of physical safety.

Adolescents in a normative sample appear to be more involved in the less serious forms of antisocial behavior[2]: 34% reported having committed at least one act of aggression in the last six months, 38% had committed at least one act of theft or vandalism, and 78% admitted to having lied to or disobeyed their parents or teachers at least once in the last six months. The level of involvement in antisocial behavior by the adolescents in our sample was slightly lower than the levels of involvement found in other European countries and in the United States. In various studies conducted in these countries, the percentages of adolescents involved in one or more categories of antisocial behavior ranged from 50% to 80% (Emler and Reicher 1995; Rutter et al. 1998).

In addition to the fact that the three types of antisocial acts considered here involve different percentages of subjects, involvement also differs in terms of gender, type of school attended, and tendencies over time. For this reason, it would seem more appropriate to refer to multiple forms of antisocial behavior rather than antisocial behavior as a whole.

Fairly strong correlations exist between the three categories of acts (Fig. 5.3), which could lead us to imagine a progression in the antisocial career, beginning with less serious behavior and leading up to more serious acts.

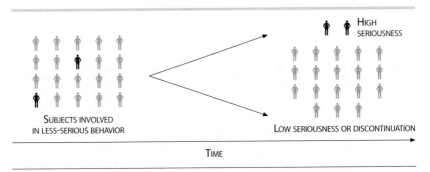

Fig. 5.4. Possible paths of involvement in antisocial behavior[3].

---

[2] Note that all the results reported in the figures are statistically significant, with $p<0.05$. In Chap. 2, Sect. 2.4, Presentation of Results and Statistical Analyses, the criteria for the presentation of results and for the use of statistics are explained.

[3] The diagram of the possible paths of involvement in antisocial behavior is based on empirical evidence and statistical analyses. Based on these findings, the high-involvement group represents about 10-15% of the total sample.

However, research has found that this progression only occurs for certain adolescents. In our sample as well, only a small number of boys and girls reported having committed serious acts only (5% of boys and 1% of girls reported having committed acts of aggression only and 2% of boys and 3% of girls reported acts of theft and vandalism only), which can indicate that antisocial behavior in these adolescents is preceded and accompanied by other less serious behavior. However, in most cases, this type of progression toward delinquency is not found (in our sample 22% of boys and 38% of girls), and antisocial behavior goes no further than lies and disobedience (Fig. 5.4).

5.2.1 Gender Differences

Consistent with the wealth of literature on various Western countries (Loeber 1990; Moffitt et al. 2001), boys are generally more involved than girls in antisocial behavior and other types of "externalized" behavior. However, the degree of this greater involvement varies based on the type of conduct considered: more specifically, 50% of boys reported having committed at least one act of aggression in the last six months compared with 21% of girls; 42% of boys were involved in acts of theft and vandalism compared with 35% of girls. As for lies and disobedience, 78% of both boys and girls reported having committed acts of this kind.

Analyzing the degree of involvement for each type of act, it emerged that boys are more involved in persistent forms of aggression than are girls (Fig. 5.5) and are also more involved in persistent forms of theft and vandalism while there are no gender differences for experimentation with these types of behavior or, rather, for committing these acts only once.

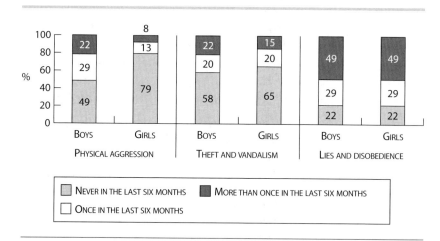

Fig. 5.5. Involvement in types of antisocial behavior for gender (chi-squared).

Finally there are no gender differences for lying and disobedience; the percentage for low involvement was 29% while 49% of the sample reported persistent involvement.

The greater implication by boys in aggressive behavior can be traced to differences in male and female socialization patterns as well as a greater need by boys to prove themselves through physical force. Various studies have demonstrated that aggressive behavior is interpreted and tolerated in different ways when acted out at an early age by boys or by girls (Björkqvist and Fry 1997). During adolescence, this same type of behavior is tolerated and in some contexts even valued in boys. As we will see more clearly over the course of this chapter, aggression performs functions that are associated more with male identity and relationships between boys.

5.2.2 School Differences

Students who attend technical secondary schools, followed by those who attend vocational secondary schools, are more involved in acts of aggression than students who attend humanities, science, or teachers' lyceums (Fig. 5.6). There are no differences between students of different types of schools for involvement in theft and vandalism and lies and disobedience.

These same trends are also found when comparing boys only from different types of schools while for girls, there are no significant differences. However, the different levels of involvement in different types of schools cannot be simply traced back to gender distribution in different schools. Nor can it be explained by other sociodemographic and sociocultural variables, such as place of residence, family composition, having an intact or separated family, and par-

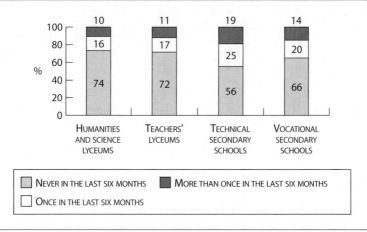

Fig. 5.6. Percentages of involvement in physical aggression for type of school (chi-squared).

ents' academic background or employment status. It was also found that differences in involvement do not emerge during the first year of secondary school and that significant differences appear only in later years. It should be noted, however, that adolescents who undertake different educational paths have different personal resources: lyceum students, compared with their peers who attend technical and vocational secondary schools, have higher expectations for success, a greater sense of academic self-efficacy, and less feelings of depression. The various school contexts also differ in terms of length of time required before students enter the workforce and for different types of training offered. Lyceum students generally foresee a lengthy educational path and a later entrance into the workforce. While this longer period of time in a way limits the autonomy of these adolescents, it also puts them in a condition to be able to negotiate their position within a family and school context. Also, especially through study of the humanities - subjects covered more frequently in lyceums - students have the opportunity to reflect on ideas that are closely related to the construction of personal identity and ways of relating to others. This kind of reflection has been found to be an excellent protective factor against aggressive behavior and other antisocial behavior (Bonino and Cattelino 2002).

5.2.3 Age Differences

The three forms of antisocial behavior considered here have different frequencies in different age groups: at the age of 14, the number of adolescents involved in forms of physical aggression is the highest, while the number of ado-

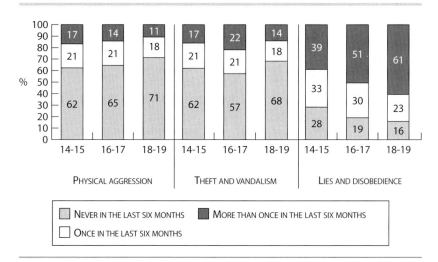

Fig. 5.7. Percentages of involvement in types of antisocial behavior for age group (chi-squared).

Table 5.1. Major sociodemographic characteristics of the adolescents most implicated in the three forms of antisocial behavior (chi-squared).

Physical aggression	Theft and vandalism	Lies and disobedience
The most heavily involved adolescents are mainly: • Boys • Between the ages of 14 and 15 • Students of technical and vocational secondary schools	The most heavily involved adolescents are mainly: • Boys • Between the ages of 16 and 17 No significant differences in terms of type	The most heavily involved adolescents are mainly: • Between the ages of 18 and 19 Boys and girls are equally involved. No significant differences in terms of type of school attended

lescents who tell lies and committ acts of disobedience is the lowest. Acts of theft and vandalism are more numerous at the age of 16-17 (Fig. 5.7). Therefore there seems to be a progressive abandonment of the most direct and detrimental forms of antisocial behavior as well as an increase in the more indirect forms - forms that are clearly symptomatic of difficulties in communicating as well as immaturity in relating to others.

Table 5.1 summarizes the main sociodemographic characteristics (gender, age, type of school attended) of the adolescents most heavily involved in the three forms of antisocial behavior.

5.3 Functions of Antisocial Behavior

The question that guides this entire book is why some adolescents behave in ways that compromise their health and personal fulfillment while others do not. The response to this question lies in the functions a particular behavior performs in the eyes of those who act it out (Silbereisen and Noack 1988). Antisocial behavior can serve multiple functions, which can change over the course of development. Here we will analyze the main functions, which are tied to self-affirmation, social desirability, and acceptance and transgression.

5.3.1 Experimentation and Identity Affirmation

From our data, it emerges that the adolescents who are most involved in forms of physical aggression are more satisfied with themselves and have more faith in their ability to confront difficulties than their nonimplicated peers (Table 5.2).

This finding shows how aggressive behavior can be perceived by some adolescents as useful in reinforcing a sense of personal identity, which would otherwise be lacking. This interpretation is consistent with Kaplan's studies (1980), which theorized that values associated with antisocial behavior are

Table 5.2. Means for various characteristics of adolescents grouped by level of involvement in the three categories of antisocial behavior (MANOVA).

	Physical aggression			Theft and vandalism			Lies and disobedience		
	Never	Once	More than once	Never	Once	More than once	Never	Once	More than once
Overall satisfaction with self	+[a]	++	+++	=[b]	=	=	=	=	=
Self-confidence in coping	+	++	+++	+	++	+++	=	=	=
Value on independence	=	=	=	+	++	+++	+	++	+++

[a] A greater number of plus signs (+) corresponds to a higher mean
[b] (=) A nonsignificant difference between means

often tied to self-defense. Physical force, which can be demonstrated through aggressive acts, can be an important - yet purely external and damaging - way to affirm oneself and to acquire self-confidence.

Self-affirmation through action, and aggression in particular, is only associated with a more positive self-image for the youngest adolescents (Table 5.3). While for these boys and girls aged 14 to 15 physical aggression is a highly visible way for them to affirm themselves, to confront difficulties, and to feel

Table 5.3. Characteristics of adolescents most involved in the three categories of antisocial behavior based on gender and age (MANOVA).

Physical aggression	Theft and vandalism	Lies and disobedience
The most involved adolescents: • Are more satisfied with themselves • Have more confidence in their coping skills • Place a greater value on their autonomy in making decisions These characteristics are stronger in girls in the low involvement group and adolescents in the youngest age group (14-15 years old)	The most involved adolescents: • Have more confidence in their coping skills • Place a greater value on their autonomy in making decisions A high value on autonomy in decision-making is characteristic of boys and girls in all age groups. Heavy involvement is accompanied by greater self-confidence in coping for the youngest group only while the most involved boys reported low confidence in their coping skills	The most involved adolescents: • Place a greater value on their autonomy in making decisions This aspect is characteristic of boys and girls in all age groups

autonomous and independent, these functions do not apply to older adolescents. Most likely, as adolescents get older, they realize that self-affirmation through opposition and aggression is only superficial and often disappointing, and they therefore seek other ways to establish themselves - ways that involve self-reflection, ideas, planning, and respect for others. The oldest and least-involved adolescents spend a good part of their free time studying, reading, or talking with friends. They communicate openly with their parents, have a high tendency toward prosocial behavior, and have detailed plans for their future. For some adolescents, this passage from external, superficial strategies to other more internal, mature strategies does not occur; these are the individuals who are most at risk for persistent involvement in antisocial behavior.

As far as gender is concerned, the statistical model, tested through variance analysis, was found to be significant for girls but not for boys; girls who have behaved aggressively on one occasion only in the last six months have more confidence in their coping skills. Also, as involvement increases, so does the value they place on autonomy in decision making.

While in physical aggression the prevailing aspects are tied to self-affirmation, the abuse of power, direct attack, and the need to feel capable of confronting difficulties through a display of force and are often connected to poorly developed social skills, the main aspect involved in theft and vandalism is indirect attack. Here, the object of the attack is not the person but the goods or property they possess. The adolescents who are most involved in these acts are characterized by a strong value on autonomy in decision making (Table 5.2). For this reason, the violation of property rights, damage to public property, and possession of goods appear to be, for some young people, a means of affirming their identity and will. Generally, their actions are directed at symbolic targets; because the family and school are the primary institutional contexts in which adolescents seek to affirm their autonomy, acts of theft and vandalism usually occur within the family and inside or against the school building. Apart from allowing for an indirect attack and an exaggerated affirmation of will, vandalism, and writing on walls and property in particular, come to represent a way of establishing one's identity through ostentatious behavior, making a display of oneself and leaving a mark that can be seen by everyone.

Examining the three age groups separately, it appears that the model tested through variance analysis is significant only for the youngest adolescents, while for all age groups, although to a lesser degree in older adolescents, the value placed on autonomy in decision making remains significant. The youngest adolescents, besides feeling more independent, are also more confident in their ability to confront difficulties; it is as if experimenting with antisocial behavior and challenging and attacking social norms and property reassures these adolescents of their strength and identity. For these adolescents in particular, in a society where appearances are what count, leaving one's sign on a wall or object or stealing to obtain objects that have symbolic value may appear to be among the few ways these adolescents have of being recognized either as individuals or as a group.

Our analyses revealed some differences between boys and girls: the most heavily implicated boys reported being satisfied with themselves and valuing highly their autonomy in decision making, but they have low confidence in their ability to confront difficulties. For girls, involvement in theft and vandalism mainly performs the function of affirming their autonomy in making decisions but is not connected to other aspects of their self-perception.

Furthermore, the fact that the most involved boys lack confidence in their ability to deal with difficulties is evidence of the fact that, even in the eyes of adolescents themselves, theft and vandalism are inadequate means by which to affirm themselves and are ineffective strategies for resolving problems.

Lies and disobedience, while more indirect forms, share some of the characteristics and functions of the other manifestations of antisocial behavior. Like those implicated in property offenses, the adolescents most involved in lying and disobedience place a higher value on autonomy in decision making than their less implicated peers (Table 5.2). This model, tested with variance analysis, is statistically significant not only for the entire sample but also for each of the gender and age-group subsamples, with the exception of the 16- to 17-year-olds.

The widespread nature of violations of the norms of honesty and obedience toward adults and the association of these types of behavior with a high value on autonomy are evidence of the difficulties experienced by most adolescents in integrating into the adult world and establishing relationships with adults on equal terms. Lies and deception are childish ways of opposing the will of others and affirming one's own will.

Summary 5.1 provides an overview of characteristics of the most involved adolescents. These data were extracted through a variance analysis on the sample stratified by gender and age group. These findings clearly show that all three categories of antisocial behavior respond to a need by adolescents to affirm themselves and their will. In the youngest adolescents, this need for self-affirmation is carried out mainly through action, abuse of power, displays of physical force, and direct aggression; subjects aged 16-17 use the damage of property to affirm themselves, while the oldest adolescents rely primarily on

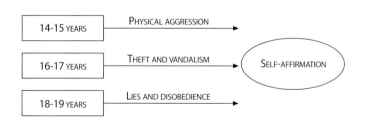

Summary 5.1. Type of antisocial behavior most closely tied to self-affirmation for subjects' age.

lies and disobedience. Thus, self-affirmation through antisocial behavior becomes gradually less detrimental, passing from more direct, blatant forms that have clear, visible effects on reality, to more indirect, private forms.

It should also be noted that, for the youngest adolescents, physical aggression and theft and vandalism take on a more pervasive function in the reinforcement of identity, increasing an overall sense of self-satisfaction and confidence in one's ability to confront difficulties. It is as if control and physical dominance over both objects and peers reassures these adolescents of their ability to control themselves and situations.

For older adolescents, self-affirmation is carried out through the achievement of independence. However, here as well, the antisocial methods of achieving this goal are very immature. Indirect opposition through striking symbolic targets or through deception are evidence of the difficulties young people find in actually achieving autonomy and affirming themselves and their will through making plans, making well-informed choices, and comparing ideas with others.

5.3.2 Social Visibility, Acceptance, and Desirability

In addition to reinforcing personal identity, antisocial behavior also performs functions that are tied to social relationships. Antisocial acts can allow adolescents to gain visibility, to feel accepted by their peers, and in some cases, to feel desirable. The adolescents who are most involved in acts of aggression believe themselves to be very attractive to the opposite sex, reported having numerous dates with someone of the opposite sex, and spend a great deal of time with friends or playing team sports (Table 5.4).

Table 5.4. Means for various characteristics of adolescents grouped by level of involvement in the three categories of antisocial behavior (MANOVA).

	Physical aggression			Theft and vandalism			Lies and disobedience		
	Never	Once	More than once	Never	Once	More than once	Never	Once	More than once
Believe oneself to be attractive to the opposite sex	+[a]	++	+++	+	++	+++	+	++	+++
Number of dates	+	++	+++	+	++	+++	+	++	+++
Time spent weekly with friends	+	++	+++	+	++	+++	+	++	+++
Time spent weekly playing team sports	+	++	+++	+	++	+++	+	++	+++

[a] A greater number of plus signs (+) corresponds to a higher mean

The model, tested with variance analysis, is significant, and the results coincide with those of the total sample for all the subgroups analyzed, except for girls (Table 5.5).

For boys, aggression appears to be more a display of strength than an act meant to cause harm. These types of displays make boys feel more attractive, and these subjects reported a greater number of dates with girls. In girls, on the other hand, strength and physical aggression are considered unattractive, as our culture requires women to be sweet and at times even submissive, disapproving of any behavior that puts the traditional roles of women - tied to procreation and caring for others - at risk.

Adolescents who are most involved in aggressive behavior spend a great deal of time with their friends. Therefore, it would seem that aggression is a group behavior or that the peer group provides an audience for acts of aggression, which are accepted, or at least tolerated, by these friends. Furthermore, aggressive behavior finds fertile ground in team sports and "contact sports" in particular. Aggression in sports is accepted and at times required or promoted and can therefore lead to the internalization of behavior that, when repeated outside of the context of the game or match, can become ways of relating to others. These findings show that sports, although offered as a solution for numerous troubled young people, can also be a source of risk where physical strength is used to compensate for internal weaknesses rather than actually seeking to overcome these weaknesses.

Theft and vandalism are closely tied to relationships with peers. Involvement in these types of acts is linked to greater success in relationships with

Table 5.5. Characteristics of the adolescents most involved in the three categories of antisocial behavior based on gender and age (MANOVA).

Physical aggression	Theft and vandalism	Lies and disobedience
The most involved adolescents: • Believe themselves to be more attractive to the opposite sex • Have more dates • Spend more time with friends • Dedicate more time to team sports These characteristics are stronger in boys	The most involved adolescents: • Believe themselves to be more attractive to the opposite sex • Have more dates • Spend more time with friends • Dedicate more time to team sports These characteristics are stronger in boys and subjects between the ages of 14 and 17	The most involved adolescents: • Believe themselves to be more attractive to the opposite sex • Have more dates • Spend more time with friends • Dedicate more time to team sports Except for time dedicated to team sports, which is not significant influence for the female sample, the other aspects are characteristic of both boys and girls in all age groups

people of the opposite sex and a greater acceptance within the group (Table 5.4). Time spent with friends appears to be a central element and is tightly linked to theft and vandalism. These behavior types take on a social connotation, as they are often carried out in groups and are ways of acting together and leaving a mark (Emler and Reicher 1995). In a circular relationship, sharing in actions - transgressing together, in particular - and thus sharing in emotions such as excitement and fear, serves to solidify relationships between those who carry out these actions. This model, tested with variance analysis, is significant for all subgroups analyzed, except for the oldest adolescents (Table 5.5). For these adolescents, spending time with friends is probably tied more to sharing thoughts and plans than to carrying out acts of antisocial behavior together. Adolescents over the age of 18 who commit acts of theft and vandalism seem to do so for other reasons unrelated to gaining the acceptance or admiration of their peer group. Again, playing on a sports team is associated with theft and vandalism for boys only, and these forms of antisocial conduct make boys and young adolescents (14-17 years old) feel more appealing to the opposite sex.

Finally, as far as lies and disobedience are concerned, implication in these types of behavior is accompanied by believing that one is attractive to the opposite sex, having had a greater number of dates with people of the opposite sex, spending a great deal of time with one's friends, and playing team sports (Table 5.4). Tested with variance analysis, the model is significant for all subgroups analyzed, although time spent weekly playing team sports is associated with lying and disobedience for boys only (Table 5.5). These results illustrate that lies and disobedience toward adults are an important aspect of social relationships between peers as well: adolescents who dare to challenge and oppose the rules imposed by adults, even through deception, are considered more attractive to their peers of the opposite sex and have a secure place in their group of friends, with whom they spend most of their free time. The fact that adolescents who spend a great deal of time with their peers are more often implicated in episodes involving lies and disobedience could also be an indicator of the difficulties these boys and girls find in negotiating for their autonomy. For this reason, hiding the truth and disobedience are easy ways to do what one wants while escaping the surveillance of parents and teachers.

Table 5.5 summarizes the characteristics of adolescents most involved in the various forms of antisocial behavior. Data were extracted through a variance analysis of the sample stratified for gender and age group. Based on these data, it is evident that physical aggression, theft and vandalism, and lies and disobedience perform functions related to gaining visibility, feeling accepted by one's peer group, and making oneself attractive to the opposite sex by affirming oneself and one's will and opposing the adult world and its rules. For boys and the youngest adolescents in particular, these functions are performed by all forms of antisocial behavior, including physical aggression and theft and vandalism while for girls and older adolescents, lies and disobedience gain importance at the expense of the other manifestations.

In general, boys and girls who demonstrate their ability to affirm themselves are seen as having strong characters, and their peers accept them and seek them out. Thus, antisocial acts have functions linked to sociability and are not merely symptomatic of socialization problems. Antisocial acts in a normative sample are carried out in groups or with the group as an audience. These actions are often norms, shared and accepted by the group (Reicher and Emler 1986; Emler et al. 1987; Hagell and Newborn 1996; Reiss 1998; Rutter et al. 1998). Emler and Reicher (1995) demonstrated that for both boys and girls, the group not only provides support for displays of opposition (or acceptance) of societal norms, it is also a context of coherent expression for their behavior, which allows them to manage their social reputation and affirm their identity. Furthermore, the acting out of certain behavior in the company of others offers protection by limiting the possibility of being identified and punished and encourages mechanisms of moral disengagement by spreading responsibility. In a circular process, transgression and self-affirmation that occur through antisocial behavior serve more to solidify a bond between those who share the action than to cause harm to others or to oppose those who are not part of the group, such as adults, for example.

However, while it is true that adolescents who are most involved are also well integrated into their group of friends and enjoy a certain level of prestige that makes them attractive and interesting to their peers, it is also true that these young people have some sociocognitive characteristics that can be obstacles in their relationships. In particular, from our data, it emerged that adolescents who are most involved in forms of aggression, theft, and vandalism have a low tendency toward prosocial behavior, have difficulties making short- and long-term plans (these adolescents spend a great deal of time doing nothing or in public places, and they are uncertain about many aspects

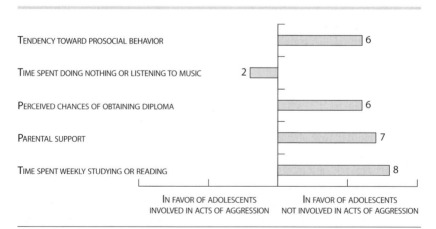

Fig. 5.8. Comparison of the proportional means for adolescents involved and those not involved in aggressive behavior.

of their future, including finishing high school), have a low perception of risk, and tend to underestimate the consequences of their actions (Box 5.1). They make little use of dialogue or reflection (not even through reading) and do not generally share with adults or peers (they make decisions alone and reported having ideas about life that are different from those held by both their parents and their friends). Therefore, these adolescents are very similar to those described in Box 3.2. Some of these characteristics have been reported in Figs. 5.8, 5.9, and 5.10.

Furthermore, numerous other studies have shown that adolescents most involved in antisocial behavior are highly egocentric (Cattelino 2001), have difficulties in decentralizing, and display low levels of empathy (Dodge 1986). What is most striking about these adolescents is their lack of cognitive ability to consider the consequences of their actions for themselves and others.

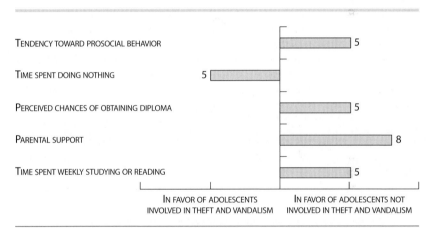

Fig 5.9. Comparison of the proportional means for adolescents involved and those not involved in theft and vandalism.

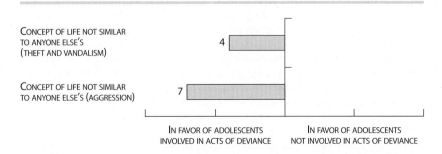

Fig. 5.10. Comparison of the proportional means for adolescents involved and those not involved in acts of aggression, theft, and vandalism.

Their actions are based on momentary impulses and, as they are unable to assume the perspective of others, they are prisoners of circumstance and immediacy. The inability to represent experiences of others and to anticipate the consequences of one's actions constitute risk factors for social and relational development.

These aspects also lead to difficulties in communicating, as evidenced by the fact that these adolescents rarely use dialogue to confront their problems. The blatant messages expressed in acts of theft and vandalism hide an inability to communicate through more mature and symbolic means - most importantly, through verbal language.

Although they have no difficulty expressing empathy and have a ten-

Box 5.1. Self-Exoneration, Self, and External Regulation

Adolescents most involved in the various forms of antisocial behavior also display a low disapproval of antisocial behavior (Table 5.6) and particularly of those types of acts that they themselves commit. Studies of cognitive dissonance (Festinger 1957) have supplied an interpretation for the tendency of individuals to underestimate the seriousness of the actions they carry out even when these actions violate norms and principles that they consider valid. According to this theory, individuals seek coherence between cognitive and behavioral data, and consequently, when incongruent relationships surface, these adolescents seek to reduce this dissonance in order to eliminate the sense of unease that it provokes. In the case of antisocial behavior, adolescents, unable to change an action that has already been carried out, alter their attitude toward this action, therefore reducing their disapproval.

Along with cognitive dissonance, other factors also come into play. Those who are persistently involved in antisocial behavior, while they are less disapproving of antisocial behavior than their peers, still maintain a moral code. Here, we find mechanisms of moral disengagement (Bandura et al. 1996; Bandura 1999) that deactivate the role of the conscience in regulating the actions one carries out and encourages self-exoneration. Moral disengagement performs the function of justifying one's conduct and making it seem more acceptable even when it goes against one's beliefs and values. At the same time, it also allows individuals to maintain their values, separating them from their actions, which are in clear contrast to these values. Moral disengagement occurs through a number of mechanisms (Caprara et al. 1995), including advantageous comparison (comparing one's own conduct with other more serious types of behavior), the misrepresentation of consequences (which are played down), attribution of blame to victims ("he got what he was looking for" or "she was asking for it"), dehumanization of the victim, and diffusion of responsibility, which occurs through a sort of collective sharing of blame. In the three forms of antisocial behavior analyzed in our study, different mechanisms of moral disengagement were identified: for physical aggression, the prevailing factors are dehumanization, blaming the victim, and diffusion of responsibility. Aggression often occurs with one's group or with a group of sports fans in situations that allow for the diffusion of responsibility. Dehumanization

dency for prosocial behavior, adolescents most involved in violating the norms of honesty and obedience toward adults also have difficulty establishing their independence and transforming their relationships with adults in order to relate on more equal terms. These difficulties, instead of diminishing with age, increase as adolescents approach the age of legal adulthood, leading to an increase in infantile ways of relating with others. These adolescents are aware of the inadequacy of this superficial communication based on dishonesty and deception and appear to be less confident and more depressed than their less implicated peers. Box 5.1 presents some of the processes associated with self-exoneration and poor self-regulation in adolescents most involved in antisocial behavior.

Box 5.1.

allows those committing acts of aggression not to identify with the victim and therefore to feel no sense of empathy, which could prevent the behavior or lead to a sense of guilt. In the case of offenses against objects and property, we find both the diffusion of responsibility and the distortion of consequences. Acts of vandalism are generally committed in groups and are very rarely punished; this, combined with a perception that public property, which should belong to everyone, actually belongs to no one allows those who commit these acts to become increasingly convinced that their crimes are neither serious nor particularly harmful. Finally, as far as violations to the norms of honesty and obedience toward adults are concerned, the main mechanisms involved are the minimizing of consequences and advantageous comparison, mechanisms that are often reinforced by adults' weak or collusive displays of authority.

The very existence of these self-exoneration mechanisms is evidence that these adolescents are not insensitive to social values and moral principles. What appears to be missing is reflection on the coherence between actions and principles and the ability to act accordingly.

In addition to self-exoneration, researchers studying adolescent antisocial behavior have highlighted the role of internal and external regulation. For example, Jessor and colleagues (1991; 1997) linked tolerance for antisocial behavior and a low value on academic achievement and religion to a weak internal locus of control. Adolescents who are most involved in various forms of antisocial behavior also reported low parental control (Fig. 5.12). Therefore, poor self-regulation is accompanied by equally poor external regulation.

From our standpoint, internal and external regulation are not the most important factors influencing antisocial conduct in a normative sample of adolescents. These types of behavior, more than the result of a personality weakness or poor internal regulation, are put into effect in certain contexts in order to reach objectives thus acting as the means or strategy for achieving a given aim. What is certain is that self-regulating abilities, as well as external regulation, are important protective factors that allow individuals to identify other less harmful and less dangerous ways to reach their goals of self-affirmation and to construct and maintain social relationships.

5.3.3 Transgression and Relations with Authority

Antisocial behavior, as it goes against the rules and norms of society, clearly performs a transgressive function. This behavior is considered a preferred means for communicating - in a highly visible, blatant manner - something about oneself to others and showing one's criticism of society's institutions (Emler and Reicher 1995). Antisocial behavior represents a way to make an impact on society, to escape from anonymity and conformity, and to be noticed not only by one's peers but by adults too. In reality, however, this anticonformity is only an appearance, as there is a great deal of similarity between the behavior and attitudes of the most involved adolescents and their peers.

This study has focused in particular on the relationship between adolescents and the school, as the school is the social institution that has the greatest ability to strongly influence the development of an adolescent's self-image (Bandura 1997) and their introduction into and identification with society (Palmonari 2000). It has been shown that during adolescence the relationship with the school, even more so than the relationship with the family, serves as the link between the individual and the broader community, and those who have a gratifying school experience also have greater confidence in society's institutions (Palmonari and Rubini 1995).

Adolescents who are most involved in the three forms of antisocial behavior considered here are characterized by a low value on academic achievement and religion and a low disapproval of antisocial behavior (Table 5.6). They are also less satisfied with the school experience, believe school to be of little use to them both at present and for their futures, often have low marks, and want to drop out of school.

Boys involved in acts of aggression against their peers (note that boys are the highest risk group) do not differ from their peers in terms of recognition of society's values (value on academic achievement and religion) nor for the time they dedicate weekly to conventional, organized activities, such as studying, reading, spending time with the family, or working on a hobby (Table 5.7). On the one hand, these results are evidence that these adolescents cannot be labeled as delinquent and, on the other hand, they reveal the persistent nature of socialization processes that favor physical aggression in boys at the expense of other more mature ways of resolving conflicts (Björkqvist and Fry 1997). Adherence to society's values and identification with its institutions are probably strong protective factors that facilitate the discontinuation of aggressive behavior - behavior that, with age, is acted out less and less. In girls, on the other hand, physical aggression has a more transgressive function and is accompanied by a clear opposition to society, its values, and its rules.

A variance analysis conducted on adolescents from the sample aged 18 and over reveals no statistically significant differences in value on school results, satisfaction with the school experience, and school grades. For this group, different personal factors probably come into play, and the role that was at first carried out by the school is gradually taken on by other social institutions.

Table 5.6. Means for various characteristics of adolescents based on levels of involvement in the three categories of antisocial behavior (ANOVA).

	Physical aggression			Theft and vandalism			Lies and disobedience		
	Never	Once	More than once	Never	Once	More than once	Never	Once	More than once
Value on academic achievement	+++[a]	++	+	+++	++	+	+++	++	+
Value on religion	+++	++	+	+++	++	+	+++	++	+
Disapproval of antisocial behavior	+++	++	+	+++	++	+	+++	++	+
Satisfaction with the school experience	+++	++	+	+++	++	+	+++	++	+
Perceived usefulness of school	+++	++	+	+++	++	+	+++	++	+
School grades	+++	++	+	+++	+	++	+++	++	+
Intention or attempts to drop out of school	+	++	+++	+	++	+++	+	++	+++
Time spent weekly in organized activities	+++	++	+	+++	++	+	=[b]	=	=
Time spent weekly in public places	+	++	+++	+	++	+++	+	++	+++

[a] A greater number of plus signs (+) corresponds to a higher mean
[b] (=) Nonsignificant difference between means

As far as theft and vandalism are concerned, adolescents aged 16-17, the age of highest involvement, do not differ from their peers in terms of their desire to drop out of school nor for the time they spend weekly in activities such as studying, reading, spending time with the family, or working on a hobby. Also for these types of behavior, involvement in organized activities that adhere to the values of our culture and are approved by society can be a strong protective factor against persistent antisocial behavior.

Lying and disobedience are typical behavior types, even in adolescents who, in many ways, identify with the values of society and are fairly well adjusted from a social and psychological standpoint. Thus, violating the norms of obedience and sincerity is a way to affirm oneself and one's will more than a way to transgress or oppose society.

Our findings show that while antisocial behavior clearly performs a transgressive function, this function applies more to acts of aggression, theft, and vandalism, which are illegal and can be prosecuted. However, in a normative sample of adolescents, these forms of transgression are merely experimental; antisocial acts for these adolescents are part of a lifestyle in which behavior hovers between adherence to and occasional transgression of the rules of authority. This experimentation with transgression is tied to a need that is typical of adolescence. To experiment with one's relationship to society norms and the possible consequences of violations of those norms.

Table 5.7 summarizes the characteristics of adolescents most involved in antisocial behavior. The findings presented result from a variance analysis conducted on the sample stratified for gender and age group.

Adolescents who feel the strongest need to transgress are those who do not experience personal fulfillment in the school context either because they feel the curricular content does apply to their lives, because of unsatisfactory rela-

Table 5.7. Various characteristics of adolescents most involved in the three categories of antisocial behavior based on gender and age group (ANOVA).

Physical aggression	Theft and vandalism	Lies and disobedience
The most involved adolescents: • Place a lower value on academic achievement • Place a lower value on religion • Are less disapproving of antisocial conduct • Are less satisfied with the school experience • Perceive school as less useful • Have lower school grades • Have thought about or attempted to drop out of school • Dedicate less time to organized activities • Spend more time in public places A lower value on academic achievement and religion and less time dedicated to organized, conventional activities are present to a greater degree in girls. Lower school grades, less satisfaction with the school experience, and less value on academic achievement are more characteristic of adolescents aged 14-17	The most involved adolescents: • Place a lower value on academic achievement • Place a lower value on religion • Are less disapproving of antisocial conduct • Are less satisfied with the school experience • Perceive school as less useful • Have lower school grades • Have thought about or attempted to drop out of school • Dedicate less time to organized activities • Spend more time in public places With the exception of intention or attempts to drop out and time dedicated to organized, conventional activities, which is not significant for adolescents aged 16-17, the other aspects are characteristics of both boys and girls in all age groups	The most involved adolescents: • Place a lower value on academic achievement • Place a lower value on religion • Are less disapproving of antisocial conduct • Are less satisfied with the school experience • Perceive school as less useful • Have lower school grades • Have thought about or attempted to drop out of school • Spend more time in public places These aspects are characteristic of boys and girls in all age groups

tionships with teachers, or because of failures in various subjects. Numerous studies have revealed the importance of academic achievement as a protective factor for all risk behavior. Being successful in school reinforces adolescents' sense of identity and allows them to attain a positive image in the eyes of their peers and adults. For this reason, those who are unfulfilled in the school context seek other forms of fulfillment and other ways to put themselves on display, which can take the form of transgression. Summary 5.2 outlines the main functions of antisocial behavior.

Summary 5.2. Main functions performed by antisocial behavior.

Physical aggression	Theft and vandalism	Lies and disobedience
	• AUTONOMY	• AUTONOMY
• SELF AFFIRMATION, through direct attacks and displays of strength (especially for the youngest adolescents)	• AFFIRMATION OF IDENTITY AND WILL, through indirect attacks and by leaving one's mark	• AFFIRMATION OF WILL, through deception
• COPING STRATEGY, tied to self-affirmation and conflict resolution (for the youngest adolescents)		
• SOCIAL ACCEPTANCE AND VISIBILITY, through displays of strength and differentiation	• SOCIAL ACCEPTANCE AND VISIBILITY, through sharing in actions and acting in front of an audience (especially for adolescents under 18)	• SOCIAL ACCEPTANCE and IDENTIFICATION, through differentiation from adults
• BONDING AND BELONGING RITUALS, through shared actions and group attacks • EXPERIMENTATION and TRANSGRESSION (especially for girls)	• BONDING RITUAL, through the sharing of actions and the emotions associated with these actions	
	• OPPOSITION AND TRANSGRESSION, through indirect attacks, which are generally directed at the family or school	• OPPOSITION AND TRANSGRESSION, through the affirmation of will (especially in girls and adolescents 18 and over)
• ESCAPE (especially for the oldest subjects)	• ESCAPE, through actions in the absence of other coping strategies	• ESCAPE, from confrontation and dialogue

5.4 Antisocial Behavior in Context

In order to analyze risk behavior within a multicausal, interactionistic perspective, it is necessary to highlight the contribution of multiple factors, both of an individual and a social nature. These factors work in synergy and are not independent from the various contexts in which they appear (family, school, peer group) or from the developmental period to which they are related (Silbereisen et al. 1986; Silbereisen and Todt 1994a; Born et al. 1997). In the present study, four main developmental contexts are considered: family, school, peer group, and free time.

5.4.1 The Family

In the study of antisocial behavior, many factors related to the family context have been identified that can either encourage or limit the involvement of adolescents in antisocial behavior. The factors considered involve different levels of analysis (Galambos and Ehrenberg 1997). First of all, there are variables of a social nature (Bronfenbrenner 1986), which include a series of demographic and socioeconomic characteristics that define both the family structure and the family's position in the broader social context. A second group of factors includes variables related to the way the family functions, such as the characteristics of the relationships within the family and aspects related to parenting styles and practices. Finally, a third group of factors relates to personal characteristics of the parents, such as antisocial behavior, perceived stress, or depressed feelings. Aspects related to the structure and functioning of the family are considered here based on recent research that cites the relationship between adolescents and their parents as the factor most closely related and most important to adolescent involvement in antisocial behavior (Loeber 1990; Loeber et al. 1998) and adolescent developmental outcomes in general (Galambos and Ehrenberg 1997; Noack et al. 1999; Cattelino et al. 2001).

Our data reveals that education level - in other words, the years of school attended - and occupations of parents have no statistically significant influence on acts of aggression, theft, and vandalism. Furthermore, despite the fact that the literature often emphasizes the connection between the break-up of the family and involvement in juvenile antisocial behavior, especially aggression, theft, and vandalism (Werner 1990; de Wit and van der Veer 1991; Farrington 1994; Loeber et al. 1998; Rutter et al. 1998; Juby and Farrington 2001), in our sample, living in a single-parent family (due to the death of a parent, separation, or divorce) or living with both parents had no direct relationship with involvement in these behavior types (aggression, theft, and vandalism). However, there is a relationship between the wholeness of the family and episodes of lies and disobedience: a higher percentage of adolescents whose parents are separated or divorced persist in the violation of these norms (Fig. 5.11). This data

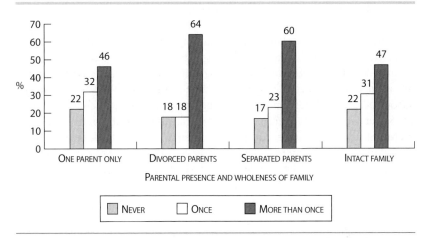

Fig. 5.11. Percentages of involvement in lying and disobedience based on family structure (chi-squared).

is confirmed by recent literature that shows that, while most children of separated or divorced parents manifest problematic behavior during the period of transition within the family, in the long run, these adolescents are psychologically and socially well adjusted.

In the sample of boys, significant differences linked to episodes of lies and disobedience emerge between boys from intact families and boys whose parents are divorced while in the sample of girls, the significant differences are between girls from intact families and girls whose parents are separated. Therefore, it seems that norm violation in girls increases in situations where there is presently conflict whereas for boys, norm violation is linked to low levels of parental control, a lack of dialogue between the two parents, and a lack of coherence in parenting styles.

Our data show that risk is tied less to living with one parent and more to situations of conflict within the family. In fact, antisocial behavior is more likely in adolescents who live with one parent only due to a divorce or separation than due to the death of a parent.

As far as parental education level is concerned, adolescents whose fathers have a university degree tell fewer lies and are less disobedient than their peers whose fathers completed primary school only. As the adolescents in our sample attended secondary school, it can be hypothesized that they are better able to relate to their parents when their parents have a higher level of education. Identifying with one's parents means being open to communication and dialogue, elements that are essential to establishing relationships based on honesty and reciprocal respect.

Consistent with other studies (Farrington 1990), the analyses we conducted show that socioeconomic factors as well as factors related to the family structure have little or no significant relationship to antisocial behavior when inserted into a hierarchical regression model that takes into account variables related to the quality of the relationships between parents and children. Therefore, it is the way the family functions that plays a central role. The main protective factors utilized here - which have also been identified in the literature (Patterson et al. 1992; Marta 1997; Scabini et al. 1999) - are control, support, and quality of communication between parents and children. Discipline and control were examined separately, as discipline that is overly severe, including coercive, hostile, and punitive methods or, on the contrary, inconsistent methods that fail to provide clearly defined rules or to assign punishments that are appropriate for the violation committed, can be risk factors for antisocial behavior in childhood and adolescence and predictors of involvement in antisocial behavior in adulthood (Loeber and Stouthamer-Loeber 1986; Farrington 1990, 1994; Patterson et al. 1992). Control refers to parents' interest in and awareness of what their children do when they are out and who they spend their time with. This factor can limit involvement in various forms of antisocial behavior (Farrington 1990, 1994; Galambos and Ehrenberg 1997; Jacobson and Crockett 2000).

The mechanisms of risk tied to inadequate discipline begin to take effect in early childhood and are related in particular to early antisocial behavior - generally taking the form of aggression - and the persistence of this behavior with increasing age (Patterson 1982; Rutter 1985; Eron et al. 1991; Rutter et al. 1998). The importance of parental control appears to increase at the onset of adolescence, in relation to the increased autonomy of boys and girls and the increase in time spent taking part in activities outside the control of adults.

Other studies (Dishion et al. 2004) have shown that parents of antisocial boys - in whom the antisocial behavior started early and persisted - decreased family management around the time their sons entered puberty. This is in comparison with parents of well-adjusted boys who maintained high levels of family management through adolescence. Adolescent males involved in deviant friendships and whose parents decreased family management were most likely to use marijuana and commit antisocial behavior.

In addition to and interacting with control, parental support - which is expressed through willingness to listen, discuss problems, and communicate openly - also appears to be a strong protective factor. Figure 5.12 reports the results of a multiple regression analysis, the predictors for which were parental control and support perceived by adolescents.

The same regression analysis, conducted on a stratified sample for gender and age group, confirms the protective role played by parental support for all groups. The possibility to speak openly with one's parents makes adolescents feel loved and accepted and aids in the development of a positive self-perception (Juang and Silbereisen 1999); at the same time, the opportunity to freely express their thoughts and feelings also appears to reduce stress (Seiffge-Krenke 1995) and is an important resource for dealing with problems tied to developmental tasks (Palmonari et al. 1993).

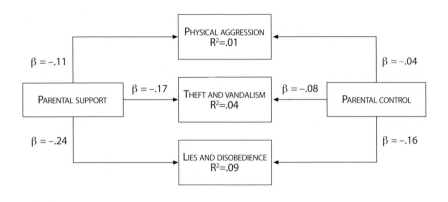

Fig. 5.12. Parental support and control and various forms of antisocial behavior (multiple regression).

Control combined with support, which forms an authoritative parenting style, also plays an important, although slightly weaker, protective role (the β values are lower), and this protective role is limited to certain groups (Table 5.8 and Fig. 5.13). While open lines of communication and dialogue with parents is a variable that maintains a high degree of continuity over time for children between the ages of 6 and 18 years, control in this same time period decreases (Cattelino et al. 2001; Loeber et al. 2000). This change is a function of adolescents gaining an ever-increasing degree of autonomy. Table 5.8 summarizes the protective factors tied to the family context. The findings presented here result from a regression analysis conducted on a sample stratified for gender and age group.

Table 5.8. Protective factors tied to the family context based on gender and age group (multiple regression).

Physical aggression	Theft and vandalism	Lies and disobedience
The protective factors are: • Parental support • Parental control Support is not protective for adolescents 18 and older, and control is only protective for the youngest adolescents (14-15 years old)	The protective factors are: • Parental support • Parental control Control is not protective for girls and adolescents 18 and older while support has a protective function for girls and boys in all age groups	The protective factors are: • Parental support • Parental control Control is only a protective factor for the youngest adolescents (14-15 years old) while support plays a protective role for boys and girls of all age groups

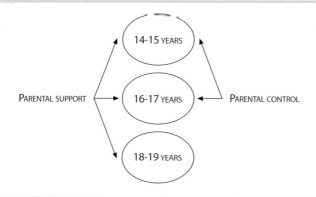

Fig. 5.13. Protective factors related to the family context for different age groups (multiple regression).

The results displayed highlight the family's role as an important developmental context that can prevent and reduce the risk of involvement in various forms of antisocial behavior (Deković 1999). The most important aspects are related to the way the family functions and the relationships between adolescents and parents. Parental control and support not only play a direct role by reducing the opportunities available to adolescents for involvement in groups at risk for criminality (Patterson et al. 1992) and by controlling adolescents' activities, they also play an indirect role that is closely tied to the functions of antisocial behavior. Willingness to listen and share are ways of relating to others that can be internalized by adolescents and transferred to other contexts, thus eliminating the need for adolescents to resort to forms of aggression and violence to affirm themselves and their will. Dialogue with adults also encourages adherence to the values of society, empathy, respect for others, and the development of an ability to take on the perspective of others.

Support also helps adolescents to see that difficulties and differences can be confronted and resolved through dialogue. Adolescents whose parents listen and provide support feel that their thoughts and feelings are valued and, through the equal relationships they have established with adults, are able to acquire the greater independence they need to confront the transitional period of adolescence and learn to identify with the adult world instead of opposing it. It should also be noted that dialogue and support from parents, teachers, and other educators are excellent instruments by which adults can help adolescents recognize that they are responsible for their actions. In this case, dialogue and support from adults takes the form of requesting, expecting, and allowing adolescents to take responsibility.

Boys and girls who have little dialogue with their parents and receive little control and support from them may be at greater risk for using displays of strength as a means of self-affirmation, for using lies and deception in order to avoid problems instead of confronting these problems within a deep and reassuring affective relationship, and for opposing the adult world rather than internalizing its rules.

5.4.2 The School Experience

Like the family, the school context also plays an extremely important role in adolescents' growth and development. At school, boys and girls are required to achieve certain results, and it is in this context that a number of other intersecting aspects, all tightly linked to the developmental tasks of adolescence, come into play. One of the most important of these aspects is the establishment of relationships with peers and adults. As we have already mentioned in the course of this chapter, school in Italy today, as in other Western countries (Emler and Reicher 1995), plays an important role in moulding the adolescent's self image and mediating the relationships between adolescents and their peers and between adolescents and society's institutions.

Figures 5.14, 5.15, and 5.16 display the results of multiple regression analyses where the variables presented as predictors of the different forms of antisocial behavior are related to the experience of success in school, the perception of oneself as a student, and relationships with teachers and classmates.

Based on these analyses and consistent with findings presented in the literature (Garnefski and Okma 1996), it was found that the school context can have a highly protective role and that this protective role is stronger for boys than for girls (Table 5.9). Girls have higher grades, experience fewer failures, and are more involved in the school experience (Cattelino et al. 2002), all of

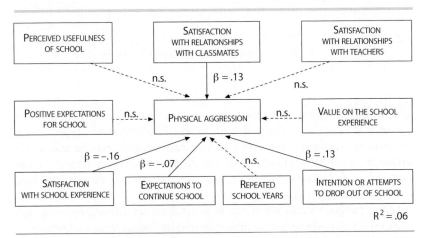

Fig. 5.14. School-related variables and physical aggression (multiple regression).

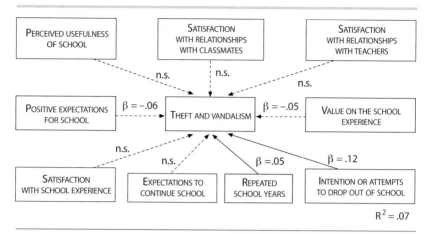

Fig. 5.15. School-related variables and theft and vandalism (multiple regression).

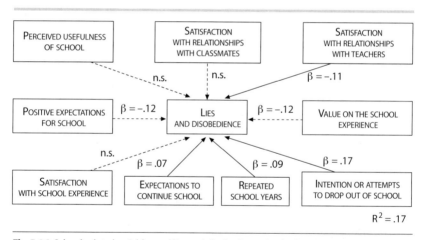

Fig. 5.16. School-related variables and lies and disobedience (multiple regression).

which constitute protective factors. However, in a multiple regression model in which the joint impact of the family and school on various types of risk behavior is examined, it appears that for girls the family has a greater effect (especially parental support), while for boys the school experience is more important. Table 5.9 summarizes variables tied to the school experience. These findings were obtained through a regression analysis conducted on a sample stratified for gender and age group. In general, adolescents who place a high value on the school experience, who reported having satisfying relationships with their teachers, who experience success in the educational context and

Table 5.9. Factors tied to school experience based on the gender and age of the adolescents (multiple regression).

| Protective factors | | |
Physical aggression	Theft and vandalism	Lies and disobedience
The protective factors are: • Satisfaction with the school experience • Satisfaction with relationships with teachers • Expectations to continue school These aspects are more protective for boys and adolescents under the age of 18	The protective factors are: • Value on the school experience • Satisfaction with relationships with teachers • Perceived usefulness of school • High positive expectations for school • Value on the school experience Satisfying relationships with teachers are protective for all age groups and are even more important for boys. The perceived usefulness of school is only protective for boys aged 14-15. Value on the school experience and high expectations for school are more protective for the female sample	The protective factors are: • Value on the school experience • Satisfaction with relationships with teachers • High positive expectations for school All these aspects are equally protective for boys and girls. For adolescents 18 and older, the only protective factor is value on the school experience, which is significant for all age groups

| Factors that increase the probability of involvement | | |
Physical aggression	Theft and vandalism	Lies and disobedience
The factors that increase the probability of involvement are: • Quality relationships with classmates • Repeated school years • Intentions or attempts to drop out of school Intentions or attempts to drop out of school are a risk factor for adolescents 16 and older. A higher number of repeated school years is not significant for adolescents 18 and older	The factors that increase the probability of involvement are: • Repeated school years • Intentions or attempts to drop out of school Intentions or attempts to drop out of school are a risk factor for younger boys and girls (14-15 years old) and for adolescents 18 and older	The factors that increase the probability of involvement are: • Expectations to continue school • Repeated school years • Intentions or attempts to drop out of school Intentions or attempts to drop out of school are a risk factor for boys and girls in all age groups. Repeated school years and expectations to continue school are more significant for boys

who have high expectations for school are less involved in forms of antisocial behavior. These individuals are probably able to affirm themselves and their identities through commitment to study and success in school. This success in turn reinforces a personal self-efficacy and affects social relationships, particularly in terms of satisfying relationships with teachers.

On the contrary, adolescents who are most unsatisfied with a school experience that they see as unimportant to their lives, who repeatedly experience failure, who have the greatest doubts about their cognitive abilities, and who are unable to establish constructive relationships with adults, may be at greater risk for frustration, distrust, and indifference toward authority. These adolescents feel a greater need for self-affirmation in other contexts and other ways, often through opposition to authority. These alternative methods generally move to forms of antisocial behavior, as it is easier to send a clear and specific message about oneself by breaking the rules than by respecting them (Skowronski and Carlston 1989; Palmonari 2000). It is important to note here that the school is the first social institution that young people come into contact with (Emler and Reicher 1995); thus, dissatisfaction tied to the school experience often results in distrust and an attitude of opposition toward other institutions.

Within the school experience, the teacher assumes an important role (Borca et al. 2002): satisfaction with the school experience depends not so much on good relationships with classmates as on positive relationships with the adults in the school who perform an educational role. Having positive relationships with adults outside the family context allows adolescents to accept the rules of the institution instead of opposing them and to feel that they are valued within the broader social context. In this way, the same objectives are reached that, in the absence of a favorable school context, could also be achieved through antisocial behavior.

5.4.3 Peers

It is mainly within the context of peer relationships that antisocial conduct develops and is put into effect (Jessor and Jessor 1977; Loeber 1990; Lyon 1996; Rutter et al. 1998; Brendgen et al. 2000). Adolescent antisocial behavior usually occurs in groups, is recalled within the group, and is talked about with other members of the group. Even antisocial behavior carried out alone is not usually kept hidden but is communicated to friends (Emler and Reicher 1995). Figures 5.17, 5.18, and 5.19 show that perceptions of the quality of relationships with friends and the support they offer are similar for adolescents who are involved and those who are uninvolved in the various forms of antisocial behavior. The variables that do have an influence are the degree compatibility between friends and parents and the models for conventional behavior offered by friends. Antisocial behavior increases when adolescents are more oriented toward their friends in making decisions and there is a low degree of agreement

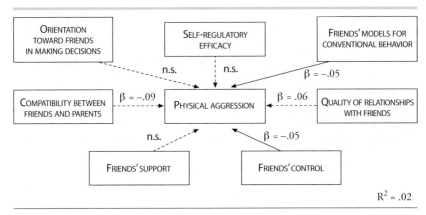

Fig. 5.17. Variables related to peers and physical aggression (multiple regression).

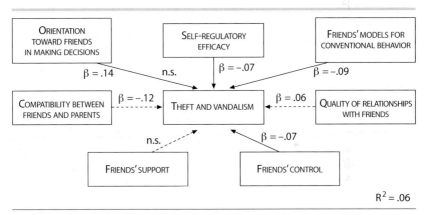

Fig. 5.18. Variables related to peers and theft and vandalism (multiple regression).

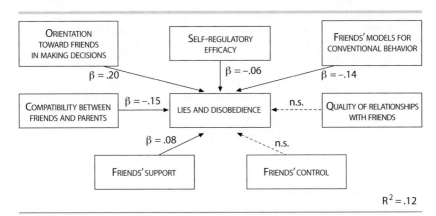

Fig. 5.19. Variables related to peers and lies and disobedience (multiple regression).

Table 5.10. Factors tied to the peer experience based on gender and age group (multiple regression).

Physical aggression	Protective factors Theft and vandalism	Lies and disobedience
The protective factors are: • Friends' control • Self-regulatory efficacy • Compatibility between friends and parents • Friends' models for conventional behavior Self-regulatory efficacy is only protective for boys, as are friends' models for conventional behavior. The latter, along with friends' control, is only protective for the youngest adolescents (14-15 years old). For girls and adolescents over the age of 16, compatibility between friends and parents is protective	The protective factors are: • Friends' control • Self-regulatory efficacy • Compatibility between friends and parents • Friends' models for conventional behavior Self-regulatory efficacy and friends' models for conventional behavior are more protective for boys. With the exception of self-regulatory efficacy, which is a protective factor for adolescents 18 and older, all aspects are protective only up until the age of 17	The protective factors are: • Self-regulatory efficacy • Compatibility between friends and parents • Friends' models for conventional behavior Compatibility between friends and parents is protective for boys and girls in all age groups. Friends' models for conventional activities are not significant for adolescents 18 and older while self-regulatory efficacy is more protective for girls and adolescents 16 and older

Physical aggression	Factors that increase the probability of involvement Theft and vandalism	Lies and disobedience
The factors that increase the probability of involvement are: • Quality of relationships with peers • Friends' support • Orientation toward friends in making decisions These aspects are stronger risk factors for boys and younger adolescents (aged 14-15)	The factors that increase the probability of involvement are: • Quality of relationships with peers • Orientation toward friends in making decisions Being oriented toward friends in making decisions is a risk factor for both boys and girls of all age groups. However, the quality of relationships with peers is only significant for subjects aged 16-17	The factors that increase the probability of involvement are: • Quality of relationships with peers • Friends' support • Orientation toward friends in making decisions These aspects are risk factors for boys and girls. The quality of relationships with peers is significant for adolescents 18 and older only

between parents and peers. This result is consistent with the dominant literature that underscores the relationships between the family and peer relations and the complexity of their possible influences (Deković and Meeus 1997; Kiesner and Kerr 2004; Deković et al. 2004). Antisocial behavior also increases when adolescents have poor self-regulatory efficacy and their friends offer weak models for involvement in conventional activities such as studying, spending time with the family, or taking part in a religious activities. In these cases, antisocial behavior comes to represent a way in which to act around others, to experiment with new types of behavior, to feel strong sensations, to feel like part of the group, and to differentiate oneself from adults and more conventional classmates by opposing them and breaking the norms of peaceful coexistence.

Friends who carry out a protective function have values that are coherent with those professed by adults - and the adolescent's parents in particular, offer control against transgression, and provide models for socially acceptable behavior (Table 5.10). Table 5.10 summarizes the variables tied to the peer experience. These findings result from a regression analysis of the sample stratified for gender and age group.

5.4.4 Free Time

Today, it is fairly clear that, in addition to the type of relationships adolescents have with their peers, it is the contexts and activities carried out with peers that constitute risk or protective factors (Emler and Reicher 1995; Garnefski and Okma 1996). Therefore, the way free time is used comes to play a central role. The activities one takes part in outside the school and family are intrinsically motivated, are perceived as a challenge, and provide an opportunity to plan and manage one's own personal development (Larson 1994). Not all environments in which adolescents choose to spend their free time are able to provide productive experiences that help them to develop a mature identity (Silbereisen and Todt 1994b).

As we have already seen in this chapter, more time spent with time friends outside the home and away from the control of parents or other adults is generally tied to greater involvement in antisocial behavior while spending more time at home with the family or studying has a protective function. Other studies have revealed the same findings (de Wit and van der Veer 1991; Hagell and Newborn 1996; Rutter et al. 1998). In the figures that follow (Figs. 5.20, 5.21, 5.22), the results displayed confirm this finding, especially as far as violating norms in relationships with adults and property offenses are concerned. In the case of aggression, on the other hand, time spent with friends is not significant while time spent with the family is only significant for girls and the youngest adolescents (Table 5.11).

The places that appear to be associated with risk are public places, such as coffee bars, video arcades, and discotheques. In these places, adolescents spend time together without any kind of specific plan, often experimenting with other types of risk behavior, such as the use or abuse of alcohol and psychoactive substances while deafened by the urgent rhythms of loud, pulsating music or lost in a virtual world of video games. This use of free time, accompanied by little time spent studying and reading, can act as an obstacle to reflection and rules out a more constructive use of one's time and resources. In these contexts - in which adolescents tend to be passive participants - exag-

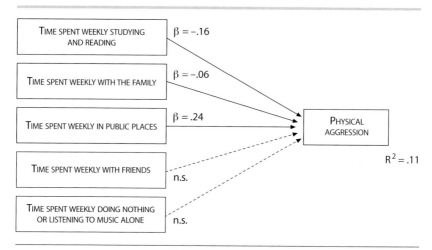

Fig. 5.20. Variables related to the use of free time and physical aggression (multiple regression).

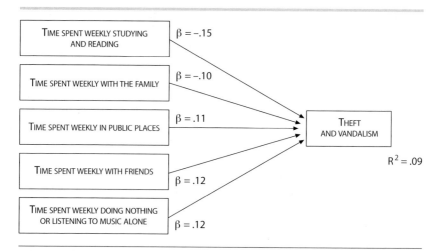

Fig. 5.21. Variables related to the use of free time and theft and vandalism (multiple regression).

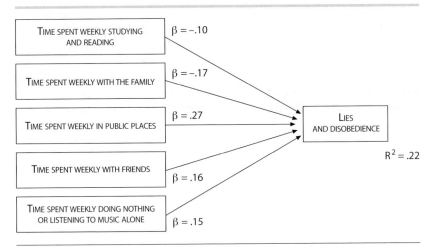

Fig. 5.22. Variables related to the use of free time and lies and disobedience (multiple regression).

gerated actions, transgression, and excessive boldness are used by adolescents to make them feel like part of the group and to gain visibility. The virtual absence of dialogue in these contexts also prevents the comparison of different points of view and blocks the processes of empathy. It follows that these adolescents tend to focus on the present and use infantile, violent means of conflict resolution.

In the case of theft and vandalism, as for lies and disobedience, boredom also seems to play a central role. In fact, spending the majority of one's time sitting around doing nothing is highly related to difficulties in planning one's time. Therefore, acts of vandalism, skipping school, and staying out at night without permission probably become easy ways to escape apathy and boredom and to experience strong sensations.

Using time passively and unproductively can be even more risky when uncompensated by time spent with the family. Contact with adults can encourage the assumption of responsibility and commitment to more structured and constructive activities and self-affirmation through less egocentric and destructive means. Contact, exchange, and time spent with adults gain importance as adolescents grow older, and they are linked to young people's ability to establish increasingly equal relationships with their parents and achieve their independence. Table 5.11 summarizes the variables tied to the use of free time. These findings are based on a regression analysis of the sample stratified for gender and age group.

In addition to the more individual use of leisure time, free time can also be spent in collective, organized activities through involvement in formal groups. Involvement in these groups is related to involvement in antisocial behavior. In considering various kinds of formal groups, it was found that only religious groups play a protective role for antisocial conduct (Fig. 5.23), while participation on sports teams and in politically affiliated groups are risk factors.

The religious group plays a protective role not only because it offers moral teachings and clear rules for behavior but also because it encourages reflection, self-regulation, and organizational capabilities and helps adolescents to develop plans for their lives. Spent in this way, free time is no longer an empty space to be filled with ostentatious actions but, rather, a meaningful time that

Table 5.11. Factors tied to the use of free time based on gender and age (multiple regression).

Physical aggression	Protective factors Theft and vandalism	Lies and disobedience
The protective factors are: • Time spent studying and reading • Time spent with the family Time spent studying is protective for boys and girls in all age groups. Time spent with the family is more protective for girls and the youngest adolescents (14-15 years old)	The protective factors are: • Time spent studying and reading • Time spent with the family Time spent studying is protective for boys and girls in all age groups. Time spent with the family is more protective for girls and adolescents 16 and older	The protective factors are: • Time spent studying and reading • Time spent with the family Time spent with the family is protective for boys and girls in all age groups. Time spent studying is more protective for boys and adolescents under the age of 18
Physical aggression	Factors that increase the probability of involvement Theft and vandalism	Lies and disobedience
The factors that increase the probability of involvement are: • Time spent doing nothing • Time spent in public places Time spent doing nothing is only a risk factor for adolescents 18 and older while time spent in public places is a risk factor for boys and girls of all age groups	The factors that increase the probability of involvement are: • Time spent doing nothing • Time spent in public places • Time spent with friends With the exception of time spent with friends, which is not significant for adolescents 18 and older, the other variables are risk factors for boys and girls in all age groups	The factors that increase the probability of involvement are: • Time spent doing nothing • Time spent in public places • Time spent with friends These factors are significant for boys and girls in all age groups

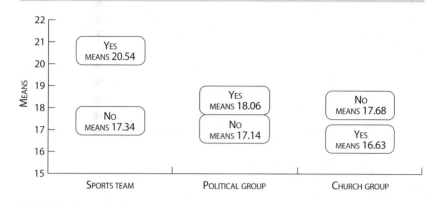

Fig. 5.23. Means for involvement in antisocial behavior (general scale) and belonging to organized groups.

offers opportunities for personal fulfillment as well as social visibility. Summary 5.3 outlines theoretically the main protective factors related to the family, school, peer group, and free time contexts. These protective factors have been linked to the various functions that antisocial behavior can perform for adolescents.

Summary 5.3. Main protective factors related to the family, school, friends, and free-time contexts in relation to the functions of antisocial behavior.

Protective factors	Related functions
FAMILY • Support • Control	The right combination of support and control encourages: • SELF-AFFIRMATION, through dialogue and exchange • SELF-ENHANCEMENT, through the sharing of ideas, feelings, expectations, and plans • INDEPENDENCE, through establishing relationships on equal terms • The use of COPING STRATEGIES, based on verbalization and exchange • Internalization of rules and values rather than OPPOSITION to them
SCHOOL EXPERIENCE • Value on academic achievement • Satisfaction with the school experience • Good relationships with teachers • Perceived usefulness • Expectations to continue school • High positive expectations	Viewing the school experience as meaningful and satisfying encourages: • SELF-AFFIRMATION • REINFORCEMENT of a POSITIVE IDENTITY • Involvement in society's institutions rather than TRANSGRESSION and OPPOSITION to them

Summary 5.3. Cont.

Protective factors	Related functions
PEERS • Models for conventional behavior • Degree of agreement (compatibility) with parents	A perception of one's peers as nontransgressive, involved in ordinary daily activities, and as having values similar to those held by one's parents encourages: • Formation of a BOND based on the sharing of ideas and activities that are organized and constructive as opposed to destructive or oppositional • Perception of SOCIAL ACCEPTANCE that is not dependent upon involvement in antisocial behavior • EXPERIMENTATION with safe, socially accepted roles and behavior • Perception of continuity with the values of the adult world and society at large instead of TRANSGRESSION or OPPOSITION to these values
FREE TIME • Time spent studying and reading • Time spent with the family • Belonging to a religious group	Time spent per week reading, studying, or with the family and belonging to a religious group encourage: • SELF-AFFIRMATION and IDENTITY CONSTRUCTION, through reflection, ideas, exchange, and prosocial behavior • Consolidation of a SENSE OF BELONGING to the community • Reflection on one's existence and on how one's actions affect oneself and others • PLANNING SKILLS and COMMITMENT • Use of effective COPING STRATEGIES • Internalization of values rather than OPPOSITION to them • SOCIAL VISIBILITY, through constructive actions

CHAPTER 6

Sexual Behavior, Contraception and AIDS

I mean... it's like... for me, this year, I came maybe closer to this problem. Probably because, growing up, and because there are more people who have done it... and so it seemed like sometimes it was too important for kids - who had done it and who hadn't, and so it comes almost... for a while, before, when we were younger, it was almost a competition... who had done it was privileged, was better... now a lot of people who have done it say... if they could go back... maybe they would think twice.

[Girl, science lyceum, fifth year]

6.1 Sexual Activity in Adolescence: A Transition Toward Adulthood

Unlike many other types of behavior discussed in this book, sexual behavior differs in that it cannot be examined solely in terms of risk. The ability to establish relationships that successfully combine affectivity and sexuality, and to be involved in sexual relationships where the individuality of each partner does not submit to physical or psychological coercion but is respected and freely expressed, is recognized by Western society as one of the characteristics of adulthood (Brooks-Gunn and Paikoff 1997). This recognition results from a changing attitude toward sexuality by society at large. Although attitudes about sexuality differ in regard to the two genders and across various cultures, sexual experiences - even when occurring outside of marriage - are generally more accepted today than in the past (Graber et al. 1998; Smith 1994). Learning to take part in an affective relationship with a partner of the opposite sex and to discover one's adult sexual capabilities can therefore be considered one of the fundamental developmental tasks of adolescence (Coleman and Roker 1998) although, in reality, the process of redefining oneself as a sexual being can last a lifetime (Buzwell and Rosenthal 1996).

Acquiring the ability to experience one's own sexuality without anxiety represents a complex challenge, in particular, for those adolescents who have not yet developed the social, affective, and cognitive capabilities necessary to have sexual experiences that encourage the development of one's identity and the acquisition of greater emotional autonomy from the nuclear family (Zani 1993; Dowdy and Kliewer 1998). Having positive sexual experiences requires the ability to recognize and guard against attempts at manipulation, as well as the ability to control one's impulses and emotions, integrating them into an affective relationship that respects the needs of one's partner. One must be able to use interpersonal negotiation strategies even in emotionally charged contexts and to comprehend and evaluate the consequences of one's behavior in both relational and reproductive terms (Byrne 1983; Tschann and Adler 1997). One must have the resources to seek out and utilize an effective contraceptive method and, finally, to accept new genital sensations and enjoy the sexual experience (Beyth-Marom and Fischhoff 1997). Therefore, a great number of cognitive, affective, and social capabilities together can contribute to experiencing the transition to sexuality in a positive or negative way. These abilities do not come automatically with the possession of an adult body that is capable of procreating but, rather, are constructed over the course of each adolescent's development based on a combination of both individual characteristics, such as the level of sexual and cognitive maturity, and environmental opportunities, such as education, which can lead to the acquisition of superior cognitive capabilities.

When these abilities are lacking - and when sex occurs at an early age it is more probable that they will be lacking - sexuality can be experienced in the context of an unsatisfactory situation or relationship and can be linked to various types of risk (Mitchell and Wellings 1998). In general, these risks, which are often interrelated, can be rather serious for both the present and future well-being of the individual and can take the form of physical risks, linked to sexually transmitted diseases (STDs) and early pregnancy; psychosocial risks, constituted by the greater difficulty of an adolescent mother to raise a child and the reduced opportunity for personal fulfillment in the mid- to long term caused by school dropout, which is often a consequence of pregnancy; and finally, psychological risk, linked to unequal, dependent, or violent relationships. Unfortunately, scientific knowledge of these themes is still quite limited. Research has tended to focus more on the incidence and prevalence of the phenomenon, dedicating less attention to risk and protective factors (Jackson et al. 1997). In addition, this knowledge is often fragmentary, as physical risk has mostly been examined separately from psychological and social risk (Ciairano et al. 2000; Ciairano 2004).

It is only recently that the various types of risks involved in early and unprotected sexual activity have begun to be investigated from a systemic, interactionistic, and constructivistic viewpoint discussed in the first chapter. From this perspective, involvement in sexual activity ceases to be described simply as an event that is the consequence of sexual development and influenced by various environmental factors, such as the inadequacy of school and family to exercise control of the behavior. Instead, by assuming an interactionistic and systemic perspective, we are allowed to conceptualize sexual behavior as a transition, carried out in different ways based on differences in limitations and resources and on the interaction between individual and context. An essential role is played by the personal choice to anticipate or delay this transition. Although it occurs at different levels of control and readiness, like other behavior types, the transition to sexuality assumes the characteristics and dignity of a motivated and self-regulated action (Bandura 1997), which the adolescent chooses and puts into effect to respond to specific needs of the developmental tasks he or she must face within a specific context (Silbereisen et al. 1986). Some peculiarities of today's Western social context can contribute to making this sexual transition even more complex. Many of these characteristics have already been considered in the introduction and are re-examined here in a limited way in terms of their implications on sexual activity by adolescents.

First, in contemporary society, adolescence has come to be understood as an increasingly lengthy period of transition. Sexual maturity, with the profound modifications and structural changes that it imposes on the adolescent, occurs at an earlier age while the assumption of adult social status tends to occur at a later age, and its definition is less clear (Crockett and Silbereisen 2000a; Juang and Silbereisen 2001; Bonino et al. in press). Being a part of this "in-between" age group means having less precise points of reference, tasks, and aims, which are not as clearly defined as they were in the past, even in terms of the transition to sexuality (Peterson 2000). Unlike in the past, sexuality is no longer prohibited before or outside of marriage, gaining economic independence from one's family is no longer a task that must be accomplished quickly, and marriage is no longer mandatory. The increased flexibility of the "social clocks" that regulate society's expectations offers greater opportunity for personal fulfillment and greater freedom to construct one's own path to development. Today, it is possible to test oneself both emotionally and sexually without being forced to make definitive choices prematurely (Brooks-Gunn and Chase-Lansdale 1995; Graber and Brooks-Gunn 1996; Schulenberg et al. 1997). On the other hand, to fully act on the greater possibilities available for personal development and fulfillment, adolescents must be able to live in the present, enjoying the advantages that their position within this "suspended social status" allows them without feeling the need to grow up too fast. The premature realization of adulthood can be detrimental on a personal and social level in terms of the limitations it may place on more advanced self-development (Silbereisen and Noack 1990; Silbereisen and Kracke 1997).

Along with lack of clearly defined tasks and objectives, contemporary society is characterized by some widespread and - for the most part, widely approved - tendencies, which can constitute for the adolescent an incentive to anticipate some of the behavior characteristic of adulthood through sexual behavior. Here we refer to cultural tendencies, such as an emphasis on immediate gratification and personal success at any cost; consumer trends, such as the desire to assume adult behavior and appearance prematurely in terms of clothing; and multimedia trends, such as the clear sexual connotations that characterize many television programs, even those directed at a very young audiences. The potential risk of hypersexualization of Western contemporary society has been highlighted both by academics in the field of adolescence (Furman et al.1999) and others (McNair 1996).

Also, contemporary society is characterized by a plurality of values, norms, and models, which range from heterosexuality to homosexuality, from which it is possible to choose those we find most befitting. The path that leads from experimentation with the first dating relationships to the construction of a new family unfolds in very different ways and in different lengths of time (Brooks-Gunn and Paikoff 1993) and, in general, allows for the possibility to reverse the choices made (Smith 1994). On the one hand, this plurality constitutes a precious resource, as it can ensure greater individual freedom. On the other hand, rapidly changing models and values can also represent a difficult challenge, as they require the individual to make more decisions and take on more responsibility (Hendry and Kloep 2002). Consider, for example, all of the choices involved in relationships and reproduction; and these choices are not always reversible, at least not completely. A breakup with a partner is an option, but it too has costs, while having a child constitutes a definite commitment for the future. For some adolescents, and in particular those with fewer resources, the lack of clear frames of reference could contribute to generating even greater confusion about the priority they should place on the various outcomes and objectives to be reached and the most adequate means by which to reach those objectives.

Finally, as was recently highlighted in the field of personality psychology, the ego of a contemporary, postmodern individual appears fairly weak, or "light," caught between motivation toward self-fulfillment, which can legitimize any form of individualism or the demeaning of others, and an equally strong motivation to conform, i.e. the unquestioning and uncritical adherence to the values and lifestyles presented in the media, including the consumption of objects, goods, and even other people (Heinz 2002). These pushes can make the task of constructing a rich and satisfying affective and sexual relationship more difficult, especially for younger girls and boys.

6.2 Experimenting with Affection and Sex: Age and School Differences

Parallel to other recent studies (Brooks-Gunn and Paikoff 1997), our results[1] show that involvement in sexual activity increases progressively with age: the percentage of those who have already had sexual intercourse increases from roughly 15% at age 14-15 years to 55% at 18-19 years (Fig. 6.1). However, considering solely the percentage of sexually active adolescents does not take into account the complexity of the affective and sexual lives of adolescents (Montgomery and Sorell 1998; Ciairano 2004).

---

[1] Note that all the results reported in the figures are statistically significant, with $p<0.05$. In Chap. 2, Sect. 2.4, Presentation of Results and Statistical Analyses, the criteria for the presentation of results and for the use of statistics are explained.

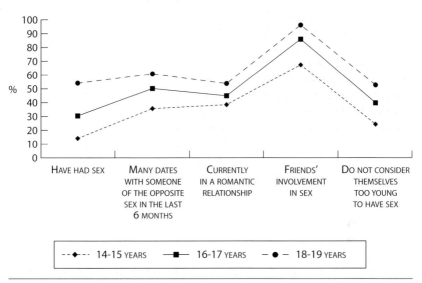

Fig. 6.1. Involvement in sexual activity, dating relationships, friendships, and attitudes about sex (chi-squared).

Adolescents adopt different patterns of sexual behavior, and they modify this pattern over time (Fig. 6.2)[2]: they may have had only one partner in their life ("high faithfulness," found to be by far the most frequent pattern) or more than one partner ("low faithfulness"); they might suspend sexual activity for extended periods of time ("stopped" for at least one year), or they may move from a pattern of promiscuous behavior to having one partner only in the past year ("ex-low faithfulness - now high faithfulness"). Observing the patterns of behavior adopted by adolescents in different age groups, some trends emerge. Between the ages of 14-15 years old and 16-17 years old, the percentage rises both of those who suspend sexual activity after having only briefly experimented with sex as well as those who adopt a low faithfulness pattern. Contemporarily, the percentage of adolescents who adopt a high faithfulness pattern is lower. This period is a critical stage for sexual experimentation in the form of either brief forays into sexuality or the adoption of promiscuous behavior patterns. The percentage of adolescents with more than one partner is higher at 16-17 years while the percentage of those who pass from a low faithfulness to a high faithfulness pattern is higher at 18-19 years. Therefore, some of the adolescents who have adopted patterns of promiscuous behavior eventually opt for a relationship with a single partner. These results display

---

[2] The questionnaire also contains questions on homosexual activity, which concerned 1% of the sample and was not analyzed here. The questions on the questionnaire and their relative answers used to construct the typologies for patterns of sexual behavior can be found in the "Appendix."

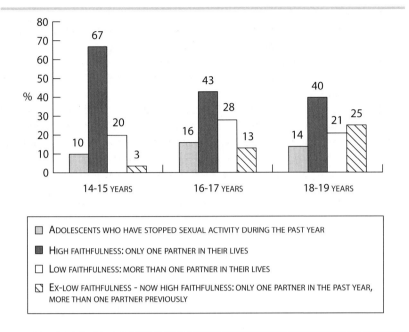

Fig. 6.2. Sexual behavior patterns at different ages (chi-squared).

how the sexual behavior of adolescents is an extremely diverse phenomenon and can scarcely be comprehended by looking only at percentages of sexually active adolescents in different age groups.

Furthermore, with age, attempts to establish intimate relationships with the opposite sex become more frequent (to have at least a few dates), and it is more likely that an adolescent succeeds in creating a special bond with another adolescent (Fig. 6.1). Adolescence appears to be, therefore, a period of experimentation with affection and sexuality and not only a progression toward increasing sexual involvement (Furman et al. 1999).

Finally, older adolescents have more friends who are sexually active and, in general, appear more receptive to engaging in sexual activity. As one progresses through adolescence, sexual activity appears to gain the characteristics of a normal, socially accepted activity. However, when it occurs well before the average age of initiation (which in our sample was roughly 15 $1/2$ years), it is less socially legitimized and can also take on a transgressive quality[3]. In general, social acceptance of a transition (such as having sex, leaving

---

[3] This behavior also has a legal aspect. Article 609 of the Italian penal code states that: (i) A minor who commits a sexual act with another minor under the age of 13, or when there is an age difference of more than 3 years, is punishable by law. (ii) An adult who commits sexual acts with a minor of less than 14 years of age is punishable by law while over 14 years, each case is evaluated singularly.

school, becoming independent, getting married, becoming a parent) is tied to how commonly that transition occurs within a given age group. An individual can count on greater support when he or she confronts the transition "on time," that is to say, not too early and not too late with respect to others of the same age group and with the same social expectations (Silbereisen and Kracke 1997).

However, considering the age of initiation alone is not sufficient, as a wide variety of often interrelated individual and situational characteristics can contribute to the connotation of sexual behavior as a positive experience and an opportunity to develop one's personal identity and become more autonomous or, rather, as a negative experience. Therefore, an investigation of the characteristics of a precocious initiation is essential (Fig. 6.3). First of all, precocious sexual activity occurs for the most part within the context of a relationship

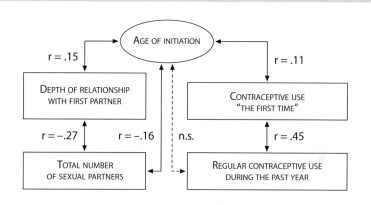

Fig. 6.3. Aspects connected to age of initiation of sexual activity (correlation analysis).

marked by superficiality and a weak emotional attachment and is linked successively to promiscuous behavior. The strong association between the degree of affective involvement with the first sexual partner and successive sexual behavior has also been encountered in other studies (Durbin et al. 1993). The majority of adolescents who initiate within a stable relationship go on to assume a pattern of high faithfulness while the inverse is true of those who initiate with a casual encounter. Furthermore, early initiation of sexual activity is linked to less frequent contraception use the first time one has sex, a characteristic that carries over to irregular use of contraception during successive sexual activity.

Adolescents who initiate sexual activity early are therefore at greater risk from an affective and relational standpoint due to the fact that, for the majority of these adolescents, sexual activity begins in the absence of an emotional connection. But they are also at greater risk from a physical and psychosocial point of view, as they tend to have a greater number of partners and to protect themselves less from the risk of STD and pregnancy.

Differences linked to age are interrelated with other differences tied to the type of school attended (Fig. 6.4). At the same age, students of vocational secondary schools, followed by those who attend technical secondary schools and teachers' lyceums, are more involved in affective and sexual relationships than are students of science and humanities lyceums. Differences exist both in terms of the rate of sexual involvement and age of initiation (younger for students of technical and vocational schools) as well as in general for affective relationships. It is more probable that students of schools other than science and humanities lyceums have had at least a few dates in the past six months and that these dates have led to the creation of a bond of some kind. Sexual activ-

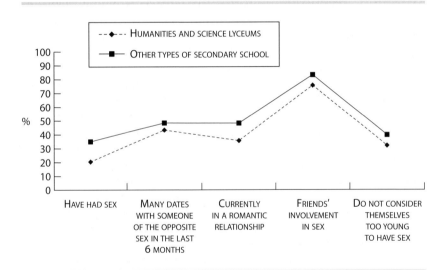

Fig. 6.4. Involvement in sexual relations, affective relationships, friendships, and attitudes about sex (chi-squared). Students of humanities and science lyceums were compared with students of all other types of schools because no significant differences were found between technical schools, vocational schools, and teachers' lyceums.

ity is more common among these adolescents' friends as well, and they are more likely not to perceive themselves as too young to be sexually active.

As has been highlighted by other authors (Silbereisen and Noack 1990), the ability to establish relationships with the opposite sex seems to be a more urgent developmental task for students who have chosen a shorter scholastic career and who, at least on paper, are more oriented toward an early entrance into the workforce. The greater urgency with which these students seem to feel the need to have sex, anticipating some of the steps toward adulthood, could be connected to differences in the type of life plans they have made (choosing to invest in a less prolonged school career) and the length of time necessary to carry out those plans (Bonino and Cattelino 2002). These adolescents are, in fact, more oriented toward the workforce and, in turn, toward the world of adults - a world that they hope to reach as soon as possible. Interrelated with the type and timing of their plans for the future, other aspects arise, such as the current school experience - in which adolescents are developing their identities - and the previous school experience. In both cases, their experiences may be less than satisfactory. In fact, the vocational school they attend holds less social prestige today compared with other schools, and its programs are still in an adjustment phase after having undergone a number of changes in recent years. Furthermore, it is more likely that their previous school experiences were marked by failure, evidenced by the fact that few students choose to enroll in this type of school because they feel they have a particular ability or strength in the subject matter. More often, adolescents enroll who have been told they are not cut out for other types of schools. Such judgments can have a strong negative effect on adolescents' perceptions of themselves and their abilities, giving way to a vicious cycle of failure that is difficult to break, disinvestment, and further failure (Steinberg and Avenevoli 1998; Borca et al. 2002).

Students of humanities and science lyceums - who, in Italian society today, represent the model of a successful student and are aware that they have a long road ahead of them before finishing their scholastic career - appear to be more willing to postpone assuming adult behavior and are, in general, less oriented toward adulthood. Being less focused on entering the workforce and the prospect of a longer period of self-actualization are linked to a greater acceptance of the waiting and "in-between" social position - not yet adults and no longer children - that characterizes contemporary adolescence and emerging adulthood (Schulenberg et al. 1997). Countering a still widely held belief, our results show that differences between students of different schools are in no way linked to their economic and cultural family background. In fact, no direct correlation exists between adolescent sexual involvement and parental education level and occupation.

6.3 Sexuality in Boys and Girls

Along with differences in age and type of school, gender differences, connected in particular to the way in which sexual activity occurs, also emerged (Fig. 6.5). Boys initiate sexual activity earlier than girls of their age and, for the most part, outside of an affective relationship. In fact, it is less likely that boys have had dates with someone of the opposite sex in the past few months or that they are involved in a stable relationship. In addition, although they have fewer friends than do girls who are already sexually active, they perceive more pressure by these friends to be sexually active and are more receptive to being so. A higher percentage of boys than girls do not feel that they are too young to have sex nor that it is right to avoid having sexual relations so as to avoid the risk of pregnancy.

The results of our research confirm that boys have more difficulty connecting sexuality with affection (Ciairano 2004), and girls have a greater tendency to have early experiences with affective and sexual relationships based on the model of a stable adult couple. Boys more frequently adopt low faithfulness behavior patterns or initiate sexual activity and then suspend it (Fig. 6.6) while girls, on the other hand, tend to follow a pattern of high faithfulness, which implies having sexual intercourse more frequently.

These results confirm what has already been revealed by previous research: despite the apparent standardization of sexual customs, male and female behavior remains quite different (Zani 1993; Coleman and Roker 1998). Many factors are at the root of this phenomenon. First of all, socialization processes encourage a greater need for autonomy and personal achievement in boys, and these needs are satisfied in part through exploration and experimentation. In girls, on the other hand, greater dependence and submissiveness are encouraged, along with a greater need for reciprocity and familiarity within social and intimate relationships (Palmonari et al. 1989; Palmonari 1997). Furthermore, the Italian culture is permeated by attitudes that promote active male sexuality while opinions on female sexuality remain, to a large degree, contradictory or negative (Ciairano 2004). All of these reasons can contribute to girls' preference for the high faithfulness pattern, which in adults is commonly considered irreproachable.

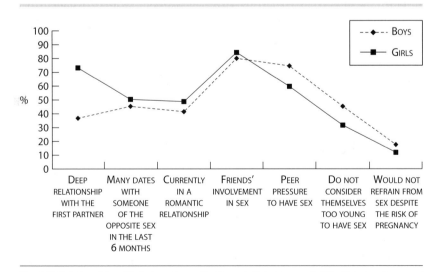

Fig. 6.5. Relationship with first partner, affective relationships, and attitudes about sex and friends (chi-squared).

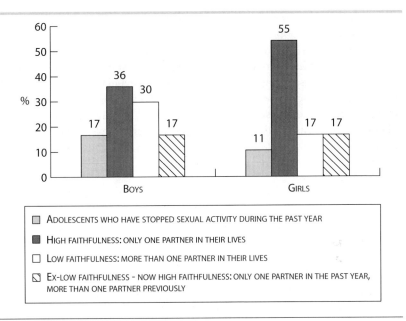

Fig. 6.6. Sexual behavior patterns for both genders (chi-squared).

On the contrary, boys seem to have a greater need, as well as greater authorization, to demonstrate that they know how to do things that children do not, testing themselves with different partners without any kind of commitment. Boys also resort more often to substitute forms of sexuality, such as pornography, especially in their peer groups (Fig. 6.7). The way in which sexual activ-

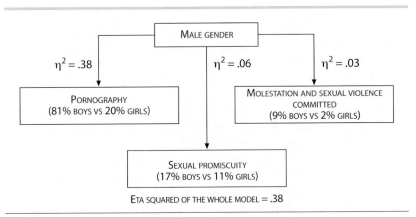

Fig. 6.7. Male gender and pornography, promiscuity, molestation, and sexual violence (MANOVA and chi-squared).

ity occurs for many boys does not seem to make use of the cognitive, affective, and social capabilities that are required to build a stable, equal, emotionally involving relationship with a partner. Furthermore, the high correlation values found in the total sample between promiscuity and pornography, on the one hand, and resorting to molestation and sexual violence on the other hand (Fig. 6.8) are causes for reflection. It appears that when there is a lack of interest by the other person or when one does not possess the resources to establish a relationship, the easiest method is to inappropriately exert one's power over the person (Rabaglietti et al. 2005).

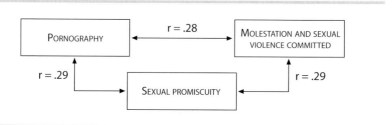

Fig. 6.8. Correlation between pornography, promiscuity, molestation, and sexual violence (total sample - correlation analysis).

6.4 Contraception and the Prevention of Sexually Transmitted Diseases. Behavior, Relational Conditions, Attitudes, and Knowledge: Which Is Most Important?

6.4.1 Contraceptive Behavior

Contraceptive use is fairly common among adolescents although 32% in our study did not use any form of contraception the first time they had sex, and 36% have not used contraception regularly over the past year. Furthermore, not all adolescents use a secure method, such as the pill or condoms, every time (Fig. 6.9).

Behavior with regard to contraception tends to remain constant over time: there is a strong association between use of contraception the first time and regularity of use during the first year and in the type of contraception used the first time and the type used thereafter. Finally, regularity of use and use of a secure method are also correlated (Fig. 6.10).

Despite the often inconsistent use of contraception or the use of unsafe methods, such as withdrawal, only thirteen cases of pregnancy were recorded (five boys and eight girls; of these, only two chose to have and keep the child) out of 2,273 adolescents (6‰ of the total sample). This proportion is almost the same as the incidence of teen pregnancy in the Italian population as a whole and is one of the lowest in Europe - around 5‰ of total birth and abor-

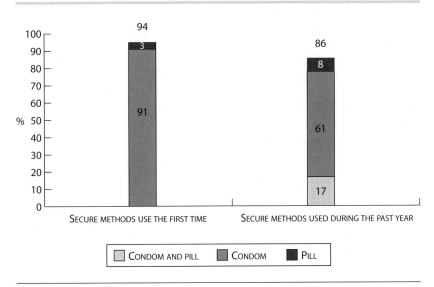

Fig. 6.9. Contraception (chi-squared). The sum of the percentages is less than 100 because only the pill and condoms were considered because they are, compared with other forms, the most common and most secure.

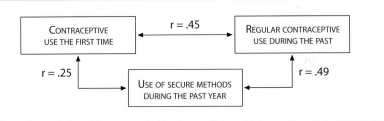

Fig. 6.10. Correlation between contraceptive use the first time, regularity of use, and secure methods (correlation analysis).

tion rates (ISTAT 2004; Bonino et al. in press). These percentages are extremely low in comparison with other countries, such as the United States or Great Britain where the percentage can range from 25‰ to 55‰. The problem seems to be more marked in some schools than in others; in fact, the percentage drops to 1‰ in humanities and science lyceums and rises to 1% in vocational schools. In general, however, this is a phenomenon that cannot be overlooked due to the serious repercussions it poses in terms of physical and psychosocial health, as we will see later.

As far as the conditions related to a more regular and effective use of contraception are concerned (Fig. 6.11), the ability to assume responsibility for

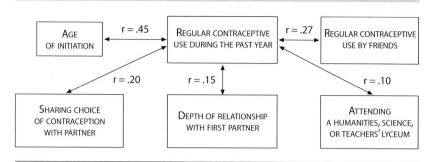

Fig. 6.11. Aspects connected to regularity of contraceptive use (correlation analysis).

contraception appears to be tied, first of all, to age: adolescents who become sexually active later are more able to make use of some method of contraception starting from the very first time. In addition, as they get older, they are able to share decisions about contraceptive use with their partner, which is in turn tied to greater regularity of use. Second, assuming responsibility for contraception is also tied to the conditions in which sexual activity takes place: contraception is used more frequently in a stable relationship with the first partner while regularity of use over the past year is greater when adolescents have had sex with only one partner. The use of contraception requires, in fact, that a contraceptive be available or ensuring that it is available to one's partner. Adolescents must also be able to agree to use contraception, and therefore, they must not be afraid to make it known to their partner that they are open to having sex. This fear, especially for girls, can be reduced when a trusting, intimate relationship has been established with the partner (Holland and Thompson 1998; Meeks et al. 1998).

Along with differences connected to the personal and relational conditions in which sexual activity occurs, other differences related in particular to the regularity of contraceptive use also exist. These differences appear to be connected to the presence or lack of a plan for long-term self-actualization through schooling. Regular use of contraception is more frequent among students of humanities, sciences, and teachers' lyceums than students of technical and vocational schools. Furthermore, humanities or science lyceums students differ from the others for having a greater number of friends who use contraception, a factor that was also revealed to be strongly associated to regular contraceptive use.

Only a minority of adolescents identified some possible reasons for irregular use of contraception, and among these, the most common were practical reasons (such as cost or unavailability) rather than psychological reasons (such as trust in partner or embarrassment); the adolescents who specified these reasons were also those who seemed at greater risk, as they were more likely than the others not to have used contraception in the past year (Fig. 6.12).

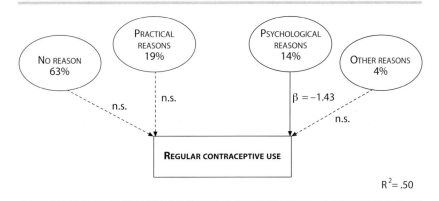

Fig. 6.12. Reasons for not using contraception and their relationship with behavior (percentages and logistic regression analysis). The "practical reasons" category includes laziness, inconvenience, cost, unavailability; the "psychological reasons" are trust in partner, embarrassment, awareness of having insufficient knowledge; the "other reasons" are violence, refusal by male partner, menstruation, pregnancy.

6.4.2 Information and Attitudes Toward Contraception

Lack of knowledge about sexuality and contraception is one of the least frequently cited reasons given by adolescents to justify failure to use contraception. In reality, the majority, especially girls, have access to sources of information on contraception: 31% have at least one source of information, 23% have two, and 12% have three. The most common source is the family, followed by friends, school, mass media, newspapers, and informational pamphlets. Few have received advice from health workers (Fig. 6.13). The opportunity to talk to adults and peers instead of having to rely on mass media has a positive relationship with an efficient contraceptive behavior: adolescents who have this opportunity appear to have a more complete understanding of contraception and are aware of the psychological risks as well as the physical risks involved in having unprotected sex (Ciairano 2004; Roggero et al. 2005).

Adolescents generally possess a good deal of knowledge about contraception, and they are aware that they are well-informed (Fig. 6.14). Furthermore, adolescents' views on contraception are more positive than negative. A positive attitude toward contraception along with increased opportunity to seek sources of information were more common in girls, older adolescents, and adolescents from families with a higher level of education, such as students from humanities and science lyceums. Despite their positive attitudes toward sexuality, adolescents - especially girls and humanities and science lyceum students - reported a fairly high level of embarrassment in purchasing contraception.

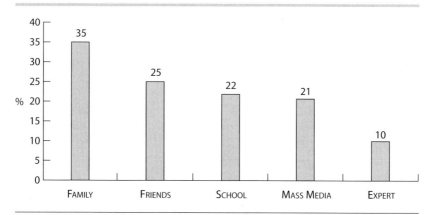

Fig. 6.13. Sources of information on sexuality and contraception. The sum of the percentages of the five main sources considered is greater than 100 because a large percentage of adolescents identified more than one source.

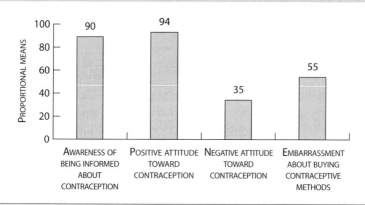

Fig. 6.14. Contraception: awareness of being informed, attitudes, and embarrassment. Negative and positive attitude toward contraception are considered separately, as they reveal different aspects and are not mutually exclusive.

6.4.3 Knowledge on the Prevention of Sexually Transmitted Diseases such as AIDS

In general, adolescents are also fairly well informed about STDs and AIDS: the mean for knowledge of STDs and AIDS is 85/100. Greater knowledge is more common in girls, older adolescents, and adolescents from families with a higher level of education, such as students from humanities and science lyceums. More precisely, adolescents' have a good degree of knowledge on how

STDs are transmitted (such as the possibility of contracting AIDS by having sex without a condom with someone who is infected) and on strategies for prevention (such as reducing the probability of contracting AIDS by using a condom). This knowledge is most common among lyceum students (knowledge about transmission: 98% in humanities and science lyceum students vs 95% in students from all other types of schools; prevention strategies: 97% in humanities and science lyceum students vs 94% in students from all other types of schools) and among those who adopt nonpromiscuous sexual behavior patterns (the difference is significant only for knowledge about transmission: 97% vs 93% of those who have had more than one partner).

Other types of knowledge, however, are less common, such as an awareness that the possibility of contracting AIDS is not by any means limited to homosexuals and that some contraceptive methods, such as the pill, can protect against pregnancy but not against STDs. About 20% of adolescents either think that AIDS can only be spread among homosexuals or have no precise opinion on how it is spread. Having accurate information is more common among girls, older adolescents, and lyceum students who have had only one partner.

About 80% of adolescents are aware of the seriousness of AIDS (perceived seriousness of AIDS). Greater awareness is more common among girls, older adolescents, adolescents who have not had sex, and lyceum students (87% humanities/science lyceum vs 77% other types of schools); 60% of the adolescents worry at times about contracting AIDS. This worry increases with age and is stronger among adolescents from vocational secondary schools and adolescents who have already had sex, particularly those who have adopted a promiscuous pattern of sexual behavior (70% of those who have had more than one partner vs 55% of other adolescents). Therefore, adolescents seem to be quite aware of the seriousness of the phenomenon and the possibility of contracting AIDS. Having more accurate knowledge and being aware of the seriousness of AIDS are generally correlated.

Almost all adolescents feel that the subject of AIDS should be covered in school (90% of those who have had more than one partner vs 95% of other adolescents). Despite this strong conviction, only about one third have dealt extensively with the subject of AIDS at school. Vocational and technical secondary school students feel that the subject of AIDS has already been covered at school more frequently than do other students (37% vs 30%). However, there does not appear to be any relationship between having dealt with the subject in school and the accuracy of the knowledge possessed. As has already been pointed out by other studies (Bakker et al. 1997; Bakker et al. 1998; Buunk et. al 1998; Yzer et al. 2000), it is difficult to evaluate the effectiveness of information provided on the subject of STDs, and particularly AIDS, due to both the numerous sources of information, which are not always accurate and up to date, and because of the possibility for misunderstanding and confusion caused by the fact that the topic involves a number of psychological dimensions, such as affectivity, relationships with others, sexuality, and death.

6.4.4 Knowing Is Essential, but Is It Enough?

In general, the results indicate that information and knowledge, while they are necessary, are not enough to promote more effective and regular contraceptive use (Fig. 6.15). The availability of information sources has no direct tie to contraceptive use. However, although it has no a direct relationship with use the first time, the accuracy of adolescents' knowledge on STDs, such as AIDS, seems to promote more regular use of contraception. It is likely that the context of the first experience with sexual intercourse is too emotionally charged for adolescents to make solid use of the knowledge they possess (Mitchell and Wellings 1998; Ciairano 2004). Information and knowledge play an important indirect role, however, in that they might mediate the effects of a negative attitude toward contraception that, although uncommon, is a risk factor.

The degree to which contraception is used regularly and effectively is also not related with the embarrassment an adolescent experiences when purchasing contraception. Rather, more regular use of contraception seems to be influenced by a complex interaction of multiple factors. These factors include the

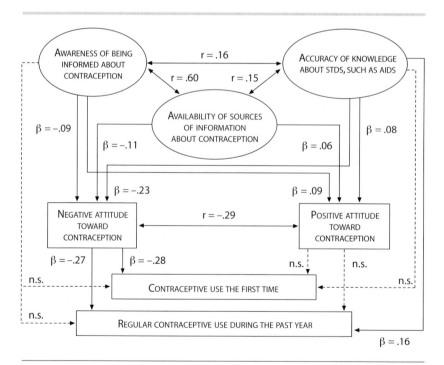

Fig. 6.15. Correlation between knowledge and information sources and their relationship with attitudes and behavior linked to contraceptive use (correlation analysis and linear and logistic regression analysis). The figure is a concise representation of correlation analyses and six separate regression models (linear or logistic), which have R2 values ranging from .02 to .10.

maturity of the individual, the ability to establish effective lines of communication with a partner on the subject of contraception and to negotiate its use within the realm of a real sexual experience, the different prospects for self-fulfillment in the short or long term; and finally, the social norms that define some types of behavior as more or less appropriate for boys and for girls.

As far as more specific knowledge of STDs, such as AIDS, is concerned, we have already observed that the level of interest in dealing with this subject in school is quite high, especially among adolescents who are less involved in sexual activity despite the fact that they are less worried about personally having to deal with problems of this kind. Second, we have already observed that AIDS is considered a less serious problem by students who have already dealt with the subject in school and by those who attend schools other than humanities and science lyceums. Finally, the knowledge that they can reduce the probability of being infected with the AIDS virus by using a condom is less common in students of technical and vocational schools and among those who are sexually promiscuous. Thus, it appears that simply spreading information, is insufficient to promote greater knowledge and that knowledge on this subject is less common among adolescents who are most at risk. Therefore, perceived seriousness and worry about contracting AIDS and about condom use are not related (Fig. 6.16). Nor is there any significant relationship between knowledge of the possible ways of contracting AIDS and strategies for preventing it and the actual use of condoms during sex.

These results call for reflection on the actual effectiveness of the various sexual education courses taught in schools and on how to promote the motivation to seek out and to acquire basic knowledge on the main prevention strategies. In fact, of all the aspects considered, the only one that is related with regular use of condoms is this last one: an interest in reflecting on and discussing these subjects. The desire to know and understand is likely related to the individual's greater maturity.

Young people are therefore aware of the seriousness of AIDS, they are convinced that the problem concerns them personally, and that it is useful to cover the topic of AIDS in school - although in many schools this has not yet happened. They possess fairly accurate knowledge on AIDS both in terms of how it is transmitted and how it can be prevented. However, this knowledge does not seem to have any direct relationship with condom use (Fig. 6.16), although it is connected to more regular use of contraception in general (Fig. 6.15).

Therefore, the case of AIDS and other STDs sheds light on some relevant aspects. First, the construction and reworking of knowledge by adolescents is a much more complex process than just the simple transmission of information. As revealed by the fact that there is no relationship between having covered AIDS in school and having accurate knowledge, more information is not always transformed into greater knowledge. Second, having accurate knowledge on the precautionary measures recommended for AIDS and STD prevention does not guarantee that these measures will actually be taken. Various factors can keep adolescents from protecting themselves (Beyth-Maron and

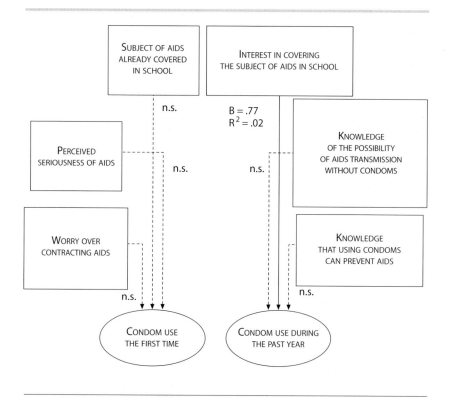

Fig. 6.16. Aspects connected to condom use (logistic regression).

Fischoff 1997); some factors identified by adolescents themselves for failing to use contraception in general, and condoms in particular, were tied to the lack of planning for the sexual encounter or to emotional aspects such as embarrassment or disgust.

In health prevention and promotion of psychosocial well being, in order for information to become preventative action, knowledge must be associated with the conviction of "knowing that one knows," or perceived self-efficacy (Bandura 1997), as these convictions are connected to the control that a person responsibly exercises over their own conduct.

6.5 Functions of Sexual Behavior in Adolescence

Sexual behavior seems essentially to perform three major functions over the course of adolescent development: the first is connected to the acquisition of *adulthood* and the integration of sexuality into personal identity; the second involves the need to *explore* and *experiment* to test oneself, and to *transgress*;

and the third is a *ritual* and *emulation* function. These functions, which were also underlined by the adolescents themselves in individual interviews (Giannotta et al. 2004; Settanni et al. 2005), can acquire greater or lesser relevance and, at times, different nuances, depending on the pattern of sexual behavior chosen by the adolescent.

6.5.1 Adulthood: Realization, Anticipation and Exasperation

The integration of sexuality into identity seems to respond, above all, to the need to feel like an adult, encouraging in this way a more positive self-perception and greater autonomy accompanied by other types of behavior characteristic of adulthood, such as work (Table 6.1). Many adolescents, however, seem driven in large part by a need to accomplish the more visible, tangible aspects of adulthood. Among the youngest boys and girls (see also Table 6.2), involvement in sexual activity corresponds to a need for *anticipation of adulthood*. This was shown by the presence of a strong connection to cigarette smoking, a behavior that is socially accepted in adults and can be used as an unequivocal sign of the acquisition of adult status (Engels 1998). For adolescents who adopt a promiscuous behavior pattern (low faithfulness), or who had adopted this pattern in the past (ex low faithfulness - now high faithfulness), sexual activity corresponds instead to an *exasperated need for adulthood*, evidenced by the correlation with high value placed on independence, the acquisition of which is an essential aspect of adulthood. Having a great number of sexual partners allows some adolescent boys to feel "macho" and to live up to an aggressive,

Table 6.1. Aspects connected to the adulthood function (MANOVA).

	Means for the characteristics of adolescents with different sexual behavior patterns				
	Nonsexually active adolescents	Adolescents who have stopped sexual relations over the past year	High faithfulness: only one sexual partner in their lives	Ex-low faithfulness – now high faithfulness: one partner only in the past year, more than one partner previously	Low faithfulness: more than one partner in their lives
Positive self-perception	+[a]	++++	+++	++	+++++
Value on independence	+	+++	++	++++	+++++
Having a job	+	+++	+++	+++	+++
Cigarette smoking	+	++	+++	+++++	++++

[a] A greater number of plus signs (+) corresponds to a higher mean; eta-squared = .04.

Table 6.2. Main characteristics of sexually active adolescents compared with others for both genders and various ages (MANOVA).

	Boys	Girls	Up to 16 years	Over 16-17 years
Positive self-perception	+[a]	–		
Value on independence	+	++		
Having a job	++	+	+	++
Cigarette smoking			++	++

[a] The + and – signs indicate the presence of a significant difference between sexually active adolescents and others and the direction of the difference. The number of signs indicates the degree of difference: ++ much higher value, + higher value, – lower value.

predatory pattern of male sexuality, which is quite common and, for the most part, appreciated in Italian society. Taking on exterior adult characteristics such as these is combined at times with other indicators of the acquisition of adult status, such as working. For girls, on the other hand, promiscuous sexual behavior is more widely used as an attempt to achieve much-desired independence that cannot be obtained in other ways.

The anticipated or exasperated acquisition of adult status is not without risks, however. Not all adolescents who are already sexually active are characterized by greater psychological well-being than adolescents who are not sexually active (Table 6.3). Among girls and younger adolescents, a certain degree of discomfort is quite common: most perceive a greater sense of alienation, more depression, and more stress. On the contrary, boys and older adolescents are characterized by a degree of discomfort only when they have not yet had sexual relations.

The link between discomfort and age could be tied to the age deemed appropriate, both by adults and peers, for the initiation of sexual activity. As was mentioned previously, a transition that occurs "on time" lets the individual feel adequate with respect to others of his or her age and guarantees greater support and social acceptance. The discomfort of the very young who have

Table 6.3. Main characteristics of sexually active adolescents compared with others for both genders and various ages (MANOVA).

	Boys	Girls	Up to 16 years	Over 16-17 years
Sense of alienation	–[a]	+		
Depressive feelings	–	++	+	
Stress	– –	+	+	

[a] The + and – signs indicate the presence of a significant difference between sexually active adolescents and other adolescents and the direction of that difference. The number of signs indicates the degree of difference: ++ much higher value, + higher value, – – much lower value, – lower value.

initiated a behavior that is considered not yet entirely appropriate for their age is, therefore, understandable. Such behavior also entails responsibilities that they or their partners may not be able to assume, demonstrated by the relationship between precocious initiation and lesser use of contraception. Similarly, older adolescents suffer who, unlike the majority of their friends, have not yet had sexual relations. In the absence of other parameters by which to judge their maturity, a comparison with others can have a strong negative impact; this is true to an even greater degree in a society as hypersexualized as today's. A similar psychological process seems to come into play in the majority of boys regardless of age and, in particular, for those who have adopted patterns of low faithfulness. For these adolescents, having sex is a decisive element of their positive self-perception while not having sex is connected to negative self-perception and a higher sense of alienation.

Integrating sexuality into identity appears to be more conflictual for girls, as their involvement in sexual activity is accompanied both by a more negative self-perception and greater discomfort. It is likely that there are multiple causes for this phenomenon. Differences in socialization processes, in social acceptance of female sexuality, and in responsibility for contraception can contribute to making the integration of sexuality into their identity a complex and uncertain event for girls that they therefore relate to ambivalent or contradictory feelings.

Furthermore, it is useful to reflect on the connection, also evidenced elsewhere (Ciairano et al. 2000) between stable, affective relationships - in which girls are more frequently involved than their male counterparts - and discomfort. In the first place, stable relationships are more difficult to manage in the present. Unlike casual, impromptu encounters, they require boys and girls to "put themselves out there," to be willing to negotiate and accept the ups and downs of a relationship and reconcile the time and energy devoted to the relationship with other needs. Second, a stable relationship implies a commitment for the future that may be experienced, in particular by girls, as a potential limitation to their future personal and professional achievements. As women generally have greater difficulty than men in obtaining success professionally due to the double strain of families and careers to sustain, this is not such a remote possibility (Bandura 1997). Therefore, even a stable relationship with a sexual partner presents aspects of risk, as it requires the adolescent to confront emotional costs and psychological difficulties that are usually confronted at a later time and with other capabilities in adulthood.

Finding oneself a step ahead of one's peers on the path to adulthood can also contribute to discomfort in another way. For example, it can weaken the value attributed to the school dimension, which is absolutely central to present lives of adolescents, and diminish educational expectations (Table 6.4). Compared with the entire sample, adolescents who have only experimented with sexuality fall somewhere between those involved in high-faithfulness relationships and those who have adopted a pattern of promiscuous behavior. In some ways, they seem to share the advantages tied to the integration of sexuality into personal iden-

Table 6.4. Value on and expectations for school (MANOVA).

	Means for the characteristics of adolescents with different sexual behavior patterns				
	Nonsexually active adolescents	Adolescents who have stopped sexual relations over the past year	High faithfulness: only one sexual partner in their lives	Ex-low faithfulness – now high faithfulness: one partner only in the past year, more than one partner previously	Low faithfulness: more than one partner in their lives
Value on academic achievement	+++++[a]	+++	+++	+	++
Expectations to continue school	+++++	++	++	++++	+

[a] A greater number of plus signs (+) corresponds to a higher mean.

tity (better self-perception and higher value on independence) without experiencing much of the negative psychological impact. They too, however, end up paying a price in terms of expectations for achievement: although they attribute almost as much value to results in school as do adolescents who are not yet sexually active, their expectations for academic success are much lower (Cattelino et al. 2002). The strategy of attempting to reconcile an investment in the sexual and affective realm with an investment in school - more commonly employed by girls who have adopted the high-faithfulness pattern - does not appear to be particularly successful cither. Such an attempt, probably due to the degree of responsibility it entails, is connected, as we have seen, to greater psychological discomfort. Among boys and younger adolescents, on the other hand, the need to demonstrate that they are grown up also increases their expec-

Table 6.5. Main characteristics of sexually active adolescents compared with others for both genders and various ages (MANOVA).

	Boys	Girls	Up to 16 years	Over 16-17 years
Value on academic achievement	– –[a]	–	– –	–
Expectations to continue school			– –	–
Expectations for success	++	–	++	+

[a] The + and – signs indicate the presence of a significant difference between sexually active adolescents and other adolescents and the direction of that difference. The number of signs indicates the degree of difference: ++ much higher value, + higher value, – – much lower value, – lower value.

tations for success - expectations that could potentially be completely unrealistic if they choose not to complete their studies (Table 6.5).

Sexual involvement, therefore, brings adolescents closer to the adult condition, serving the function of achievement of adulthood and contributing to the satisfaction of an important need. However, it can also serve to discourage the accomplishment of other developmental tasks, which are perhaps even more important and urgent than this first, namely, the development of the competencies and capabilities that can be obtained in the school context. Some adolescents either do not value these capabilities or do not believe in their ability to attain them, and they could be useful in the future in order to achieve their aspirations for social and professional success. This serves as further evidence that anticipation of adulthood can have negative consequences, both in the short term with respect to their well-being and individual adjustment and subsequently in terms of diminished opportunities for future development (Graber et al. 1998; Weichold et al. 2003).

Adolescents who are not yet sexually active appear to be slightly behind others of their age in the transition to adult life, but their condition is more favorable: although they do not have an extremely positive self image nor a strong desire for independence, they are less afflicted by discomfort, they place a higher value on the main activity they are involved in - school - and above all, they believe that school will have a positive effect on their future. These results suggest that the pause taken by these adolescents before becoming sexually active has a positive effect both on their present well-being and indirectly on their future personal accomplishments. Adolescents who enjoy the greatest psychological well-being - greater than those who are not sexually active and those in the high-faithfulness category - are those who are currently involved in an affective, nonsexual relationship with a partner of the opposite sex. These boys and girls appear to be more able to recognize their current status as adolescents, drawing on the advantages this can offer in terms of experimentation with affection and confirming their self-perception without rushing toward adulthood through involvement in a sexual relationship (Ciairano et al. 2000).

6.5.2 Adolescent Sexual Activity as Transgression, Experimentation and Exploration

In addition to the function it serves in the acquisition of adulthood in all its forms, sexual behavior can serve other functions as well, such as transgression of social norms, which are reluctant to approve of female promiscuous behavior, and the exploration of and experimentation with new sensations and new roles or types of behavior.

The *transgressive function* of sexual behavior is confirmed largely by the presence of a strong negative correlation with certain attitudes - in particular, disapproval of antisocial behavior and value on religion - that are considered to be indicators of willingness, or lack thereof, by adolescents to transgress social norms or to share the values that are common to society at large (Jessor et al. 1991). These attitudes are less common among adolescents who are already sexually active (in particular, among adolescents in the low-faithfulness group, boys, and the youngest adolescents; see Tables 6.6 and 6.7). The transgressive function is further evidenced by a correlation with involvement in other behavior types that entail both physical and psychosocial risks, such the violation of social norms of honesty and coexistence in relationships with adults (skipping school, staying out all night without permission, or lying to hide something they have done) and the use of illegal psychoactive substances such as marijuana. Sexually active adolescents, especially girls and those in the low-faithfulness group, are more likely to do both of these. It is important to note that for young adolescents and girls, even smoking cigarettes can be considered transgressive, as it is commonly held to be a normal activity for adults but not for women or for the very young.

The tie between norm violation, represented by lies, disobedience, and marijuana use, and other types of risk behavior, such as heavy alcohol consumption and disturbed eating, indicates how sexual behavior can be another possible way to fulfill a need to explore new sensations and test one's lim-

Table 6.6. Aspects connected to the transgressive and exploring functions (MANOVA).

	Means for the characteristics of adolescents with different sexual behavior patterns				
	Nonsexually active adolescents	Adolescents who have stopped sexual relations over the past year	High faithfulness: only one sexual partner in their lives	Ex-low faithfulness – now high faithfulness: one partner only in the past year, more than one partner previously	Low faithfulness: more than one partner in their lives
Value on religion	+++++[a]	+++	++	++++	+
Disapproval of behavior	+++++	+++	++++	+	++
Lies and disobedience	+	++	+++	++++	+++++
Marijuana smoking	+	+++	++	++++	+++++
Purging behavior	+	+++	++	+++++	+++
Risk-taking behavior	+	++	+++	++++	+++++
Risky driving	+	++	++	+++++	++++
Heavy alcohol consumption	+	++	+++	++++	+++++

[a] A greater number of plus signs (+) corresponds to a higher mean; eta-squared = .05.

Table 6.7. Main characteristics of sexually active adolescents compared with others for both genders and various ages (MANOVA).

	Boys	Girls	Up to 16 years	Over 16-17 years
Value on religion			– –	–
Disapproval of behavior	– –	–[a]	– –	–
Lies and disobedience	+[a]	++	+	++
Marijuana smoking	+	++	+	++
Purging behavior	+	+	++	+
Risk-taking behavior	++	+	++	+
Risky driving	++	+	+	++
Heavy alcohol consumption	+	+	++	+

[a] The + and – signs indicate the presence of a significant difference between sexually active adolescents and other adolescents and the direction of that difference. The number of signs indicates the degree of difference: ++ much higher value, + higher value, – – much lower value, – lower value.

its and capabilities (Molinengo et al. 2004; Giannotta et al. 2005). The behavior of sexually active adolescents, especially boys, is aimed more at externalized types of exploration and experimentation (risk-taking behavior, heavy alcohol consumption, and risky driving) while the types of behavior girls adopt are more internalized (disturbed eating). This is further evidence of the potential negative impact, both in terms of poorer psychosocial adjustment and greater discomfort, that an overly demanding relationship can have on an adolescent even though morally this kind of relationship is considered irreproachable.

In general, both the transgressive function and the explorative function are less relevant in adolescents who adopt the high-faithfulness pattern. The explorative function seems to be more important for adolescents who have had only brief encounters with sexual activity while the transgressive function is more important for adolescents who are, or were, promiscuous. With regard to age, sexual activity assumes a transgressive and explorative significance for younger adolescents while for those 18 and older, only promiscuous sexual behavior assumes this significance. As for the type of function, transgression seems to be more important for girls (evidenced by a strong association with lying, disobedience, and marijuana use) while exploration and experimentation have greater relevance for boys (showed by a stronger association to risk behavior, such as heavy alcohol consumption and risky driving).

Low-faithfulness adolescents in particular use sexual behavior, generally in connection with other types of risk behavior, to carry out various interrelated functions: to explore their limitations and possibilities, to experience new sensations, and to transgress social norms. In the case of these adolescents, promiscuity seems to belong to a larger constellation of risk conduct and seems to serve another function as well: an *escape* from social and rela-tional difficulties that they lack the resources to deal with in a more mature way.

The need to transgress social norms and experience new sensations or new roles is generally stronger when the adolescent's current situation, par-ticularly in the school context, is troubled. In general, sexually active adoles-cents are less satisfied with the scholastic experience: they fail to see its use-fulness and feel less certain of succeeding; in fact, they have less success in school than others their age. For these adolescents, school is not a context in which they feel they can put their abilities to the test and be successful but, rather, a place from which they want to escape as quickly as possible (Table 6.8). Their present troubled situation does not seem to leave much for the devel-opment of more far-reaching plans, which foresee more gradual personal accomplishments through dedication and work for the future (Silbereisen and Noack 1990; Steinberg and Avenevoli 1998).

In this rather negative general view, there are, however, some differences tied to behavior pattern. High-faithfulness adolescents and those who have

Table 6.8. Well-being and discomfort at school (MANOVA).

	Means for the characteristics of adolescents with different sexual behavior patterns				
	Nonsexually active adolescents	Adolescents who have stopped sexual relations over the past year	High faithfulness: only one sexual partner in their lives	Ex-low faithfulness – now high faithfulness: one partner only in the past year, more than one partner previously	Low faithfulness: more than one partner in their lives
Overall satisfaction with school experience	+++++[a]	++++	+++	+	++
Perceived usefulness of school	++++	+++	+++++	+	++
Positive expectations for school	++++	+++	++	+++++	+
Grades	++++	++	++	+++++	+
Intentions and attempts to drop out of school	+	++++	++	+++	+++++
Repeated school years	+	+++++	+++	++	++++

[a] A greater number of plus signs (+) corresponds to a higher mean.

experienced only a brief foray into sexuality occupy an intermediate position compared with both non-sexually-active and promiscuous adolescents. It is above all this first group who try, unsuccessfully, to reconcile personal accomplishment across various sectors. They are characterized, in fact, by low expectations to continue school, and many have at times thought of or tried to drop out. Their early initiation into a pattern of sexual behavior deemed irreproachable in adults can contribute to dissuading them from the fulfillment of other objectives more appropriate to their age.

The situation of ex-low-faithfulness - currently high-faithfulness adolescents appears more complex. While they are fairly unsatisfied with the school experience and report intermediate values on intention and attempt to drop out, their expectations to continue school are high, and they appear able to live up to these expectations. It is possible that these adolescents, in the middle-upper age bracket, fulfilled the need for sexual exploration by taking on a promiscuous behavior pattern and then, although not without difficulty, succeed in finding the personal or environmental resources necessary to successfully confront the school experience.

The most worrying situation again appears to be that of low-faithfulness adolescents who have a highly negative view of the school experience - an experience that has been marked by repeated failure. It is not surprising that these adolescents are characterized by a greater need to transgress and explore, as they are more troubled by their current situation - a situation in which they seem unable to foresee opportunities for personal achievement, at least as far as an important dimension such as school is concerned.

These differences, tied to behavior patterns, are also interrelated with other differences linked to gender and age Table 6.9). Discomfort in the school dimension translates into failure more frequently for boys than for girls. In regard to age, however, the connection between negative school experience and sexual activity is stronger in the case of younger adolescents. These results,

Table 6.9. Main characteristics of sexually active adolescents compared with others for both genders and various ages (MANOVA).

	Boys	Girls	Up to 16 years	Over 16-17 years
Overall satisfaction with school experience			– –	–
Perceived usefulness of school			– –	–
Positive expectations for school			– –	–
Repeated school years	++[a]	+	+	+

[a] The + and – signs indicate the presence of a significant difference between sexually active adolescents and other adolescents and the direction of that difference. The number of signs indicates the degree of difference: ++ much higher value, + higher value, – – much lower value, – lower value.

once again, highlight the central role of school in adolescent development and evidence some of the possible short- and long-term negative consequences of failing in school and even of being dissatisfied with the school experience.

6.5.3 Ritual and Emulation Functions

Adolescents' sexual behavior can also serve a *rite of passage* function, demonstrating to themselves and their peers that they have surpassed child status and can be accepted by a group of peers who are already sexually active, thus gaining greater acceptance and prestige. In fact, adolescents who have had sex, particularly low-faithfulness boys, spend more time with and receive greater support from their friends (Table 6.10).

The ritual function of sexual behavior is felt more strongly when the adolescent has limited social resources. For example, those who adopt a promiscuous behavior pattern can count less on their friends to express disapproval toward the behavior of others, depriving them of the opportunity to compare their point of view with others. Especially during adolescence, this comparison of view points can represent an important opportunity for the development of an individual's cognitive, affective, and social capabilities (Meeus et al. 2002). Consider, for example, the ability to remove themselves from the present situation and their own point of view, to anticipate the possible results of their actions, and to attempt

Table 6.10. Aspects connected to the ritual function (MANOVA).

	Means for the characteristics of adolescents with different sexual behavior patterns				
	Nonsexually active adolescents	Adolescents who have stopped sexual relations over the past year	High faithfulness: only one sexual partner in their lives	Ex-low faithfulness – now high faithfulness: one partner only in the past year, more than one partner previously	Low faithfulness: more than one partner in their lives
Time spent weekly with friends	++[a]	++++	+++	+	+++++
Friends' support	++	++++	+++	+	++++
Friends' control	+++	++++	++++	+	+
Compatibility between friends and parents	+++	++++	+++++	+	++
Parental support	+++++	+++	+++	++	+
Parental control	+++++	+++	+++	+	++

[a] A greater number of plus signs (+) corresponds to a higher mean; eta-squared = .04.

to put themselves in another person's shoes. These abilities appear to be particularly lacking in boys who resort to molestation and violence against their peers.

Furthermore, sexually active adolescents perceive a low level of compatibility between their friends and their parents on important objectives to accomplish in the future. This can bring them to choose one at the expense of the other, significantly reducing the possibility to receive help and support in case of difficulty or need (Meeus et al.1996).

In the choice between friends and parents, it is girls and younger adolescents in particular who tend to choose their friends (Table 6.11). Early and excessive orientation toward friends, however, reveals itself to be rather disadvantageous, as it deprives the adolescent of the fundamental contribution of their parents in terms of opportunity for dialogue and emotional support and con-

Table 6.11. Main characteristics of sexually active adolescents compared with others for both genders and various ages (MANOVA).

	Boys	Girls	Up to 16 years	Over 16-17 years
Time spent weekly with friends	++[a]	+	++	+
Friends' support	+	+		
Compatibility between parents and friends	–	– –		
Orientation toward friends in decision making	+	++	+	+
Parental support	–	– –		
Parental control			– –	-

[a] The + and – signs indicate the presence of a significant difference between sexually active adolescents and other adolescents and the direction of that difference. The number of signs indicates the degree of difference: ++ much higher value, + higher value, – – much lower value, – lower value.

trol of the adolescents' behavior. In fact, adolescents feel the need to renegotiate their relationships with their parents on a more equal level although they continue to require the support and encouragement of adults as they identify the objectives they need to accomplish and develop plans and strategies for reaching these objectives (Juang and Silbereisen 2002; Scabini et al. 2005, in press). Sexually active girls in particular seem to be more affected by the lack of parental support while younger adolescents are more affected by the lack of control. These results confirm the positive role played by parental control over behavior (Cattelino and Bonino 1999; Aunola et al. 2000; Juang and Silbereisen 2002): requiring respect of adolescents for norms and rules can promote the development of individual responsibility and self-control - characteristics that, as we have seen, are central to sexual behavior as well, especially in terms of choosing when and how it is carried out.

Lacking more mature ways to express one's identity and differentiate oneself from others, for some adolescents, sexual behavior becomes the favored grounds on which to measure themselves against their peers and establish themselves and their abilities. For these adolescents, sexual activity and promiscuity, in particular, like other types of risk behavior, carry out an emulation and reciprocal surpassing function: they not only want to act like and imitate their peers but, rather, to prove themselves by attempting to surpass their peers. Previous studies have demonstrated that the relationship between an adolescent's behavior and that of their friends cannot be interpreted merely as the effect of peer influence on the adolescent but, rather, as the result of a process of reciprocal selection and influence (Engels and Knibbe 2000). Adolescents are not inclined to take part in certain types of behavior only because they are commonly practiced within the group they belong to; they choose as friends the peers who most correspond to their needs in terms of sharing activities, ideas, and feelings. Finding others who are similar to oneself constitutes an important acknowledgment of one's identity, and the chance to engage in activities together is useful in obtaining cognitive consonance.

Therefore, it is probably no coincidence that sexually active adolescents,

Table 6.12. Aspects connected to the emulation function (MANOVA).

	Means for the characteristics of adolescents with different sexual behavior patterns				
	Nonsexually active adolescents	Adolescents who have stopped sexual relations over the past year	High faithfulness: only one sexual partner in their lives	Ex-low faithfulness – now high faithfulness: one partner only in the past year, more than one partner previously	Low faithfulness: more than one partner in their lives
Friends' risk behavior	+ᵃ	++++	+++	++	+++++
Friends' conventional behavior	+++++	+	+++	+++	++
Time spent weekly in nonorganized activities	+	++++	+++	++	+++++
Time spent weekly in organized activities	+++++	+++	+	+++	+
Belonging to a church group	++++	++++	+++	+	+

ᵃ A greater number of plus signs (+) corresponds to a higher mean.

especially those who are promiscuous, have friends who are more involved in risk behavior, less involved in conventional activities, and spend more of their free time in nonorganized activities, which can be characterized as "empty time" for the lack of planning they involve (Table 6.12). Involvement in this type of activity brings us to reflect on the superficial characteristics of adulthood that these adolescents seem to aspire so strongly to.

On the other hand, adolescents who are not yet sexually active spend a greater portion of their time in organized activities, and it is more likely that they attend a church group. It is probable that the protective role carried out by the church derives not only from the application of moral precepts connected to religious principles but also from the presence of a specific educational purpose, proposing activities that serve to meet that purpose. The aim of the church group transcends that of spending time together and implies the sharing of values within a clear and well-defined life plan. As other research has demonstrated (Wallace and Williams 1997), religion is a protective factor that is too often underestimated by prevention programs. It carries out its role in a largely indirect way by providing the possibility to take part in meaningful activities marked by important moral and social principles, such as respect for others and their rights.

Table 6.13. Main characteristics of sexually active adolescents compared with others for both genders and various ages (MANOVA).

	Boys	Girls	Up to 16 years	Over 16-17 years
Friends' conventional behavior			– –	–
Time spent weekly in nonorganized activities	++[a]	+	+	++
Time spent weekly in organized activities	– –	–		
Time spent weekly in sport-related activities	+			+

[a] The + and – signs indicate the presence of a significant difference between sexually active adolescents and other adolescents and the direction of that difference. The number of signs indicates the degree of difference: ++ much higher value, + higher value, – – much lower value, – lower value.

Differences related to behavior patterns are interrelated with gender and age differences (Table 6.13). Boys, and in particular those who follow a promiscuous behavior pattern, are less involved in organized activities and more involved in disorganized and sports-related activities. These adolescents are likely those who are most affected by social comparison with their peers and feel the greatest need to emulate and surpass. An athletic group can be a good context in which to express these needs, as a comparison between physical performance is institutionalized in sports, and body size is central.

Girls, and in particular those in the high-faithfulness group, find themselves in a similar position to adolescents who have not had sexual relations - that is to say, they do not spend much time in nonorganized activities and are fairly involved in organized activities. The need to appeal to the emulation function does not seem as strong in girls while the need to maintain a "double investment" - on the one hand an affective and sexual relationship with a partner and on the other hand the family, school, and other activities - appears stronger. The psychological costs of such an endeavor, as we saw previously, can be quite high for a person of this age.

The youngest boys and girls seem more sensitive than older adolescents to not sharing conventional activities with their friends, such as a commitment to studying or helping others and spending time with the family. As shown by previous research, social comparison with friends who have already distanced themselves from activities common for adolescents, such as attending school, for example, encourages a need to emulate and surpass their friends' behavior, especially at younger ages (Magnusson et al. 1986; Silbereisen and Krache 1997).

Finally, the correlation between a sexually promiscuous pattern and nonorganized activities increases over time. During adolescence, a lifestyle initiates characterized by a greater propensity for immediate satisfaction of one's needs and a lesser willingness to work hard and assume responsibility. When an adolescent lacks, or fails to see more significant opportunities for, personal achievement, only the image of themselves that they are able to communicate to others, or simply spending time together, seems important. This view is perfectly compatible with today's current image-based society where everything is a show and, often, superficiality rather than depth is encouraged in relationships. The possible effects of such a condition on the development of cognitive, relational, and affective capabilities remains, in large part, unexplored (Petersen 2000).

6.5.4 One or More Partners: What Is the Difference?

Research has revealed consistent differences between adolescents who are not yet sexually active and those who are, but differences in the type of behavior patterns they adopt also exist within the sexually active group. Under numerous, although not all, aspects, the line that appears to determine the particular value or meaning assigned to sexual behavior is constituted by the number of partners these adolescents have had in their brief sexual lives. For this reason, we wanted to examine, through a discriminant analysis, which of these various aspects connected to the functions considered in the previous paragraphs would allow us to best differentiate between these adolescents. Two dimensions were revealed. Intentions and attempts to drop out of school, participation in nonorganized activities, and marijuana smoking were positively correlated to the first dimension (*exploration-transgression function*) while a negative correlation exists with value on religion and parental control. On the other hand, cigarette smoking, having a job, positive self-perception, failed school years, depressive feelings, and friends' risk behavior are positively correlated to the second dimension while models of friends with conventional behavior is negatively correlated. These aspects are linked in part to the *anticipation of adulthood function* and in part to the *emulation function*. Figure 6.17 demonstrates how the first dimension separates all three groups. It appears to be less relevant for those who are not yet sexually active, slightly more relevant for those who have had sexual relations with only one partner, and much more relevant for those who had more than one partner. Adolescents who have had multiple partners differ from all other groups for the transgressive significance their behavior assumes at this age. The second dimension differentiates between sexually active adolescents and those who have not yet had sex. Precocious sexual activity during adolescence carries out an anticipation of adulthood function and can represent a way of exploring and proving oneself and emulating the behavior of peers.

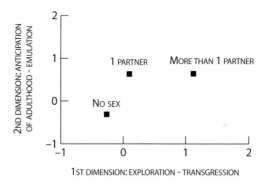

Fig. 6.17. Differences in groups of sexually active and non-sexually-active adolescents (discriminant analysis). Percentage of correct classification: 71%.

6.5.5 Different Functions of Sexual Activity in Relation to the Way It Is Carried Out

Involvement in sexual activity during adolescence can fulfill various functions (summarized in Table 6.1), depending on the way it is carried out. Boys and girls who adopt the low-faithfulness pattern use their sexual involvement to carry out a plurality of functions: transgression, experimentation, ritual-emulation, escape from difficulty, and a heightened need for adulthood. They seem to feel particularly trapped between a completely unsatisfactory present - so unsatisfactory, in fact, that they want to escape from it - and a future that seems so far away and vaguely defined that they are unable to imagine it. The strong sense of discomfort they feel is connected to a greater need to transgress the values and expectations of adults, to experiment with new sensations, and to emulate new behavior types in order to signal the difference between themselves and their peers who, on the other hand, are fairly content in their present situation and identify more closely with the behavior and attitudes that are socially accepted in adolescents.

While recourse to sexual activity as an escape from difficulties is a characteristic exclusive to low-faithfulness adolescents, the heightened need for adulthood is also shared by a smaller group of older adolescents who, following a period of promiscuous behavior, are currently involved in a relationship with a single partner. Although they are not as discontent in their present situations, these adolescents, many of whom are already old enough to actually be considered adults in all respects, seem to continue to feel a strong need to demonstrate to themselves and others that they have reached adult status. This need is also felt, although to a lesser degree, in adolescents - especially girls - who seek to achieve the model of a stable couple. Although adults judge this model irreproachable, it can bring with it the difficulty of assuming respon-

Summary 6.1. Main functions carried out by different sexual behavior patterns.

Sexual behavior
• ADULTHOOD, through having sex, a behavior considered normal for adults
• ANTICIPATION OF ADULTHOOD, through achieving a stable relationship, considered morally irreproachable in adults: "high-faithfulness" behavior pattern (especially in girls and younger adolescents)
• EXASPERATION OF ADULTHOOD, through adopting a promiscuous behavior pattern: "low-faithfulness" behavior pattern (especially in boys and younger adolescents) and "ex low faithfulness"
• TRANSGRESSION, of social norms that consider precocious sexual behavior and promiscuity unacceptable: "low-faithfulness" behavior pattern (especially in younger adolescents and girls)
• TESTING ONESELF AND ONE'S ABILITIES, "low-faithfulness" behavior pattern and "experimentation with sex" (especially up to 16-17 years and in boys)
• EXPLORATION, of new sensations: "experimentation with sex" behavior pattern (especially up to 16-17 years and in boys)
• RITE OF PASSAGE, by demonstrating that they are no longer children (especially in younger adolescents and boys)
• ACCEPTANCE AND SOCIAL RECOGNITION, through entering into the adult community (especially in younger adolescents)
• EMULATION and SURPASSING, of the behavior of others to measure oneself against peers and affirm oneself (especially in boys)
• COPING STRATEGIES and ESCAPE, tied to establishing oneself and problem solving: "low-faithfulness" behavior pattern

sibility and the necessity to reconcile the demands of different dimensions: school, sentiments, and family.

Adolescents who have experienced only a brief foray into sexuality seem to have used their sexuality above all as a means of experimentation, to experience new sensations, try out new roles, or emulate the behavior of their peers. These adolescents do not feel the need to transgress and are less affected by the need to show that they are grown up.

6.6 Adolescents and Pregnancy

Adolescents who adopt a promiscuous behavior pattern are in many ways the group that is at greatest risk of all sexually active adolescents: they appear to be less equipped to confront the transition to adulthood both in terms of individual resources and environmental opportunities, and for this reason, they want to race ahead to reach adulthood as quickly as possible (Ciairano et al. 2005). One may pose the question whether anything changes - and eventually what - with respect to this already less-than-satisfactory condition when adolescents must confront a pregnancy.

Numerous differences exist between low-faithfulness adolescents and those, both boys and girls, who have had to deal with either their own or their partner's pregnancy. Those in the low-faithfulness group who have not had to deal with pregnancy are in better condition than adolescents who have had to deal with pregnancy (Fig. 6.18). Adolescents who have had to deal with pregnancy have a negative self-perception and are, for the most part, unsuccessful in school, leading to setbacks in their school careers. Furthermore, these adolescents cannot rely on control from their peers, and they are heavily involved in internalized risk behavior, such as disturbed eating. They are also involved in other types of risk behavior, such as the use of psychoactive substances and other externalized behavior (antisocial and risk-taking behavior) although in this way, they do not differ significantly from low-faithfulness adolescents.

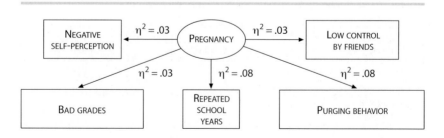

ETA SQUARED OF THE WHOLE MODEL = .15

Fig. 6.18. Variables linked to dealing with pregnancy during adolescence (MANOVA).

The picture that emerges of adolescents who have had to confront pregnancy is decidedly negative, especially considering that the comparison was made with another high-risk group of adolescents who have adopted a pattern of promiscuous behavior. It is impossible to establish if the poor condition of these adolescents existed prior to the pregnancy and therefore may have predisposed them to it, if it began after the pregnancy, or if - the most likely answer - it is the result of an interaction between a negative preexisting condition and the pregnancy. What emerges is that pregnancy in adolescence clearly places major limitations on individual development, both in terms of present adjustment and the possibility of future adjustment. At this age, pregnancy can represent a critical event that is difficult to endure and overcome, regardless of the outcome.

6.7 Family, School Experience, and Friends as Protective and Risk Factors

The results displayed in the previous paragraphs offer numerous indications of the complex interactions between individual resources and environmental opportunities and how these interactions can have very different behavior origins, which carry out numerous functions over the course of adolescent development. Let us now look at this interaction from another perspective by examining the role that resources and opportunities can play as protective or risk factors with respect to sexual behavior. In particular, we posed the question: which aspects of the school, family, and peer environment contribute the most to reducing the probability of sexual involvement (Fig. 6.19), to making

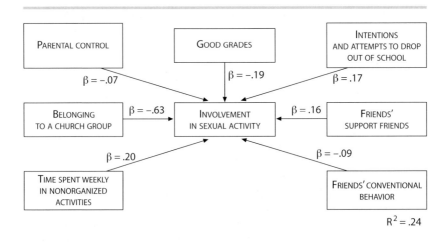

Fig. 6.19. Protective and risk factors related to involvement in sexual activity (logistic regression).

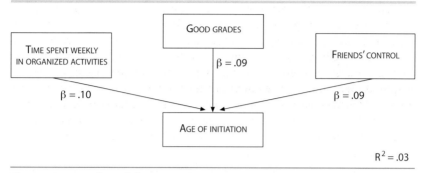

Fig.6.20. Protective factors linked to age of initiation of sexual activity (linear regression analysis).

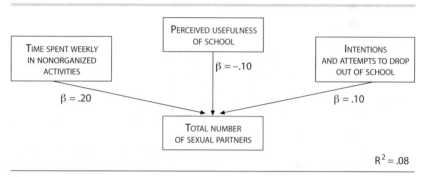

Fig.6.21. Protective and risk factors linked to sexual promiscuity (linear regression analysis).

the adolescent less inclined to initiate sexual activity precociously (Fig. 6.20), and to adopt a pattern of promiscuous behavior (Fig. 6.21)?

The most important roles seems to be played by the school and, in particular, by the type of experience the adolescent has in this context: the more an adolescent is able to be successful in school, the less likely it is that he or she will be sexually active or will begin precociously. The more adolescents perceive the school as useful to their present and future, the less likely they are to adopt a promiscuous behavior pattern. On the contrary, the more an adolescent has thought about or has attempted to drop out of school, the more likely it is that he or she is sexually active and willing to adopt a promiscuous behavior pattern. The motivation to assume ahead of time and in a highly visible way the most exterior types of adult behavior can therefore be reduced when the school promotes other ways for adolescents to express themselves as adults and test their limits, providing the possibility for a more satisfying experience. The promotion of satisfaction and interest in the school experience - along with the strengthening of those cognitive, affective, and social abilities that promote both the achievement of school success and richer, more evolved ways of relating with peers - are the fundamental objectives of any effective prevention program (Mahoney and Stattin 2000).

Family and friends play an important role as well, above all for the role of mediation carried out by the control they offer. In the case of the family, the presence of and requirement to respect a few simple rules of behavior, such as doing homework that has been assigned, helping with household chores, telling the family where they are going when they go out, and coming home at an acceptable time have a protective effect on the probability of sexual involvement.

The protective role of the family is not carried out through control alone. It is also accomplished through the ability to combine rules and control with support and affection in a flexible way, modifying parenting methods to suit the changes that take place during adolescence (Ciairano et al. 2001). An authoritative parenting style in fact seems to encourage adolescents to assume responsibilities that are appropriate for their age and to work toward long-term objectives, in this way countering a need for the adolescent's early involvement in characteristically adult behavior, such as sexual behavior (Fig. 6.22). On the contrary, a permissive parenting style is more common among parents of adolescents who were promiscuous in the past. Parents who adopt a permissive parenting style seem to have given up on carrying out their role as parents. Because they do not enforce rules or act as a source of support, they are not frames of

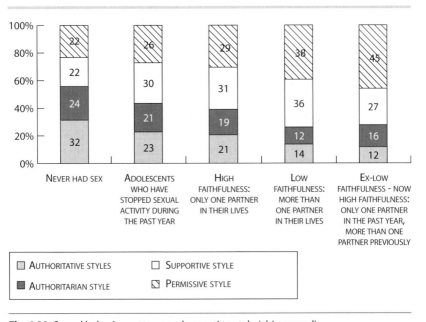

Fig. 6.22. Sexual behavior patterns and parenting style (chi-squared).

reference for their children. As for the other two parenting styles, the authoritarian style, the main function of which is that of control, is more effective in counteracting sexual involvement by younger adolescents, while the supportive parenting style, which offers support alone, succeeds in limiting the choice of a promiscuous pattern to an initial phase of experimentation in older adolescents. Therefore, the way the family functions proves to be much more important than its structure, as shown in previous studies (Jacobson and Crockett 2000; Stattin and Kerr 2000; Cattelino et al. 2001; Ciairano 2004). Other studies (Kerr and Stattin 2000) stressed that the family functioning is not only the results of parenting, but rather that of the interaction between parents and children.

As for the role of friends, their willingness to be critical, when necessary, of an adolescent's behavior can protect that adolescent from precocious sexual activity. On the contrary, having friends who are always supportive can be a risk factor in the probability of sexual involvement. Relating with friends, in particular by comparing points of view on equal terms, can also provide an appropriate context for the development of a broader view and a greater understanding of the problems to be confronted as well as the possibility to identify more mature strategies for solving these problems (Cattelino 2000).

Finally, the community can also serve as a protective factor by providing places for adolescents to meet (Silbereisen et al. 1992; Mahoney and Stattin 2000) where they can meet and participate in purposeful activities, offering an opportunity for them to test their limits and reflect on their present and future - possibly with the educational presence of some adults. The important mediating role played by taking part in a meaningful project is evidenced by the fact that participating in nonorganized activities increases both probability of sexual involvement and inclination to adopt a promiscuous behavior pattern while participation in organized activities decreases the inclination to initiate sexual activity precociously. Furthermore, belonging to a church group and the presence of friends who represent conventional models reduces the probability of sexual involvement.

In short, there are numerous personal characteristics and environmental opportunities that can promote a more gradual and less precocious entry into adulthood. Furthermore, these protective factors are similar, even in nations with different social policies on issues, for example, the prevention of STDs (Ciairano et al. 2001). These factors have been theorically connected to the main functions performed by sexual behavior in adolescence (Summary 6.2). Acting in synergy, each single protective factor is made stronger to form a broader network of resources available to the adolescent.

Summary 6.2. Main protective factors in relation to the functions of sexual activity.

Protective factors	Related functions
PERSON • Expectations to continue school • Value on academic achievement • Value on religion • Disapproval of antisocial behavior	Long-term personal goals to accomplish through school can encourage BEHAVIOR THAT IS MORE APPROPRIATE FOR ADOLESCENTS vs SEEKING ADULTHOOD EARLY. Sharing the values of religion and peaceful coexistence promotes IDENTIFICATION with the adult world and society vs TRANSGRESSION or EXASPERATION OF ADULTHOOD.
FAMILY • Parental support • Parental control • Authoritative parenting style	Living in a family context characterized by closeness, affection, and clear rules for behavior encourages the use of MORE HEALTHY METHODS OF PROVING ONESELF vs EXPERIMENTATION with alternative affective relationships and ESCAPE from difficulty. An authoritative parenting style promotes: • The expression of ADULTHOOD through dialogue, comparing points of view, and sharing. • The gradual acquisition of AUTONOMY, the ability to assume age-appropriate responsibilities, and individual characteristics vs SEEKING ADULTHOOD EARLY. • IDENTIFICATION with behavior types that are socially acceptable for adolescents and the INTERNALIZATION of rules and values that counteract the need for TRANSGRESSION. • The use of COPING STRATEGIES based on verbalization and comparing points of view. • The strengthening of REFLECTION and SELF-CONTROL abilities vs EMULATION and EXASPERATION OF ADULTHOOD.
SCHOOL EXPERIENCE • Satisfaction with school experience • Perceived usefulness of school • Positive expectations for own abilities • Good grades	Satisfaction with the current school experience and perceived usefulness of commitment to school promotes the VALUING ONESELF and one's ROLE AS A STUDENT vs SEEKING ADULTHOOD EARLY. Having high expectation for one's abilities and being successful in school encourages: • PERSONAL ACHIEVEMENT and the STRENGTHENING OF A POSITIVE IDENTITY through the opportunity to experiment and put oneself to the test in nonrisky situations. • ASSUMING RESPONSIBILITY and LONG-TERM COMMITMENTS vs TRANSGRESSION and ESCAPE.

Cont. ▶▶

Protective factors	Related functions
PEERS • Control • Conventional (non-transgressive) behavior patterns • High level of compatibility with parents • Models for use of secure contraception	The perception of friends as people who are not involved in transgressive activities, with expectations for the future and values similar to those of adults and who are willing to dissuade involvement in socially unacceptable behavior encourages: • Processes of IDENTIFICATION and DIFFERENTIATION based on the sharing of ideas and constructive activities vs SEEKING ADULTHOOD EARLY and ESCAPE. • EXPERIMENTATION with socially acceptable roles and actions rather than EMULATION of risky behavior. • Relating to the values of the adult world vs TRANS-GRESSION. • PERSONAL ACHIEVEMENT not limited to demonstrating to others that adult status has been reached through sexuality as a RITE OF PASSAGE. Friends' models for secure contraceptive use can promote, through the SHARING OF PERSONAL CONVICTIONS and processes of IDENTIFICATION, a reduction in the under-evaluation of risks and recourse to healthier conduct.
PARTNER • Deep attachment to partner	The presence of a deep connection to a partner can promote: • SELF AFFIRMATION through sharing and comparing points of view on equal terms. • DECENTERING FROM one's own point of view through sharing thoughts, feelings, and plans. • Reflection on the VALUE OF ONE'S OWN EXISTENCE AND THE EXISTENCE OF OTHERS and on the CONSE-QUENCES OF ONE'S ACTIONS on oneself and others. A deep affective relationship promotes more effective and regular contraceptive use through sharing in the planning of its use.
FREE TIME • Time dedicated to studying, reading, hobbies, and artistic activities • Time spent with family • Belonging to a church group	Time per week dedicated to study, reading, hobbies, and family and belonging to a religious group encourage: • SELF-AFFIRMATION and the CONSTRUCTION OF IDEN-TITY through reflection, exchange of ideas, comparison of points of view, and prosocial behavior • PLANNING and COMMITMENT. • Internalization of values related to the RECOGNITION OF OTHERS and their rights.

CHAPTER 7

Disturbed Eating

> Tuesday 3 January. 130 pounds… I can actually feel the fat
> splurging out from my body. Never mind. Sometimes you
> have to sink to a nadir of toxic fat envelopment in order to
> emerge, phoenix-like, from the chemical wasteland as a
> purged and beautiful Michelle Pfeiffer figure. Tomorrow new
> Spartan health and beauty regime will begin.
>
> *[H. Fielding, Bridget Jones Diary, 1996]*

7.1 Self-Perception, Social Relationships, and Eating in Adolescence

Although eating behavior is a day-to-day part of our lives and essential to survival, during adolescence, it can be associated with risk, especially in terms of two important aspects of development: self-perception and relationships with peers (Vandereycken 1996). The major physical changes that occur with biological maturation during puberty give way to a process of transition, introducing changes in self-perception and particularly in body image (Schulenberg et al. 1997). Accepting one's new body and integrating its appearance into a broader self concept, intended as the interpretive framework of personal experience and regulative foundation for behavior, is one of the main developmental tasks of adolescence (Bosma and Kunnen 2001). This process of restructuring and self-organizing, both socially and individually, involves the redefinition of relationships with adults and peers and can be carried out in different ways depending on the historical period and specific context. This task can vary in difficulty depending on the various personal and environmental resources the individual possesses, and it can be connected - to a greater or lesser degree of satisfaction - with one's physical appearance and the desire to alter this appearance by adopting a particular eating behavior. The physical processes tied to pubertal development represent a particularly difficult challenge for adolescents because they occur at precisely the same time as individuals have the greatest need to feel similar to and appreciated by their peers. In comparing themselves with their peers, weight and height can become indicators of inadequacy in development and can result in difficulties when development occurs earlier or later than normal (Silbereisen and Kracke 1997).

The restructuring of body image is a more difficult process for girls who, on average, have a more negative body image of themselves than do boys (Seiffge-Krenke 1990) and are generally more involved in disturbed eating (Attie and Brooks-Gunn 1989). Many factors contribute to the difficulty adolescents experience in adjusting to the changes in their bodies, not the least of which are the speed of physical development in puberty and the increasingly precocious initiation of these changes. An abrupt physical change provides less opportunity for the individual to gradually adapt, and an excessively early change can occur before adequate methods have been developed to deal with this change (Silbereisen and Noack 1990). Furthermore, the effects of sexual maturation on psychosocial well-being are not the same for all individuals, as these changes are intertwined with societal norms, which are more severe in their judgments of the adequacy of physical development in girls. Having a pleasant appearance, which in Western culture is strongly associated with being thin, is increasingly important to women's positive self-perception, and the desire to be thin is normative among women in Western countries today (Henderson-King and Henderson-King 1997). Women's greater discontent toward their bodies, particularly women who develop earlier than their peers, could also be tied to the physiological effects of sexual maturity, as puberty for women entails an accumulation of body fat while for boys puberty brings an increase in muscle. The fear of seeming ridiculous, cited by adolescents as one of the main sources of their anxiety, and worry over the appearance of their body on a daily basis (Rodriguez-Tomé and Bairaud 1990; Seiffge-Krenke and Shulman 1993), are an indication that, today, the need to conform to society's standard of beauty is very strong. Finally, identity construction in general appears to be a more fragmentary, ambiguous process for girls than for boys. Girls perceive greater difficulty in defining who they are, identifying goals and seeing these goals as obtainable (Nurmi 1997). These difficulties can also combine with a greater tendency toward self-limiting strategies, expectations for failure, and feelings of inadequacy that derive from the contrasting demands that are made of girls, such as having a successful career while at the same time respecting traditional values. Thus, it is not surprising that adolescents, especially those who possess more limited personal and environmental resources, can find it difficult to detach themselves from the pervasive cultural models of beauty and success. It is also not surprising that, for adolescents, dissatisfaction and anxiety originating from various sources become concentrated on the body (Buysse 1996).

In order to better understand the adoption of healthy or unhealthy eating behavior during adolescence, it is necessary to consider the aspect of peer relationships not only in terms of social comparison and identity development but also in terms of the sharing of actions and the possibility of experimenting with eating behavior and foods that are unlike those of the adolescent's family. From this point of view, relationships with peers and the need to acquire greater independence from the family appear to be equally important both for boys and girls. It is within the peer group and network of friends that new criteria and new values develop; it is here that new roles and behavior types are tried out, including unhealthy eating behavior, such as dining on fast food or other snacks and beverages that are so widely available today (Braet 1996). In contemporary Western society, the consumption of a wide variety of highly caloric prepared foods is by no means only characteristic of young people. Recent studies have pointed to changes in eating habits shared by people of all ages (Brown and Bentley-Condit 1998). On the one hand, more calories and fat have been introduced into our diets - which is due in part to the reduction of time dedicated to the preparation and sharing of food within the family, the availability at any time of day of prepared foods, and the disappearance of physical space and time dedicated specifically to consumption of food. On the other hand, caloric requirements have decreased significantly due to a reduction in physical activity and to the fact that our homes are climate controlled. The interaction of these two trends has led to a higher proportion of obesity in Western populations and increased risk for cardiovascular problems linked to excess weight and a diet that is rich in fat and poor in fiber.

It is within this complex framework that numerous adolescents resort to different types of eating behavior that are more or less disturbed and widely varying in nature and in the seriousness of the consequences they entail in the short and long term. These are types of behavior that, except when they reach the level of actual anorexic and bulimic behavior - phenomena that, in Italy, concern less than 1% of the adult and adolescent female population (Cuzzolaro 1997) - have drawn little attention from the public and even from researchers, most likely because they involve neither criminal activity (as do some types of antisocial behavior, illegal psychoactive substance use, and risky driving) nor moral judgments, such as promiscuous sexual activity. In general, these behavior types are scarcely noticeable outside of the close circle of the individual's family and friends, and for this reason, they have been classified, along with anxiety and depressive feelings, as internalized problems. However, the discomfort they express is no less serious than that which is expressed through other more outward, visible behavior (Wade and Lowes 2002). Both internalized and externalized behavior are used to respond to specific developmental tasks that the adolescent is unable to confront in a more well-adjusted way. For adolescents who have no alternative means of personal fulfillment, the easy availability of food is actually part of the reason they choose it as a testing ground for their limits and an area in which they can achieve their need for independence without risking too much in terms of social disapproval (Spruijt-Metz 1999). However, the negative effects of even slightly disturbed eating behavior on health and psychological well-being in the long term can potentially be more serious than those of other more visible types of behavior, as these behavior types are very common and tend to persist. Dissatisfaction with one's weight and the pursuit of thinness continue throughout the transition to adult life (Fairburn 1995) while the probability of assuming other types of risk behavior decreases drastically (Schulenberg et al. 1997).

Recent studies have also shown that internalized behavior, when accompanied by other forms of risk behavior, give way to poor overall functioning both socially and academically, characterized by poor coping skills, lack of self-control, low self-esteem, and a poor sense of competency (Compas et al. 1998). Because it is carried out alone, internalized behavior tends to increase the social isolation of those who carry it out. This aggravates a condition that already exists as a result of these individuals' negative self-perception and body image, thus leading to a vicious cycle (Vandereycken 1996).

7.2 Body and Body Image: Gender Differences

As eating is necessary first and foremost to allow for development and to permit the body to function properly, we used the body mass index (BMI) to examine whether body measurements of the adolescents in our study were consistent with the image they have of their bodies. The average height and build[1] of the boys and girls in our sample were compared with the standards of Italy's adolescent population and were found to be normal (Centro Studi Auxologici 2004). Through the relationship between weight and height (or more precisely, between weight in kilograms and the square of the height in meters), the BMI was calculated for each subject. This value, compared in turn with various parameters, allowed us to divide subjects into the following groups: seriously underweight, underweight, normal weight, overweight, seriously overweight. We found that the majority of our sample of boy and girl adolescents is of normal weight (Fig. 7.1)[2] while a relatively small percentage is overweight. The total percentage of underweight adolescents is higher among boys while the seriously underweight group includes a high number of girls.

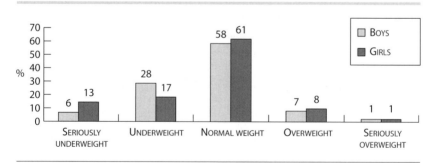

Fig. 7.1. Body mass index for the two genders (chi-squared).

---

[1] The questions and scales included in the questionnaire, along with their related responses and main psychometric characteristics, are reported in the "Appendix."

[2] Note that all the results reported in the figures are statistically significant, with $p<0.05$. In Chap. 2, Sect. 2.4, Presentation of Results and Statistical Analyses, the criteria for the presentation of results and for the use of statistics are explained.

Because of the fact that the adolescent body is subject to marked and sudden changes, especially in the case of boys, we also investigated the occurrence of weight and height increases over the past year. Relationships were found between current body measurements and a recent change in weight for individuals in the seriously overweight group and a recent change in height for those in the seriously underweight group. Therefore it appears that some "abnormal" physical conditions can likely be considered temporary. With age, the situation appears to normalize significantly (Fig. 7.2) for boys more so than for girls.

Despite the fact that their measurements are absolutely within the norm, satisfaction with body appearance was found to be very low among the adolescents in our sample. The girls are more dissatisfied with their bodies than are the boys, especially in terms of weight (Fig. 7.3), and while desire to be tall is lower in older boys (40% at 18-19 years vs 61% at 14-15 years), dissatisfaction with their body measurements is characteristic of girls in all age groups.

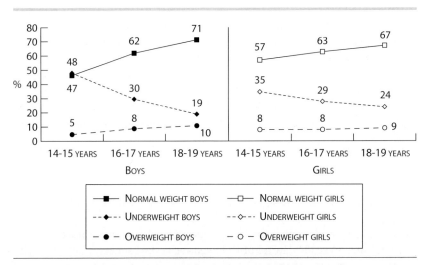

Fig. 7.2. Body mass index for age group for the two genders (chi-squared).

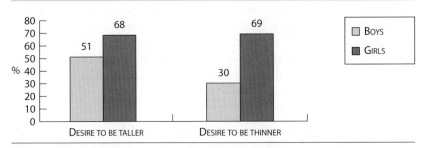

Fig. 7.3. Desire to be taller and to be thinner for the two genders (chi-squared).

In general, adolescents appear to have a fairly distorted image of their bodies, especially girls. A considerable percentage of underweight girls would like to weigh less, as would the great majority of normal-weight girls (Fig. 7.4). Among girls, the desire to conform to the standards of excessive thinness, even at the expense of their health, is fairly common.

Overweight boys, on the other hand, particularly those who are seriously overweight, appear to be at risk for the opposite reason. A good percentage of these individuals have no desire to lose weight; in fact, they consider their weight to be ideal or would even like to gain weight. Therefore, in the case of these boys, we see an underevaluation of the possible risks of excess weight.

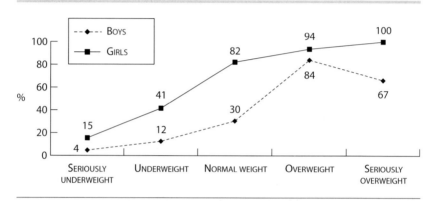

Fig. 7.4. Desire to weigh less for the two genders with respect to body mass index (chi-squared).

7.3 Knowledge of the Risks Involved in an Unhealthy Lifestyle

We asked ourselves whether the adolescents interviewed who wanted so badly to be thinner were also aware of the negative consequences associated with being underweight and, in more general terms, of an unhealthy, sedentary, or relatively inactive lifestyle that can lead to excess weight gain. Although numerous studies have underlined the absence of a direct relationship between knowledge and behavior (Savadori e Rumiati 1996; Spruijt-Metz 1999), increased awareness may at least reduce the most severe risks.

Our results show that an awareness of the possible negative consequences of being overweight is actually quite common in our sample (Fig. 7.5)[3]. Girls appear to be more aware than boys of both the negative physical and psychological consequences that can occur together.

---

[3] The questions from the questionnaire and their related responses, which were used to construct the "awareness of the negative consequences of being overweight" typology, as well as the methods used to construct this typology, are reported in the "Appendix."

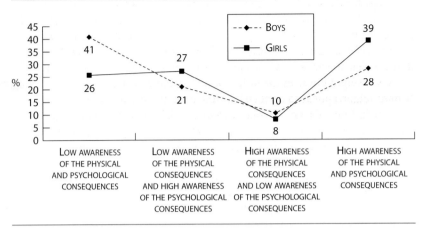

Fig. 7.5. Awareness of the negative consequences of being overweight for the two genders (chi-squared).

Awareness of the negative consequences is even higher among overweight girls while the opposite is true of overweight boys, who have relatively little knowledge of the risks (Fig. 7.6). In the case of boys, psychological mechanisms of cognitive consonance can come into play, or in other words, the tendency to perceive one's own behavior or conditions as less dangerous than they actually are and to perceive any information or knowledge that contrasts with their actions as dissonant. This phenomenon can be extremely dangerous, as it leads individuals to underestimate the actual risks they face (Mendelson and White 1985; Pierce and Wardle 1997).

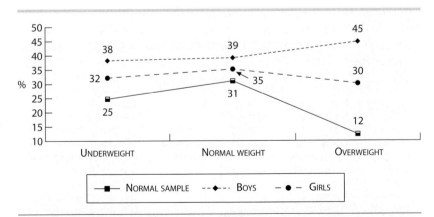

Fig. 7.6. High awareness of the negative consequences of being overweight with respect to body mass index for the total sample and for the two genders (chi-squared).

Through their responses to an open-ended question on the questionnaire (Table 7.1), about half the adolescents demonstrated that they are not only aware of the existence of negative consequences associated with being over-weight but also that their knowledge of these risks is accurate. Boys more fre-quently identified problems of a physical or psychological nature, particular-ly with reference to relations with members of the opposite sex, while girls demonstrated a greater awareness of the complexity of the phenomenon, iden-tifying a greater number of aspects. The fact that boys worry more about the possibility of having problems with the opposite sex while girls are more con-cerned with the appearance of the body itself has been shown by other stud-ies as well (Seiffge-Krenke and Shulman 1993).

The different types of awareness about the negative consequences of being overweight and of other unhealthy behavior are strongly correlated (Fig. 7.7). Awareness of the negative consequences of not exercising regularly and sitting for long periods of time is more common among boys who, as shown previ-ously, are more concerned with problems of a physical nature. There is a stronger relationship between awareness of the negative consequences of being over-weight and awareness of the consequences of a lack of physical activity for boys than for girls. Girls, on the other hand, are very attentive to diet; they are more aware of the negative consequences both of skipping breakfast and of eating unhealthy foods, and girls' knowledge of both of these risks is higher at older ages.

In general, it can be stated that an awareness of the possible risks involved with an unhealthy lifestyle, in terms of bad eating habits and little physical activity, is very common among adolescents. However, a very weak relationship exists, especially among girls, between awareness and actual physical condition and body image. Girls, even in the normal weight group, are deeply dissatis-fied with the appearance of their bodies and have a very negative perception of the possible consequences of being overweight. They seem to be driven by

Table 7.1. Negative consequences of being overweight identified by the adolescents in the sample (chi-squared)[a].

Physical problems	Psychological problems	
	Referring to the person	Referring to relationships with others
• Different types of health-related risks (respiratory, cardiovascular, etc.) • Greater risk of developing eating-related pathologies (bulimia, anorexia, obesity) • Motor difficulties • General developmental problems	• A general state of discomfort • Discomfort over the appearance of one's body • A state of discomfort to others	• Exclusion from relationships with others • Excluding oneself from relationships with others • Excluding oneself for fear of the negative judgments of others • Difficulty in relationships with the opposite sex
Cited more often by boys than by girls: 40% vs 26%	Cited more often by girls than by boys: 24% vs 20%	Cited more often by boys than by girls: 15% vs 9%

[a] Girls more often than boys cited at least two types of problems: 41% vs 25%.

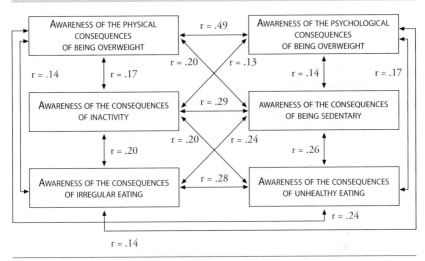

Fig. 7.7. Awareness of the negative consequences of being overweight and of various types of unhealthy behavior (correlation analysis).

an obsession with being thin in an attempt to live up to the standards of female beauty that the modern consumer society has imposed.

On the contrary, boys are more satisfied with the appearance of their bodies and perceive less negative consequences of being overweight, even when they are actually overweight. They seem to worry almost exclusively about the fact that being overweight could translate into weaker physical performance or that it could reduce their appeal from the opposite sex. For both genders, more attention was focussed on physical appearance than on health (Israel and Ivanova 2002; Wade and Lowes 2002).

7.4 Healthiness and Regularity of Eating Habits: A Controversial Relationship

7.4.1 Daily Eating Habits of Adolescents, Their Parents, and Their Friends

As far as the healthiness of daily food consumption is concerned, for example, choosing fruit or milk over sweets and fatty or fried foods, and the regularity or lack thereof of meals (Fig. 7.8)[4], boys more frequently adopt a type of eating behavior that is not very healthy but is regular (low healthiness and high regularity in eating habits) while girls tend to eat very healthily but with little regularity (high healthiness and low regularity in eating habits).

---

[4] Questions from the questionnaire and the related responses that make up the healthiness and regularity of eating habits scales, along with a description of how the "regularity and healthiness of eating habits" typology was constructed, are reported in the "Appendix."

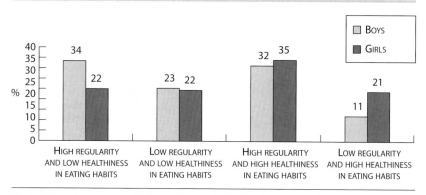

Fig. 7.8. Regularity and healthiness of eating habits for the two genders (chi-squared).

Girls' greater obsession with weight, greater awareness of the negative consequences of an unhealthy lifestyle, and greater attentiveness toward eating healthily is not always accompanied by regularity of meals, which is one of the main antidotes to weight gain (Bandura 1997). On the other hand, although boys are generally not worried about the appearance of their bodies and the consequences of bad eating habits, and pay little attention to the healthiness of their bodies, they eat with greater regularity than girls. The combination of high attention to a healthy diet and irregular eating habits is a phenomenon that, among girls, is higher at older ages. As shown in previous studies (Herman et al. 1987), over the course of time, a vicious cycle of anxiety over body weight and irregular eating habits can initiate. These results show the dissociation, more pervasive for girls, of an awareness of the principles of good nutrition and the assumption of a given eating behavior. Concern for a healthy diet is not only insufficient to alleviate risk, it is actually connected to greater irregularity in eating habits. This finding reveals a need for a more in-depth examination of the possible meanings tied to eating behavior in terms of the interaction between knowledge, emotions, affection, and social models.

In older age groups (Fig. 7.9), the percentage of adolescents characterized by high regularity and high healthiness in eating habits is lower while the percentage of adolescents who adopt irregular and unhealthy eating habits is higher. This finding can probably be seen as an indirect effect of the increased independence acquired by adolescents at this same time, which results in a greater number of meals taken outside the home, often in fast food restaurants or pubs in the company of friends.

As far as the examples for eating behavior of those with whom adolescents have the most contact - parents and best friend - the adoption of healthy eating habits is most often attributed to the mother's example, followed by the father and lastly the friend (Fig. 7.10). The perception of healthiness of parents' diet is lower at older ages, particularly after the ages of 16-17, while the per-

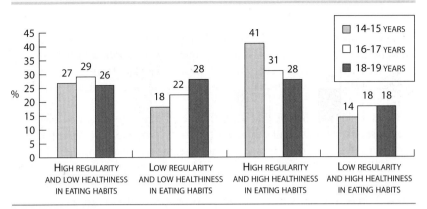

Fig. 7.9. Regularity and healthiness of eating habits for different age groups (chi-squared).

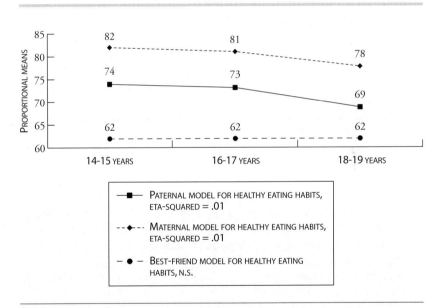

Fig. 7.10. Healthiness of parents' and best friend's eating habits for age group (ANOVA).

ception of friends' behavior remains consistently lower than that of parents for all age groups considered. With age, adolescents become more critical of their parents' eating habits; the greater independence they enjoy allows them to experiment not only with fast food but with different foods and dishes unlike those that are part of their families' normal diet, such as regional, ethnic, or organic cuisine.

7.4.2 Eating, Body Image, Knowledge, and Models

We asked ourselves which of the various factors considered previously - physical condition, body image, awareness of consequences of an unhealthy lifestyle, and the presence of positive behavior models provided by adults and peers - has the greatest relationship with the adoption of healthier or more regular eating habits.

First of all, we observe that a healthy diet is connected to an awareness of the consequences of an unhealthy lifestyle and having positive parental models and not to individual characteristics such as physical condition or body image (Fig. 7.11). However, not all types of awareness are related with healthy eating habits: for girls in particular, an awareness of the negative psychological consequences associated with being overweight is linked to less healthy eating habits, confirmation that these individuals are concerned not about their

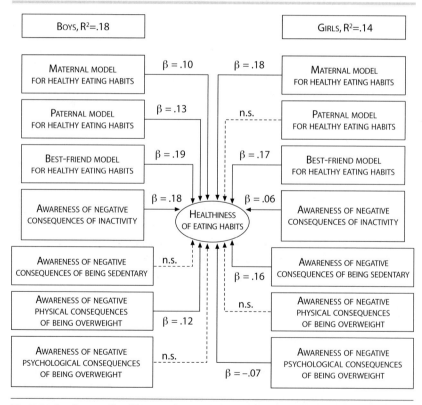

Fig. 7.11. Predictors of healthiness of eating habits for the two genders (linear regression). In the regression model, the following predictors were also inserted but were not reported here because they were not significant for either boys or girls: being of normal weight, recent weight change, and dissatisfaction with weight.

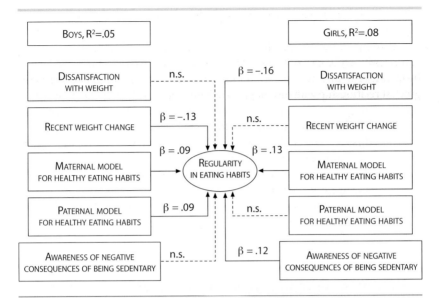

Fig. 7.12. Predictors of regularity of eating habits for the two genders (linear regression). In the regression model, the following predictors were also inserted but were not reported here because they were not significant for either boys or girls: being of normal weight, healthiness of best friend's eating habits, awareness of negative consequences of inactivity, awareness of negative physical consequences of being overweight, and awareness of negative psychological consequences of being overweight.

health but about being thin. Finally, some behavioral models, in particular paternal models, seem to encourage healthier eating habits in boys only.

Irregular eating habits, on the other hand, are mainly tied to personal characteristics, such as a recent change in weight or dissatisfaction with one's weight (Fig. 7.12). These characteristics are different for the two genders, as irregularity in eating in girls is connected to dissatisfaction with weight while in boys it is linked to a recent change in weight. The results reported in Fig. 7.12, along with those described in the previous paragraphs, suggest the presence of two different paths of involvement in risky eating behavior. The first path, characteristic of girls, originates essentially from a profound dissatisfaction with their bodies, even when their measurements are in the norm. The second path, typical of boys, is connected to an actual recent change in body measurements, which, as we saw previously (Fig. 7.2), can lead to a temporary "abnormal" physical condition. The existence of these two different paths for boys and girls contributes to explaining the greater pervasiveness and persistence over time of risky eating behavior in women; it is more difficult to modify a distorted self-perception than it is to take notice of the changes in one's body. Furthermore, dissatisfaction with the body is characteristic of the majority of girls (80% of normal-weight girls would like to weigh less; Fig. 7.4) while risk for boys applies mainly to the overweight group who are not at all interested in losing weight (Fig. 7.4) and are unaware of the negative health-related consequences associated with their physical condition (Fig. 7.6).

Healthiness and regularity of eating habits, despite the fact that the former is tied more to knowledge and models and the latter to individual characteristics, also have some predictors in common, such as the maternal model for healthy eating for both genders and the paternal model for boys in particular. The importance of the maternal model is a predictable result considering the role that this figure plays, especially in Mediterranean countries in the day-to-day organization of family life, the home, and the times and characteristics of meals. The emergence of the importance of the father's role, however, is a relatively unexpected finding (Ardone 1998). This result likely signals the gradual changes, however modest they may be, in the management of family, where fathers have become more receptive to sharing in the tasks of housework and raising children.

7.5 Disturbed Eating: A Gender Phenomenon

7.5.1 Dieting, Comfort Eating, and Purging Behavior: Many Sides of the Same Coin

The phenomenon of dieting is quite common, involving over 30% of the adolescents in our sample over the last six months. Dieting is more common among girls and older adolescents, especially girls. The term comfort or emotional eating refers to the consumption of food even after one's energy needs have been satisfied (eating when not hungry or when already satiated) or to deal with negative emotional states (eating because of depressive feelings or boredom). Once again, this phenomenon is more common in girls and is higher at older ages. The opposite is true for boys, among whom this type of behavior seems to decrease at 18-19 years old after reaching its peak at ages 16-17. Purging behavior, meaning the use of pills, laxatives, or vomiting to lose weight or stay thin, is also more common among girls and increases constantly with age.

Diets, comfort eating, and purging behavior are highly correlated with one another and also with healthiness and regularity of eating habits (Fig. 7.13), as discussed in the previous section. These relationships indicate the existence of a single dimension that can be referred to as disturbed eating and which is expressed as dieting, comfort eating, or purging behavior. The negative relationships between comfort eating and purging behavior on the one hand, and healthiness and regularity of eating habits on the other hand provide further proof that these behavior types form a single dimension.

These relationships, however, are stronger for the female sample: in girls only, dieting is positively correlated with comfort eating, which in turn is correlated with purging behavior. There is also a link between dieting and purg-

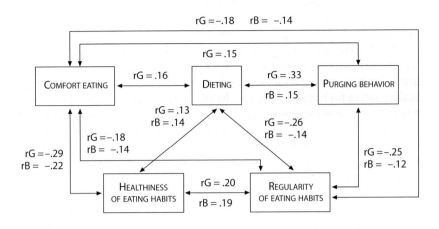

Fig. 7.13. Relationships between disturbed eating, healthiness, and eating regularity for the two genders (correlation analysis). Data contained in the figures are correlation values (r). As the analyses were carried out separately for boys and girls, the letters B and G have been used to distinguish these values.

ing behavior, which exists for both genders but is stronger for girls. Thus, disturbed eating behavior can take many forms, particularly in girls.

The results also confirm the ambiguous nature of dieting, confirmed previously by other studies (Garfinkel and Kaplan 1994): dieting is connected to other behavior aimed at losing weight, such as purging, and overeating to deal with negative emotional states, as well as greater irregularity in eating meals. The negative association between dieting and regular eating confirms that irregular eating habits, and specifically the tendency to substitute main meals with small snacks, obstructs the effectiveness of any kind of diet (Bandura 1997), just as it has been shown that there is a vicious cycle between constant nibbling and attempts to lose weight (Herman et al. 1987; De Zwaan et al. 1992).

Dieting is not always tied to a real need to lose weight: in the last six months, 50% of normal-weight girls have dieted, and 40% of all adolescents of both genders claim to be currently on a diet due to aesthetics and for health-related reasons. The motivations behind these diets limit the possibility to seek the advice of a professional, as these professionals, for ethical reasons and to safeguard patients' health, cannot prescribe diets when unnecessary. Most of the adolescents (60%) refer to a professional, such as a pharmacist, doctor or, dietitian, as the best person to prescribe a diet, and only a small percentage (10%) reported that they would not go to anyone. In reality, though, only 15% actually received advice from a specialist while the majority (60%) had not gone to anyone. However, among overweight adolescents, a higher percentage (25%) had seen a specialist about their diet.

7.5.2 Different Patterns of Disturbed Eating

Disturbed eating is a common behavior that can take a number of forms: there are those who resort to comfort eating, dieting, or purging behavior while others combine all of these behavior types (Fig. 7.14)[5]. In general, disturbed eating is a prevalently female phenomenon; girls are more involved than boys in all forms with the exception of comfort eating, and they are significantly more involved in purging behavior, which presents the most serious risks (Braet 1996; Kinzl et al. 2001). Furthermore, disturbed eating in girls, and purging behavior in particular, are higher at older ages (Fig. 7.15) and at the ages of 18-19 involve roughly one fourth of the female sample.

Intertwined with differences in gender and age are differences in the type of school the adolescents attend (Fig. 7.16): disturbed eating is more frequent and more serious in female students of vocational secondary schools and teachers' lyceums.

7.5.3 Disturbed Eating and Distorted Body Image: A Female Risk

For girls in particular, the various patterns of disturbed eating appear to be linked to negative body image and a recent weight change (Fig. 7.17 for comfort eating, Fig. 7.18 for purging behavior, Fig. 7.19 for dieting). High sensitivity to the potential negative consequences of an unhealthy lifestyle was shown to be not at all protective but actually a risk factor, as it is tied to involvement in comfort eating as well as purging behavior; in other words, the behavior

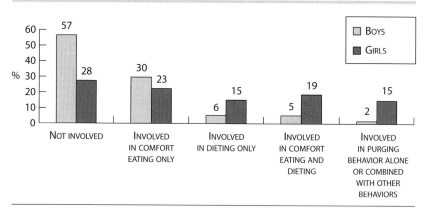

Fig. 7.14. Patterns of disturbed eating for the two genders (chi-squared).

---

[5] The "Appendix" includes a description of how the "disturbed eating" typology was constructed.

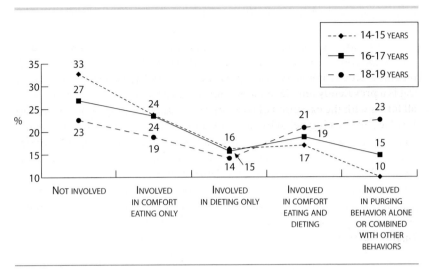

Fig. 7.15. Disturbed eating in the female sample for the different age groups (chi-squared).

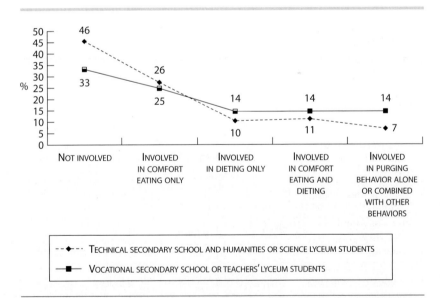

Fig. 7.16. Disturbed eating for different types of schools (chi-squared). For this analysis, the students of humanities lyceums, science lyceums, and technical secondary schools were considered together, as were students of vocational secondary schools and teachers' lyceums, as the distribution of percentages in these types of schools was found to be similar.

used to eliminate the food that has been consumed (Figs. 7.17, 7.18). The only exception is an awareness of the negative consequences of physical inactivity, which, in boys only, plays a protective role against purging behavior. An awareness of the negative psychological consequences of being overweight is strongly related with comfort eating of girls. As we mentioned previously, excessive attention to eating and, more generally, to a healthy lifestyle runs the risk of becoming an obsession with food, which in turn encourages patterns of disturbed eating behavior. This aspect must be taken into consideration when developing prevention programs in order to avoid counterproductive effects, such as the risk-provoking tactics of many magazines and television programs.

Models for positive eating habits among an individual's family members or close friends act as a protective factor, which offers further confirmation of the findings discussed earlier with regard to healthiness and regularity of daily eating habits. The fact that these positive models play a protective role may be due not only to imitation but to relational processes as well. Meals represent an important moment for dialogue and exchange within the family as well as

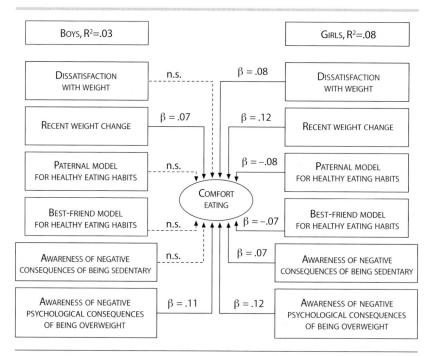

Fig. 7.17. Predictors of comfort eating in the two genders (linear regression). The following predictors were also inserted in the regression model but were not reported because they were not significant for either boys or girls: being of normal weight, maternal model for healthy eating habits, awareness of the negative consequences of inactivity, and awareness of the negative consequences of being overweight.

with friends. Dialogue can promote a more positive self-perception through the appreciation and interest shown by others while exchange with others can encourage decentralization from one's own point of view and from an excessive focus on body weight. Sharing meals with other people also signifies greater regularity and control over eating. As for the positive relationship that exists between an adolescent's behavior and the behavior of his or her best friend, the explanation can be found in the processes of reciprocal selection based on the sharing of interests, values, and activities; these processes increase the probability that adolescents will form friendships with those who are similar to themselves (Engels 1998).

As for the behavioral models within the family, the father was found to play an important protective role, in this case for girls only. Both comfort eating (Fig. 7.17) and dieting (Fig. 7.19) are reduced by a perception of one's father as a positive role model for healthy eating habits. These results evidence the need for more careful consideration of the paternal role in the development of adolescent children (Marta 1997; Scabini et al. 1999).

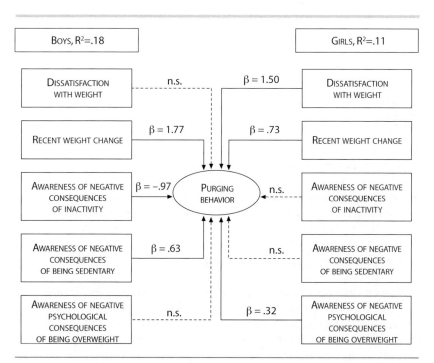

Fig. 7.18. Predictors of purging behavior for the two genders (logistic regression). The following predictors were inserted in the regression model but were not reported because they were not significant for either boys or girls: being of normal weight, maternal model for healthy eating habits, paternal model for healthy eating habits, best-friend model for healthy eating habits, awareness of the negative physical consequences of being overweight.

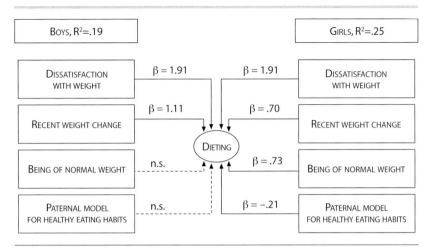

Fig. 7.19. Predictors of dieting for the two genders (logistic regression). The following predictors were inserted in the regression model but were not reported because they were not significant either for boys or girls: maternal model for healthy eating habits, best-friend model for healthy eating habits, awareness of negative consequences of inactivity, awareness of negative consequences of being sedentary, awareness of negative physical consequences of being overweight, and awareness of negative psychological consequences of being overweight.

Adolescents commonly use dieting to obtain or maintain a normal weight; this type of behavior shows no signs of diminishing with age and actually increases. This tendency exposes adolescents to various types of physical and psychological risks. The physical risks of dieting are tied mainly to an unbalanced diet, as the various diets that come into fashion exclude foods with important nutritional value. The psychological risks are related to a loss of confidence in one's self-control, which results from a vicious cycle of irregular and frequent eating, or even binging, followed by attempts to return to one's previous weight.

7.6 Functions of Disturbed Eating

Disturbed eating behavior in adolescence carries out three major functions. The first is connected to a negative self-perception and serves as an *emotional strategy for problem resolution and a way for adolescents to affirm their independence and competence*. These types of behavior are adopted particularly by adolescents who are unable to foresee other ways of dealing with the problems of daily life and demonstrating their independence and abilities. The second, related to *transgression, experimentation, and the perception of control* occurs particularly when other forms of personal achievement and other ways to test limits and take control of events are unavailable. The third function responds to a need for *communication, emulation, and surpassing* that is stronger in adolescents who have poor relationships with their family members and friends or when adolescents are unable to behave in a more responsible and committed way. These functions can have a greater or lesser importance, depending on the adolescent's gender and level of involvement in these behavior types.

7.6.1 Disturbed Eating as an Emotional Strategy for Problem Resolution and a Way to Affirm Independence and Competence

For adolescents, particularly girls, involved in purging behavior, disturbed eating is above all an emotional strategy for problem resolution. This strategy, however, is generally totally ineffective and can actually become a means of escape, further intensifying the feelings of uneasiness that are characteristic of these adolescents (Jackson and Bosma 1990; Heatherton and Baumeister 1991). Adolescents who are most involved in disturbed eating not only have a negative and distorted image of their bodies, they are also very dissatisfied with themselves in general and experience profound depressive feelings (Table 7.2); this, again, confirms the greater importance of body image for girls in the process of identity construction (Rosenberg and Simmons 1975; Kroger 2000). Also, as the construction of an individual's self-perception inter-

Table 7.2. Aspects connected to emotional strategy for problem resolution and escape (MANOVA).

	Means for the characteristics of adolescents based on eating behavior patterns					
	Boys not involved in disturbed eating	Girls not involved in disturbed eating	Boys involved in comfort eating and/or dieting	Girls involved in comfort eating and/or dieting	Boys involved in purging behavior	Girls involved in purging behavior
Overall satisfaction with self	+++++[a]	+++	+++++	++	++++	+
Perception of own academic abilities	++++	++++++	+++	+++++	+	++
Depressive feelings	+	++++	++	+++++	++	++++++
Satisfaction with relationships with peers	++++++	+++	+++++	++	++++	+
Stress caused by social life	+	++	+++	+++++	++++	++++++
Sense of alienation	+	++	+++	+++++	++++	++++++
Self-regulatory efficacy	++++++	+++++	++++	+++	+	++
Difficulty in falling asleep or sleeping	+	+++	++	++++	++++++	+++++

[a] A greater number of plus signs (+) corresponds to a higher mean; eta-squared = .07.

acts with his or her social context (Youniss and Smollar 1990), these adolescents are also dissatisfied with their relationships with peers in which they experience stress and a sense of alienation. The boys who are most involved in these behavior types are dissatisfied with their ability to control their behavior against the influence of the peer group. The discomfort and dissatisfaction that characterize those who use purging behavior are also accompanied by psychosomatic symptoms, such as difficulty in falling asleep and in sleeping regularly through the night (Noack and Krache 1997). Under these conditions of deep discomfort, disturbed eating, much like psychoactive substance use and heavy alcohol consumption, can be used in an attempt to reconstruct emotionally positive and desirable situations (Labouvie 1986).

In boys, seriously disturbed eating also represents an attempt to display their competence and good looks, evidenced by the high confidence they report in their ability to deal with the difficulties of daily life, the belief that they are attractive to the opposite sex, and their high expectations for success, which they attempt to bring about in the present through having a job (Table 7.3). This personal competence is only an appearance and is misleading not only in the present but also in the long term: in reality, expectations for high success are not accompanied by equally high expectations to continue school and acquire a secondary school diploma or a university degree.

As for girls, purging behavior is a way of affirming independence, which these adolescents aspire to highly and feel they cannot obtain in other ways (Seiffge-Krenke 1990). The girls who are most involved in this behavior lack

Table 7.3. Aspects connected to a way of affirming competence and independence (MANOVA).

	Means for the characteristics of adolescents based on eating behavior patterns					
	Boys not involved in disturbed eating	Girls not involved in disturbed eating	Boys involved in comfort eating and/or dieting	Girls involved in comfort eating and/or dieting	Boys involved in purging behavior	Girls involved in purging behavior
Believe oneself to be attractive to the opposite sex	++++[a]	+	++++++	+	+++++	+
Self-confidence in coping	++++	+++	+++++	+	++++++	++
Expectations for success	++++	+++	++++	++	++++++	+
Having a job	++++	+	++++	++	++++++	+++
Expectations to continue school	++	++++++	+++	++++	+	+++++
Value on independence	++	+++	++++	+++++	+	++++++

[a] A greater number of plus signs (+) corresponds to a higher mean.

confidence in their ability to deal with the problems of daily life and have fairly low expectations for success. They generally expect to complete their chosen academic path but are not convinced that this will lead to greater personal achievement in the future.

The fact that girls have more difficulty than boys in identifying specific plans for their future and that they feel they have little ability and little possibility of achieving their goals has also been found in other studies (Nurmi 1997). What is missing in women who decide against a greater scholastic or professional commitment is not actually the ability itself nor the value placed on these activities (Cattelino et al. 2002). These girls lack confidence in their ability to plan their actions in order to obtain success (Heatherton and Baumeister 1994; Bandura 1997). This lack of confidence has various origins, including socialization process that, still today, leads boys to develop a greater tendency toward independence and achievement and girls to develop a greater tendency toward submissiveness (Palmonari et al. 1993). Furthermore, women are more frequently required to choose between investing in either preparation for a career or interaction in affective relationships instead of being able to have both, as men commonly do. This conflict appears to be more significant for female students of vocational secondary schools, who are more involved in disturbed eating behavior. By choosing a longer educational path that opens up more opportunities for future jobs with a certain level of responsibility, lyceum students demonstrate, along with their families, that they are confident in their abilities. Their future achievements will occur in the more distant future, but it is precisely for this reason that, for these students, the future is more clearly defined and viewed more positively than it is for girls attending other schools (Silbereisen and Noack 1990). Vocational school students have undertaken a shorter educational path that, at least on paper, should lead to a more immediate introduction into the work force. However, these adolescents' plans to initiate work early risks being disregarded, as higher levels of specialization and more education are increasingly important in order to gain access to jobs in contemporary society. Also, the few jobs available for those with limited qualifications are more easily filled by men. Therefore, these girls experience greater uncertainty about their futures and how they will reach their goals; these conditions, in turn, lead to higher involvement in the various forms of disturbed eating behavior in an attempt to deal with difficulties that they are unable to confront using other resources (Crockett 1997). The different opportunities for personal fulfillment offered to boys and girls and the importance of both the professional and emotional aspect for an individual's well-being contribute to explaining the higher levels of discomfort experienced by girls, the persistence of this discomfort into adulthood, and the need to resort to disturbed eating to deal with it. In fact, for girls, disturbed eating does not tend to diminish toward the end of adolescence after reaching its peak but, rather, continues into young adulthood.

Using disturbed eating behavior as an emotional strategy for resolution and escape from problems displays serious maladjustment and actually prevents adolescents from reaching their goals of achieving independence and demonstrating their competence. Adolescents involved in this behavior can fall into a vicious cycle that is difficult to break of dissatisfaction with oneself, use of food, obsessive ritual of purging the food consumed, social isolation, and heightened dissatisfaction.

7.6.2 Disturbed Eating as Transgression, Experimentation, and a Way of Exercising Control

Disturbed eating also serves other functions, such as the transgression of adult norms, which call for well-established and, for the most part, regular eating habits. Similar to the function discussed in the previous section - disturbed eating as an emotional strategy for problem resolution - this function plays a more significant role for adolescents who are heavily involved in disturbed eating behavior; however, unlike the function discussed previously, disturbed eating as a form of transgression is more common in boys. For these adolescents, disturbed eating is a way of affirming themselves through opposition to adult rules. The transgressive function of disturbed eating is evidenced by strong relationships with low disapproval of antisocial behavior and low value on religion and on academic achievement accompanied by deep dissatisfaction with the current school experience (Table 7.4). Adolescents who feel a greater

Table 7.4. Aspects connected to the transgression and opposition function (MANOVA).

	Means for the characteristics of adolescents based on eating behavior patterns					
	Boys not involved in disturbed eating	Girls not involved in disturbed eating	Boys involved in comfort eating and/or dieting	Girls involved in comfort eating and/or dieting	Boys involved in purging behavior	Girls involved in purging behavior
Disapproval of antisocial behavior	+++[a]	++++++	++	+++++	+	++++
Value on religion	+++	++++++	++	+++++	+	++++
Value on academic achievement	+++	++++++	++	++++	+	++++
Satisfaction with the school experience	++++	++++++	+++	+++++	+	++
Perceived usefulness of school	+++	++++++	++	++++	+	+++++
Stress caused by school	+	+++	++	+++++	++++	++++++
Intention and attempts to drop out of school	++	+	+++	+++	++++++	+++++
Repeated school years	++++	+	++++	++	+++	++++++

[a] A greater number of plus signs (+) corresponds to a higher mean; eta-squared = .06.

Table 7.5. Aspects connected to experimentation and way of exercising control (MANOVA).

	Means for the characteristics of adolescents based on eating behavior patterns					
	Boys not involved in disturbed eating	Girls not involved in disturbed eating	Boys involved in comfort eating and/or dieting	Girls involved in comfort eating and/or dieting	Boys involved in purging behavior	Girls involved in purging behavior
Antisocial behavior	+++[a]	+	+++++	++	++++++	++++
Risk-taking behavior	++++	+	+++++	++	++++++	+++
Heavy alcohol consumption	++++	+	+++++	++	++++++	+++
Total number of sexual partners	++++	+	+++	++	++++++	+++++
Cigarette smoking	++	+	++++	+++	+++++	++++++
Marijuana smoking	++++	+	+++++	++	+++	++++++

[a] A greater number of plus signs (+) corresponds to a higher mean.

need to transgress through disturbed eating feel a sense of discomfort and uselessness in their daily school experience and in their current role as students. Their dissatisfaction is directed at both the quality of their social relationships within the school context, particularly with their teachers, as well as their perception that their efforts in school are useless in terms of their future achievement. This discomfort is expressed in a greater number of failed school years for girls and a greater desire to drop out of school for boys. The role of the student is the only role society recognizes for adolescents and, as a consequence, school is the favored environment in which to experiment and put one's abilities to the test (Borca et al. 2002; Moliner et al. 2004).

In this context of serious discomfort where the school experience is perceived as dissatisfying, useless, and even disastrous, adolescents resort to disturbed eating, just as they do other risk behavior (Steinberg and Avenevoli 1998; Bonino and Cattelino 2002), not only to transgress but also to experiment and test themselves, regaining a sense of having control over events (Table 7.5). Overeating because one feels depressed or simply has nothing better to do and then using various methods to eliminate the food that has been taken in can be a way of demonstrating, first and foremost to themselves, that they have control over the events in their lives. These adolescents lack this perception of control when confronting the normal developmental tasks presented by the school (Tyszkowa 1990; Määta et al. 2002).

Boys and girls have different ways of experimenting and testing themselves. Boys use more visible tactics, such as stuffing themselves with food or consuming excessive quantities of alcohol or other psychoactive substances in the company of friends, or else having promiscuous sex. These types of behavior are used both to test themselves and their ability to communicate and to temporarily assume some characteristically adult behavior, other aspects of which appear to be denied. Girls, on the other hand, favor arduous rituals, such as diets, or self-punishing rituals, such as purging behavior, in an attempt to actually conform to or to feel more similar to the models presented by the mass media. The methods used by boys respond to a need for experimentation and to test themselves in a public context in order to obtain social recognition from the peer group. The tactics used by girls, on the other hand, respond to a greater need to experiment with controlling their bodies and their physiological reactions to food, in much the same way that they test out their reactions to psychoactive substances, demonstrated by heavy involvement in smoking and marijuana use. This method of withdrawing into themselves is a regressive and ineffective way of adjusting to reality: absorbed in their own feelings, girls are unable to detach themselves from contingent situations and identify alternative ways of resolving their problems and reaching their objectives.

On the one hand, the adolescents involved in disturbed eating display a greater need to redefine their identity by differentiating themselves visibly from adults and using behavior that is disapproved of by adults, such as gorging themselves or, in the opposite extreme, refusal to eat. On the other hand, these adolescents also demonstrate a deep need to identify with the more external, evident aspects of adulthood, such as showing that they are grown up, good-looking, or thin. Their behavior expresses compliance and dependence and is evidence of an uncritical adherence to the values of contemporary postmodern society, which hold "appearing" above "being," the external above the internal, and immediate gratification of the self and one's desires above postponed gratification.

The school experience plays a significant role in influencing students' needs to resort to these strategies in order to affirm themselves. For adolescents who do poorly in school, the current negative experience, often sparked by a previous, equally disastrous experience (Fonzi 2002), entails not only personal discomfort but also poor development of critical tools that enable us to detach ourselves from advertising messages and fashions. The school curriculum itself in the various types of schools can encourage the development of these abilities. Girls who attend vocational schools, who have had less opportunity to study literature and art, and to witness and reflect on the various models of feminine beauty that have come to pass over the centuries, are significantly more likely to hold thinness as an undisputed ideal.

7.6.3 Disturbed Eating as Communication, Emulation, and Surpassing

The functions of emulation and surpassing refer to the strong symbolic ties between eating and communication within social relationships and to daily rituals in which eating is viewed in terms of sharing (Eibl-Eibesfeldt 1974) and similarity of habits. These functions apply mainly to adolescents whose social network of family and friends is lacking both in quantity and quality. In other words, when there is a condition of solitude, both subjective and objective, that is linked to a negative emotional state (Marcoen and Goosens 1993; Lo Coco et al. 2001), this emptiness may be filled by disturbed eating rituals.

Parents of adolescents who are most heavily involved with disturbed eating behavior generally communicate less with their children and show little interest in controlling the behavior adopted by their children when outside the home and encouraging shared activities within the family context (Table 7.6). Adolescents themselves judge this condition as stressful because, at this age, they still have a rather strong need to be listened to and to share in family activities, such as having meals together (Ciairano 2004). When adolescents are given small daily tasks, such as taking care of younger brothers or sisters, they feel as if they are an important resource to the family, which encourages the development of a greater sense of responsibility.

When these aspects are missing from or are insufficient in the family context, adolescents attempt to satisfy their needs for communication and sharing through other relationships, both with other adults and with peers. This is evidenced by the strong ties, particularly among girls, with references to other adults, a greater orientation toward friends, and a greater commitment to building and maintaining social relationships. However, as other studies have also found (Helsen et al. 2000), this attempt is generally ineffective, as rela-

Table 7.6. Aspects connected to the sharing and communication function (MANOVA).

	Means for the characteristics of adolescents based on eating behavior patterns					
	Boys not involved in disturbed eating	Girls not involved in disturbed eating	Boys involved in comfort eating and/or dieting	Girls involved in comfort eating and/or dieting	Boys involved in purging behavior	Girls involved in purging behavior
Parental support	+++++[a]	++++++	+++	++++	++	+
Parental control for behavior outside the home	+++	++++++	++	+++++	+	++++
Time spent weekly in family activities	++++	++++++	+++	+++++	+	++
Stress caused by family life	+	++	+++	++++	+++++	++++++
Reference to other adults	+	++++	++	++++	+++	++++++
Orientation toward friends in making decisions	+	+++	++++	+++++	++	++++++
Time spent weekly in social activities	+	+	+++	++++	+++++	++++++
Friends' support	++	++++++	+++	++++	+	+++++

[a] A greater number of plus signs (+) corresponds to a higher mean.

tionships outside the family are unable to compensate for poor relationships with family members. Actually, a synergy of effects often comes into play: those who perceive their family relationships as poor and who receive little support from their parents are also less able to build solid, satisfying relationships with people outside their family and vice versa. This is often the case for adolescents who are most involved in disturbed eating behavior. Boys, in particular, receive little support from parents and from their friends. Girls prefer to seek models to identify with outside the family. For both boys and girls, an early or excessive orientation toward other adults or peers, combined with a greater urgency to find models to identify with outside the family - a family they feel neither listens to nor appreciates them - can translate into a poorer ability to select these models and a greater probability they will be selected without proper criteria.

Adolescents who are most involved in disturbed eating behavior have a strong need for communication and exchange with others, and this need, in boys particularly, remains unsatisfied despite an active, at times even frenetic, social life that is poor in substance and lacks the planning that could lend it meaning and value. With the friends these adolescents choose, they take part in more risk behavior and fewer conventional activities, such as studying and spending time with the family (Table 7.7). Driven by a desire to avoid being excluded (Seiffge-Krenke and Shulman 1993), these adolescents, along with

Table 7.7. Aspects connected to the emulation and surpassing function (MANOVA).

	Means for the characteristics of adolescents based on eating behavior patterns					
	Boys not involved in disturbed eating	Girls not involved in disturbed eating	Boys involved in comfort eating and/or dieting	Girls involved in comfort eating and/or dieting	Boys involved in purging behavior	Girls involved in purging behavior
Friends' models for risk behavior	++[a]	+	+++	++++	+++++	++++++
Time spent weekly in public places (coffee bars, video arcades, discotheques)	++++	+	+++	++	++++++	+++++
Friends' models for conventional behavior	++++	++++++	+++++	+++	+	++
Time spent weekly studying and reading	+++	++++++	++	+++++	+	++++
Time spent weekly doing nothing	++	+	++++	+++++	+++	++++++
Time spent weekly exercising alone	++++	+++	+++++	++	++++++	+

[a] A greater number of plus signs (+) corresponds to a higher mean.

their friends, take part in activities that lack planning and in which they seek to emulate and surpass one another, evidenced by the fact that they report spending less time in reflective activities, such as studying and reading, and more time in exclusively recreational activities, such as going to pubs or discotheques. Girls who are most involved in disturbed eating spend a good portion of their time doing nothing, further evidence of the major differences between boys and girls in the ways they manifest their discomfort: in boys, discomfort is expressed through action while girls use the avoidance of action along with self-criticism (Rodriguez-Tomé and Bariaud 1990).

The relationship between disengagement or even absence of activity and psychological discomfort has been investigated further in recent studies: adolescents need to have experiences in which they can test their abilities through challenging tasks. These challenges are essential to the development of a stronger sense of responsibility, a greater interest in the activities they are involved in, and higher expectations for success (Marta et al. 1998; Csikszentmihalyi and Schneider 2000). Although they are considered pleasant because they are free from any potentially anxiety-causing content, purely recreational activities, such as spending time in bars, video arcades, or discotheques, are unable to test adolescents and provide them with a realistic evaluation of their abilities. Thus, it is the responsibility of adults to make sure that adolescents and young people have access to challenging activities instead of strictly recreational and nonorganized activities.

Finally, we observed that disturbed eating, which is often accompanied by an obsession with the body and the figure, is not related to greater involvement in sports: only boys dedicate more time to exercising alone, probably aimed at improving their physical appearance. For these boys, too, the attention they dedicate to their bodies responds above all to a need to appear, rather than to actually *be*, healthy.

7.6.4 The Highest Risk Group

The results displayed in the previous sections have shown that purging behavior are the most dangerous type of disturbed eating behavior. As some adolescents use this behavior only sporadically, we asked ourselves how these adolescents differ from those who carry out the behavior often. The results of this analysis, displayed in Fig. 7.20, show that adolescents who vomit or take laxatives frequently have the worst functioning and the worst psychological adjustment. These adolescents perceive a high degree of discomfort, expressed by a strong sense of alienation and low expectations to continue school. This discomfort is not alleviated at all by other personal or environmental resources, such as the possibility of dialogue and contact with parents or a school experience that is perceived as at least *good enough*. Furthermore, these adolescents also appear to be quite tolerant of and actually involved in antisocial behavior, just as they are involved in risky behavior and psychoactive substance use,

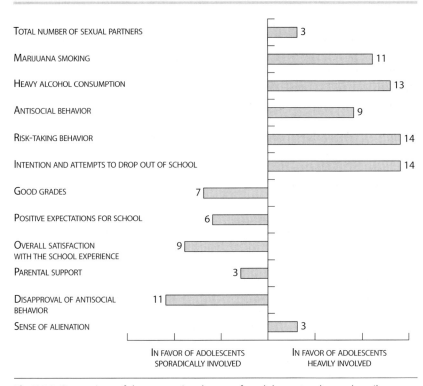

Fig. 7.20. Comparison of the proportional means for adolescents who are heavily or sporadically involved in purging behavior.

Summary 7.1. Main functions carried out by the various forms of disturbed eating.

Disturbed eating
• EMOTIONAL STRATEGY FOR PROBLEM RESOLUTION: purging behavior (especially for girls)
• ILLUSORY WAY OF AFFIRMING IDENTITY: purging behavior (especially for girls)
• ILLUSORY WAY OF AFFIRMING COMPETENCE: purging behavior (especially for boys)
• TRANSGRESSION and OPPOSITION of social norms, which call for regular, moderated eating habits
• EXPERIMENTATION, through highly noticeable eating habits (especially for boys)
• REGAINING SELF-CONTROL: through controlling one's body and eating (especially for girls)
• SOCIAL ACCEPTANCE AND RECOGNITION, through noncritically aspiring to the models of beauty presented by the media: comfort eating and dieting (especially for girls)
• EMULATION AND SURPASSING of the behavior of others to measure oneself against others and prove oneself: irregular, unhealthy eating habits (especially for boys)
• COMMUNICATION of discomfort by adopting eating behavior that is not shared by the family: irregular, unhealthy eating habits (especially for boys)

presenting both internalized and externalized behavior. For these adolescents in particular, disturbed eating is used as an emotional strategy - however counterproductive and maladjusted - for avoiding problems, as a form of transgression of society's norms, and as a way to express a deep sense of distress. As other studies have also found (Jessor et al. 1991; Jessor 1998; Ciairano 2004) our results confirm the high degree of discomfort and lack of adjustment that is characteristic of the adolescents who are seriously involved in these types of behavior. Summary 7.1 reports the functions carried out by the various, more or less maladjusted, forms of disturbed eating.

7.7 Main Protective and Risk Factors

We have seen that numerous, often intertwined, factors contribute to disturbed eating behavior. At this point, we ask ourselves which of these factors, in the different contexts of family, school experience, peer group, and free time, can play a protective role or increase risk for adolescents.

First of all, relationships with peers are more important for boys than they are for girls, which confirms the central role of these relationships in boys' development (Rodriguez-Tomé and Bariaud 1990). For boys, stress related to social life and models for unhealthy eating habits are important risk factors. Being able to rely on strong regulatory efficacy to fight peer pressure along with a high level of parental support, and participation in challenging activities that encourage the ability to reflect and make plans, such as studying and reading, are protective factors (Fig. 7.21).

As for girls, processes tied to identity construction and positive self-perception play a central role in involvement in disturbed eating behavior (Bosma and Kunnen 2001). In fact, the only protective factor for girls is an overall satisfaction with oneself while risk factors include stress related to the social life and family life, the desire to drop out of school, and time spent doing nothing (Fig. 7.22).

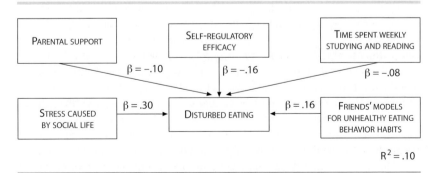

Fig. 7.21. Protective and risk factors in boys (logistic regression).

In order to further analyze the role played by overall family functioning, parenting styles were also examined. A number of factors are involved in the definition of the various parenting styles, including dialogue, emotional closeness, and control (Ciairano et al. 2001). Significant relationships with disturbed eating were found in girls only. In general, authoritative and supportive parenting styles appear to be more effective than authoritarian or permissive/nonexistent styles in countering purging behavior (Fig. 7.23). Even these two parenting styles, however, seem not to be able to prevent other disturbed eating behavior, such as dieting and comfort eating. This finding reveals that the development of body image at this age is strongly influenced by the models presented by society, which, in Western culture, elevate thinness to an ethical and not merely an aesthetic virtue (McDonald and Thompson 1992; Pinhas et al. 1999).

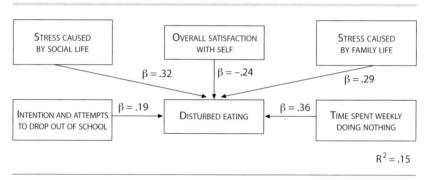

Fig. 7.22. Protective and risk factors for girls (logistic regression).

Healthier eating habits are promoted by different factors for boys and girls. For girls, a positive self-perception, also in a physical sense, should be encouraged, along with the ability to reach preestablished goals without wasting time ruminating or doing nothing. It is in this empty time that a vicious cycle of disturbed eating can be set into motion: dissatisfaction, comfort eating, attempts to regain control through purging the food consumed, overeating, dissatisfaction with appearance, attempts to diet, and so on. For boys, the most effective strategies involve promoting the ability to behave independently instead of following the crowd (Pastorelli et al. 2001) and offering opportunities to take part in meaningful activities that provide them with the chance to affirm themselves and prove their competence (Mahoney and Stattin 2000) without having to resort to gorging themselves or other risky behavior in order to measure themselves against their friends and surpass them to obtain their recognition.

The main protective factors are theorically identified in Summary 7.2. These factors have been linked to the main functions carried out by the vari-

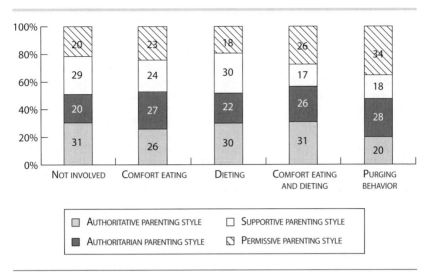

Fig. 7.23. Disturbed eating and parenting style - female sample (chi-squared).

ous forms of disturbed eating. In the face of the increasing pervasiveness and widespread nature of commercial models of beauty and the values presented by the media (Henderson-King and Henderson-King 1997; Crockett and Silbereisen 2000b), promoting these protective factors and countering the risk factors is a challenge not only for adolescents (Silbereisen 1998). The results presented in this study provide clear evidence that these models and values are unsuited to promote optimal development both during and after adolescence, particularly for individuals who lack sufficient resources and especially in terms of the ability to reflect and reason critically. In the absence of these resources, there is a risk that disturbed eating, which can be defined as an "antisocial social behavior" (Gordon 1990), may prevail.

Summary 7.2. Main protective factors and related functions of disturbed eating.

Protective factors	Related functions
PERSON • Positive body image • Positive self-perception • Expectations to continue school • Value on academic achievement • Value on religion • Disapproval of antisocial behavior	Being satisfied with oneself encourages the construction of a positive identity instead of the use of EMOTIONAL STRATEGIES FOR PROBLEM RESOLUTION (especially for girls). Personal plans and goals to achieve through commitment to school favor the adoption of HEALTHY BEHAVIOR instead of ILLUSORY METHODS of AFFIRMING INDEPENDENCE AND COMPETENCE. The sharing of religious values and peaceful coexistence encourages IDENTIFICATION with the adult world and society instead of TRANSGRESSION and OPPOSITION (especially for girls).
FAMILY • Orientation toward parents in making decisions • Parental support • Parental control over behavior outside the home • Authoritative parenting style	Parental models for healthy behavior and an orientation toward parents in making decisions encourage: • IDENTIFICATION instead of SEEKING MODELS OUTSIDE THE FAMILY. • Assuming a HEALTHY LIFESTYLE instead of EMULATION and SURPASSING. Living in a family environment where there is an orderly pace of life, rules for behavior, the possibility of dialogue, and emotional closeness favors HEALTHY MEANS OF SELF-AFFIRMATION instead of disturbed or irregular eating as a MEANS OF AFFIRMING INDEPENDENCE, TESTING SELF AND LIMITS, and COMMUNICATING a sense of discomfort. The right combination of parental support and control encourages: • The gradual acquisition of INDEPENDENCE and RESPONSIBILITY. • The use of COPING STRATEGIES based on verbalization and comparing points of view instead of ESCAPE. • The reinforcement of the ability to REFLECT and SELF-REGULATE instead of EMULATION and the need to REGAIN CONTROL.

Cont. ▸▸

Protective factors	Related functions
SCHOOL EXPERIENCE • Positive expectations of own abilities • Perceived usefulness for the future • Satisfaction with the school experience • School success (good grades)	Expectations of one's own abilities, the perception that a commitment to school will be useful for the future, and satisfaction with and success in school encourage: • THE ASSUMPTION OF RESPONSIBILITY and LONG-TERM COMMITMENTS instead of TRANSGRESSION and ESCAPE from commitment. • VALUING ONESELF and one's role as a student instead of the use of EMOTIONAL STRATEGIES FOR PROBLEM RESOLUTION (especially in girls). • The DEVELOPMENT of THE ABILITY TO REFLECT AND REASON CRITICALLY acquired by studying literature, history, and art, instead of noncritical adherence to models and behavior promoted by the media.
PEERS • Friends' models for healthy behavior • Friends' models for conventional behavior • Self-regulatory efficacy	Friends' models for healthy behavior encourage: • IDENTIFICATION and assumption of a healthy lifestyle. • Fewer occasions to share unhealthy foods. The perception of one's friends as nontransgressive encourages: • Processes of IDENTIFICATION AND DIFFERENTIATION based on the sharing of ideas and constructive activities instead of ILLUSORY WAYS of affirming oneself or escaping from problems. • EXPERIMENTATION with socially accepted roles and actions instead of TRANSGRESSION and EXPERIMENTATION with disturbed eating behavior. • The perception of the SOCIAL ACCEPTANCE AND RECOGNITION unrelated to models of beauty and fashion. Strong ability to SELF-REGULATE in the face of the behavior of others instead of EMULATION AND SURPASSING.
FREE TIME • Time spent weekly studying and reading	Time spent weekly studying and reading encourages the development of: • A SENSE OF RESPONSIBILITY and AWARENESS OF ONE'S OWN VALUE. • PLANNING SKILLS and COMMITMENT instead of the use of EMOTIONAL COPING STRATEGIES.

CHAPTER 8

Prevention: What Can We Do?

> But to the extent that teenagers have had experiences that demand discipline, require the skilful use of mind and body, and give them a sense of responsibility and involvement with useful goals, we might expect the youth of today to be ready to face the challenges of tomorrow.
>
> *[M. Csikentmihalyi and B. Schneider, Becoming Adult, 2000]*

8.1 The Health and Well-Being Myth

According to the definition in the World Health Organization (WHO) charter dated 1946, "health is a state of complete physical, mental, and social well-being and not merely the absence of disease or infirmity." This definition had the undisputed merit, in a period in which health was conceived in purely physical terms, of emphasizing the entirety of the person and therefore of moving from a narrow, limited concept to a much broader view that includes physical as well as psychological and social aspects. For this reason the WHO definition was met with a great deal of consensus, and the concept of health gradually expanded to a broader view of well-being, which it eventually came to encompass. The connection between physical, psychological, and social aspects in determining the state of one's health has been confirmed in numerous studies and is the basis for the so-called biopsychosocial approach (Engel 1977). According to this model, health and illness are the result of an interaction between psychosocial and biological factors.

The most recent research on the relationships between psyche and soma, and more specifically between mind, brain, and immune system, has clarified and defined some aspects of the relationship between psychosocial well-being and physical health although many aspects still remain unclear. With regard to adolescence in particular, studies have highlighted the specific influence of psychological well-being on physical health (Spruijt-Metz 1999) and the fact that the negative effects of risk behavior influence physical as well as psychological health both in the short and long term.

The WHO definition, which essentially identifies the broadest meaning of well-being with health, might therefore seem particularly appropriate and useful. Yet, in reality, with a more careful reading, it opens itself to a number of criticisms and poses a number of risks. As Antonovsky, a well-known scholar in the area of health observed (1979), the first misgiving derives from the impossibility of translating such a broad definition into practical terms. This, indeed, makes it useless on a concrete level, as it is so totally all-encompassing that it eludes any attempt to actually work with it. This impossibility brings us to an even more serious criticism, which in time led the author cited to assume a position that contrasts neatly with this definition of health. As developmental psychologists, we have no choice but to share these criticisms.

In the first place, this definition proposes an objective that is unrealistic and impossible to accomplish, as no one is able to achieve and maintain over time a condition of complete physical, psychological, and social well-being; if this is the definition of health, none of us, except in a few quickly passing moments, can claim to be healthy. As a consequence of this utopian concept of health - which Antonovsky reproaches as naïve - unrealistic optimism, the imbalances, discomfort, crises, and temporary maladjustment that people experience over the course of their lifetimes, both on the physical level and psychological and social levels, are viewed negatively and are seen as unhealthy. In reality, these situations are not only frequent but are actually the normal conditions under which individuals achieve well-adjusted relationships between themselves and their surrounding environment and in which living systems, particularly humankind, evolve.

A negative view of imbalance has no foundation in modern biology, which traces the emergence of vital, increasingly complex structures with higher levels of organization to situations of imbalance and disorder (Laborit 1987): in complex systems governed by the ability to self-organize, order emerges out of disorder (Kauffman 1993). A negative concept also finds no foundation within developmental psychology. Balance, which was spoken of by Piaget (1964; 1975) and Werner (1940), is not a stagnant situation but rather a dynamic condition in which individuals change in relation to their environment and the changes in this environment and, through this exchange, they improve their life opportunities. In the pursuit of a better-adjusted relationship with reality, individuals experience constant changes and imbalance that, over the course of development, lead to a new sense of equilibrium characterized by greater stability and flexibility. Modern systemic developmental theory (Ford and Lerner 1992) has resumed this concept, viewing development as an incremental change that is able to realize greater complexity, coherence, and stability in people and their relationships with the environment.

Although development gradually brings about a more complex, highly structured equilibrium, it is always achieved through imbalance. This is particularly evident in adolescence when, as noted earlier, the forms of discontinuity introduced by biological, cognitive, and social development are significant and often sudden. For this reason, times of crisis should be viewed positively and not negatively, or better yet, as normal periods of change and opportunities for growth; it should be noted that conditions of imbalance, discomfort, and uneasiness do not necessarily have a negative impact on health and development. For example, it has been shown that the process that leads adolescents to emotional independence from their parents, essential to both psychological and physical well-being, is by no means painless but rather includes periods of crisis and discomfort, indicative of the profound behavioral, cognitive, and emotional transformations this process involves (Lo Coco et al. 2000; Lo Coco et al. 2001). The development of affective and sexual relationships is also not without experiences of discomfort. An idealistic concept of health does not allow us to comprehend these times of imbalance and suffering, which are actually essential to development and thus are not to be avoided.

More generally speaking, the concept of health as a perfect state of psychological and physical well being also involves another risk: that of negatively evaluating not only times of crisis that occur throughout development but also the unavoidable deficiencies that individuals may have either on a physical or social and psychological level. In fact, these deficiencies are viewed as defects that prevent individuals from reaching a state of complete well-being instead of as the inevitably imperfect combination of strengths and limitations that individuals have to reckon with and in relation to which their development unfolds (see Fig. 1.5).

These strengths and limitations change over the course of one's lifetime (for example, an adolescent normally has greater physical strength than an elderly person); they change in terms of individual differences based on genetic inheritance and the complex interrelationship that occurs over the course of development between biological predispositions and environmental opportunities. For example, a certain adolescent may have stronger athletic abilities than another who, in turn, is more talented musically. Psychology today sees development as a process of gradual change that does not have the same predetermined targets for everyone but rather occurs over time in relation to the limitations and opportunities that derive from an individual's biological make-up and environmental context. It is in relation to these conditions that individuals seek to achieve a well-adjusted and balanced relationship with their surrounding environment. This theoretical concept leads us to evaluate well-being not in abstract, utopian, or normative terms but rather in relation to the actual possibilities and limitations that individuals meet with in their lives or that are present in a given moment of their existence. Well-being and development can therefore be considered possible, even in the presence of serious obstacles both of an environmental (for example, a family with only one parent) and biological (for example, a child with a genetic disease) nature. On a practical level, this positive view takes form in the task of guaranteeing the best possible conditions for well-being and development despite biological, psychological, or environmental limitations.

If crisis and imbalance are normal developmental processes; if limitations and obstacles are the conditions under which development occurs; if, in short, development and well-being are not defined by the absence of crises or limitations; it follows that these cannot be viewed as negative elements to refuse and to eliminate at all costs. On the other hand, as individuals are active players in their development, along the course of their lives, they must learn to recognize and confront these crises and limitations and to work through them to reach the highest possible level of well-being and development.

Here we can identify yet another negative consequence of idealistically defining health as a state of perfect well-being: the inability to confront difficulties, limitations, and imbalances and transform them into opportunities for development or, at the very least, into conditions that do not obstruct development. As we pointed out numerous times, individuals themselves play an active role in their development, and precisely from the differences in individuals' abilities to recognize and confront imbalance and negative or unexpected conditions (for example, an unexpected accident), can arise different paths of personal development as well as different opportunities to experience well-being on a physical, psychological, and social level. The result of a utopian vision of health is a total inability to adjust to situations that do not correspond to an ideal of perfection. Instead of learning to deal with illness, limitations, imbalance, and times of crisis, individuals pursue an ideal of perfection that is free of all of these aspects. Gradually, they become incapable of adjusting to these situations, which come to appear as more serious than they actually are. An example of this phenomenon can be found in those who undergo dangerous surgeries in order to correct slight physical imperfections, which they subjectively experience as intolerable. As we saw in Chap. 7, some girls in particular are victims of the myth of aesthetic perfection, which idealizes thinness at the expense of health. In terms of relationships with others, the perfection myth can lead to a refusal of those people who are affected by imbalance, disease, or imperfection. This is often the case in respect of elderly people, whose potential for development is often not considered, as there is a tendency to focus solely on the growing biological limitations that affect them. Accepting imbalance and limitations certainly does not mean assuming an attitude of passive acceptance but rather strengthening the ability - both one's own and that of others - to confront difficulty and use times of crisis as opportunities for development.

Contemporary developmental psychology guides us to a much more realistic and productive concept that recognizes both imbalance and limitations as constituent parts of the human condition. This concept is coherent with the models proposed by health psychology, which deny the existence of conditions of absolute health or well-being and affirm that health and illness, like well-being and discomfort, are not static but dynamic conditions; they are the extremes of a continuum on which people may be situated in different places at different times of their lives. Thus, the utopian, static definition supplied by WHO is replaced by a realistic, dynamic concept that Antonovsky defined with a neologism as the salutogenesis approach. This definition makes no dichotomous distinctions between health and illness but rather sees health as a continuum that ranges from maximum well-being to maximum suffering (health ease/disease continuum) (Antonovsky 1987). Contrary to the traditional pathogenesis approach characteristic of many epidemiological studies, the crucial question in this approach is not what causes illness but rather what allows people to maintain or to regain health despite exposure to risk factors.

The need to move from a static model of illness to a dynamic model of health, which identifies varying degrees of vitality and efficiency in different physiological systems, as well as different levels of physical and psychological functioning, is a central focus of health psychology today. This field also emphasizes the active role of individuals in promoting their own health and therefore preventing illness. Health is not only the result of external influences or biological conditions; it is closely tied to an individual's behavior, lifestyle, attitudes, and beliefs. In particular, studies on sense of coherence (Antonovsky 1987; Mroziak and Frączek 1999) and the perception of self-efficacy (Bandura 1997) have demonstrated that the individual constitutes a crucial variable. This has led us to modify the way we conceive the role of stress in the cause of illness and of psychosocial discomfort. The different ways in which people deal with stressful situations are much more important than the seriousness of stress itself. Thus, our attention must shift from the characteristics of the factors that provoke stress to an analysis of an individual's coping skills and degree of tolerance for stress.

8.2 Prevention Methods

In the following pages, we attempt to provide a better understanding of prevention of risk behavior in adolescence based, in the first place, on dynamic and not idealistic models, and, in the second place, on the results of our study, which conceives risk behavior as action laden with subjective meaning and that, during adolescence, performs specific developmental functions.

When studying adolescence, a utopian concept of health and well-being is particularly negative, as it is incapable of comprehending the imbalances that are entirely normal in a period that requires a great deal of restructuring and adjustment. This approach superficially diagnoses risk behavior as pathological, as it does not correspond to the ideals of health and well-being and fails to consider the positive functions this behavior can carry out in a normal process of development. Recognizing these functions does not imply justifying or making light of the seriousness of this behavior, which can have highly negative consequences both in the short- and long term, but rather, understanding what this behavior means for adolescents in their normal processes of development and making sure that adolescents can obtain the same positive objectives through actions that are less harmful to their health and less dangerous for their future development.

The model of health as a static condition of absolute well-being leads us mistakenly to view prevention as a tool to guarantee this ideal outcome, thus affirming the possibility of preventing every imbalance and problematic behavior during adolescence. As this is, in fact, impossible, it gives rise to yet another problem: adults find it difficult to deal with this period and its disharmony and come to consider adolescents as a problem and a source of discomfort for society. They are unable to see that adolescents represent the future of the community and can actually be a precious resource. The media's strong emphasis on the troubles of adolescence is tied in part to the overall tendency toward exaggeration that is characteristic of the media, which constantly seeks, in this as in other areas, to capture the attention of the public. However, this emphasis appears to be tied as well to an actual inability by many adults to deal with adolescents who do not correspond to their unrealistic, prepackaged ideal of perfection. The real adolescents that we come into contact with on a daily basis are quite different from those seen in the impossibly perfect *Mulino Bianco* ("White Mill") family from the famous Italian television advertisements. When compared with these examples, real adolescents risk seeming absolutely unbearable. As a consequence, any adolescent behavior that diverges from this illusion of perfection is considered as an anomaly or pathological (see Box 1.2).

This utopian view is often accompanied by deterministic models, on the basis of which it is believed that adolescent imbalance can be prevented by acting early, working on the assumption that the earlier an intervention occurs, the more certain we can be of its result. Thus, it is held that adolescent risk behavior can be prevented by intervening in the early phases of development, asserting more or less consciously that there is an obligatory connection between the past, particularly the early phases of development, and the age of adolescence. In this respect, it is necessary to make a distinction between the progressive development of individual cognitive, emotional, and social competencies, which occurs throughout all of development and thus begins from one's first experiences, and the appearance of specific imbalances, problems, and behavior that are tied to the developmental tasks of adolescence. The gradual development of competency allows individuals to reach adolescence with an ample supply of ability that allows them to successfully confront the specific developmental tasks of this age. However, in this case, we are referring not to the prevention of a given behavior but to the development of one's potential over the entire course of the developmental period.

The various types of risk behavior, however, are characteristic of the period of adolescence, as they represent the ways that adolescents have found to deal with the developmental tasks of this age in a certain context and with the resources that they have at their disposal *in the present*. Having a larger store of resources, beginning from early childhood, can certainly be helpful in dealing with these tasks and provides a solid foundation on which to build the particular competencies that their new condition as adolescents requires. But the prevention of a specific risk behavior cannot be confronted until the moment in which these developmental tasks are posed or begin to be posed. In other words, the prevention of marijuana use cannot take place in primary school, as we saw proposed recently in a program presented by a school authority, because substance use is a possible adolescent response to a developmental task of adolescence in a specific life context. Along these same lines, studies on the prevention of smoking tobacco have highlighted (Engels 1998) that there is no relationship between being opposed to smoking at the end of primary school and involvement in smoking in early adolescence; for children, smoking has no psychological importance or significance, and a negative attitude toward smoking at this age does not guarantee the rejection of this behavior at a later age. In general, the most opportune time for an effective intervention is when habits or a single behavior are beginning to change (Spruijt-Metz 1999) and individuals become aware of these changes. Although these times can vary widely from one adolescent to another in relation to a number of individual variables (the onset of puberty, for example) and contextual variables (the models offered by family and friends, for example), a "cohort effect" comes into play. Useful information on this phenomenon can be found in the findings of recent studies on the involvement of large groups of adolescents in various types of risk behavior. The results displayed in the previous chapters point to the existence of critical ages for approach to and experimentation with different types of risk behavior as well as for the establishment of involvement.

8.3 Risk Behavior: The Main Protective Factors

In an approach that is centered around disease, a great deal of attention was dedicated to risk factors, as it was thought to be of primary importance to identify all the elements that, both on an individual and contextual level, can put one's health at risk in order to eliminate these risks or prevent their onset. For instance, difficult temperament and chronic conflict between parents were identified as risk factors during adolescence.

In the dynamic and nondichotomous concept that, as we have seen, is characteristic of modern health psychology, the central question no longer relates only to factors that can predict negative results; it is held to be more productive to ask ourselves what can favor a positive result even in the presence of negative conditions (Rutter 1990). This is a considerable change in perspective that has significant consequences in the field of prevention. The focus is shifted from risk factors to protective factors, providing not only a more structured view of the complexity of adolescent developmental conditions but, most importantly, offering broader prospects for action in the present. Many risk factors are actually part of an adolescent's past (for example, a troubled family experience), and therefore, although interventions can alter the adolescent's representations of these experiences, the experiences themselves cannot actually be changed. Still other risk factors cannot be altered directly by educators or health workers due to both their complexity and to the fact that they are outside the competence of their field of action (for instance, financial difficulties or family conflicts). Basing our actions on protective factors, on the other hand, we are able to confront conditions of risk with interventions that can be carried out in the present and that are within the reach of a variety of figures (teachers, educators, psychologists) who work with adolescents.

In terms of preventing risk behavior, protective factors can be defined as particular characteristics or situations that decrease the probability of involvement or reduce involvement if already in course, or as factors that serve to limit the environmental risk factors in what is referred to as the "buffer effect." These factors and their characteristics were discussed at length in Chap. 3 (in the "Protective Factors" section), and it is thanks to them that even adolescents who live in disadvantaged conditions are able to successfully construct a positive developmental path and to limit - both quantitatively and qualitatively - their involvement in dangerous behavior (Rutter 1996).

As we have already noted, protective factors can relate as much to the individual as to the context, as there is constant interaction between these two aspects. Our research suggested different protective factors that could be traced to different contexts of adolescents' lives - family, school, community - as well as to the adolescents themselves and, in particular, their attitudes and actions. Here, we will discuss the most important factors, which are not specific to a single behavior but were found to be protective for all types of risk behavior studied.

The family constitutes an extremely important protective factor that acts in both a specific and general way. At a specific level, the positive adult models it poses are crucial. It should be noted that along with family members' behavior (for example, not smoking or driving safely) the family also plays a protective role in terms of other factors that are often underestimated, such as attitudes of explicit disapproval toward risk behavior (for example, of smoking tobacco or marijuana). More generally speaking, the family acts through the parenting style used by the parents. Confirming many other studies, our research indicates that the most protective is the authoritative parenting style, which combines adequate supervision of children's behavior, explicit rules that children are required to respect, and constant openness to dialogue. Protective figures are therefore parents who play a strong educational role and who consider it appropriate to impose rules and to supervise adolescent children, especially younger adolescents, but who are also able to take their children seriously and listen to and discuss the difficulties they experience. These adolescents know that they can count on their parents, who have not abdicated their educational role nor abandoned their children to a kind of freedom that borders on indifference and who are sources of advice they can always turn to.

Another very important area for achievement in the lives of adolescents is school. Here, adolescents spend a large part of their time and test their abilities in a number of tasks, which it is crucial that they overcome both at present and for their future. The main protective factors tied to school can be traced to the type of experience adolescents have in this context. Important aspects from this point of view are satisfaction with the school experience, well-being at school and being successful in school. Boys and girls who enjoy school, who make good grades, and who view school as a positive experience, which is useful at present and for their futures, are less at risk for involvement in risk behavior. The sense of accomplishment that these adolescents find in doing well in school and in responding to the expectations of society and their families prevents them from having to seek superficial ways of asserting themselves. This, combined with commitment to long-term plans that include absorbing, realistic challenges, therefore diminishes the need to seek other challenges and other forms of experimentation. These data confirm the need to invest in both school attendance - as the boys and girls at highest risk have considered or attempted to drop out of school - and in the quality of the experiences adolescents have at school (Bonino and Cattelino 2002).

Even the community, both on a global and local scale, can play a protective role, first by reducing the pressures to grow up fast - pressures that are motivated today by the market, which urges consumption. Second, the community should have a greater acceptance of the adolescent period, acting on the conviction that the entire community must be committed to the development of its citizens of tomorrow. Adolescents who feel they are accepted for whom they are and are aided in making plans for their personal success and achievement are less involved in risk behavior (Benard 1991).

This greater acceptance is protective when it is put into action by providing adolescents with opportunities for experimentation and self-actualization: involvement in risk behaviors is greater when adolescents have too much "empty time" spent primarily in recreational activities that do not include challenges capable of enhancing their identity. Being asked to act responsibly toward the local community is also protective; this request means that adolescents are considered as individuals who have something to contribute to their town or neighborhood and are not only an irritating problem that "something must be done about". Note that the results from our research indicate that adolescents are less involved in risk behavior when their communities provide gathering places where they can take part in personally significant and socially recognized activities with other young people. The kind of positive visibility found in these settings is highly protective. Even more protective are the groups that offer adolescents the chance to reflect on themselves, their lives, their future, their plans for personal achievement, their values, and their relationships with others, encouraged by the educational presence of adults. In Italy today, these experiences are provided almost exclusively by religiously affiliated groups and therefore participation in them is limited to adolescents who share the religious views professed there; however, involvement by a much greater number of adolescents in these types of groups would be desirable. Once again, this confirms the necessity of the presence of adults who play a strong educational role, who provide adolescents with opportunities for other kinds of experiences than simply gatherings with their peers, and who do not consider adolescents a strange or dangerous presence but rather as active participants who, while differently from adults, are able to contribute to society. At the same time, it is clear that adolescents also need to apply themselves in self-reflection and making plans for their lives; this appears to be particularly important in today's world where the choices - on a personal, professional, and ethical level - available to adolescents are so numerous that adolescents run the risk of becoming disoriented. The adolescents who are least prepared in terms of having the ability to reflect on themselves and their futures are the most likely to fall prey, in the midst of this confusion, to the falsehoods of the media and fashion and to resort to risk behavior to assert their independence, their personal achievement, and their identity, which they are unable to express in other ways.

Some of the attitudes held and some behavior types carried out by these adolescents can also play a protective role. As we have noted, adolescent development is the result of the adolescent's own actions, which are oriented toward goals and values. Involvement in certain activities, such as participation in religious or other organized groups, can play a protective role. The protection offered by belonging to these groups should not be seen, as it sometimes is, only in terms of a stronger orientation toward conventional behavior and ideals although a greater disapproval of deviance does play a primary role. Most importantly, though, belonging to these groups leads to an increased awareness and ability in planning one's life and in giving sense to it and, as a result, to a greater commitment into meaningful values. This interpretation is supported by the fact that higher expectations for success combined with the value placed on the school experience and health, and on the belief in one's own self-efficacy, are also protective factors: adolescents are less likely to become involved in risky behavior if they have a plan for their self-actualization that tests their abilities and if they are able to combine this plan with the academic experience - an experience that they feel they have the proper resources to confront. The personal significance of these plans guides the adolescent's actions and strengthens his or her development.

It is worth noting that the factors that were found to protect against various types of risk behavior were generally not specific. These are aspects that not only help individuals to avoid involvement in risky activities but that generally encourage optimal development as well. In other words, the factors that promote the best personal development and a more balanced social adjustment allow adolescents to confront the developmental tasks of this age without having to resort to harmful or dangerous behavior. This confirms that risk behavior is a possible adolescent response to the problems of development and adjustment that are characteristic of their age and indicates, on a practical level, that the prevention of dangerous behavior, apart from specific behavior that may require specific interventions, should fall within a broader framework that promotes the best possible development for every individual.

The various individual and context-related protective factors map out a complex yet consistent picture: that of adolescents who can rely on responsible adult figures who make demands of them; adolescents who have undertaken a project of self-actualization and identity construction and who are involved in challenges that are personally and socially relevant; adolescents who are accepted and valued by the adult world; adolescents who are developing cognitive and social abilities, which they have confidence in; and adolescents who are not pressured to act out superficial or consumer-oriented adult behavior. These results are consistent with the recent literature that has highlighted the importance of commitment to activities - both studying and free time activities - that require adolescents to apply themselves and allow them to test themselves through tasks that require ability: "Experiencing high levels of challenge and skill is part of an important dynamic in the transition from adolescence to adulthood. Whenever teenagers report being in high challenge, high skill situations, the quality of their experience is positive… Furthermore, adolescents who are more likely to experience high levels of challenge and skills have a better overall quality of experience" (Csikszentmihalyi and Schneider 2000).

Relegating adolescents to the role of noncritical consumers certainly does not help in this sense. Under the pressures of consumerism, adolescents, as well as adults, run the risk of developing an inauthentic identity based on uniformity and adaptation to the conformist demands of consumerism. Under these conditions, risk behavior can appear as a genuine, rewarding way to regain the diversity and originality that are part of another cultural imperative that is in complete opposition to standardization. This tactic is clearly an illusion, as risk behavior is actually promoted by both the legal and illegal consumer markets, which directly and indirectly draw major economic advantages from them. Thus, as forms of transgression and assertion of independence, they are totally false. It is no wonder that the boys and girls who are most involved in risk behavior are those who have the least opportunity both in school and in the community to develop capabilities of critical analysis and to test their abilities through working toward objectives for personal achievement.

8.4 Prevention Based on Functions: Direct and Indirect Action

The factors considered here perform a protective role because they constitute individual and contextual resources and opportunities that adolescents can draw on. These factors help boys and girls to choose from types of behavior that do not endanger their physical health nor their psychological or social well-being but are just as effective in reaching objectives for significant personal growth. As we have seen, these objectives are related mainly to identity development and the redefinition of social relationships, and it is in relation to these objectives that some adolescents more than others are able to find alternative, healthy, and nondangerous behavior that perform the same positive functions. These adolescents express their adulthood by assuming responsibilities, committing themselves to a plan for self-actualization, and working for the community instead of precociously assuming adult behavior, such as smoking, drinking alcohol, or having sex. The differences found between boys and girls, like the differences found between students of different types of schools, can be traced back to differences in the way they become adults and in how they confront the developmental tasks of adolescence in various contexts. Family and society in general demand greater responsibility and greater commitment from girls; girls, much more so than boys, consider school success essential to gaining independence and are therefore more committed to school. It should be noted that the school plays an extremely important role in structuring male and female identity; in fact, upon entering the first year of secondary school, no differences were found in involvement in risk behavior in adolescents, both boys and girls, attending different types of schools (Bonino and Cattelino 2002). The differences that can be found later are linked to differences in planning skills, in the quality of the school experience, and in the development of cognitive and social competencies. These results suggest that, throughout the years of adolescence, attending a certain type of school, combined with other family or social variables, plays a crucial role.

It is a question, therefore, of working through prevention to provide the opportunity for more adolescents, and especially those in high-risk situations such as many students of vocational schools, to reach their developmental objectives not through harmful behavior but through activities that are healthy both for the individual and society. This is the goal of a preventative approach centered around functions: to encourage the use of other types of behavior that perform the same positive functions but do not compromise the adolescent's health and well-being. This is an innovative approach that is centered on the actions of the adolescent and the adolescent's ability to use functionally equivalent, nondangerous behavior. We have identified two forms of preventative intervention, one *direct* and one *indirect* (Fig. 8.1), which involve the family as well as the school and the community.

In general, *direct preventative action* involves adult behavioral models and attitudes on risk behavior, as well as interventions that are targeted at specific types of risk behavior, and supply information on these behavior types and their functions in order to find strategies that include alternative behavior. This can be achieved in a concrete way through a discussion of the various types of risk behavior and their behavioral aspects and related physiological effects but, most importantly, by reflecting on the meanings these types of behavior assume for adolescents. In this way, we can reflect on the various functions of risk behavior, understand that many other types of behavior are already being used to reach the same or similar objectives, and seek out alter-

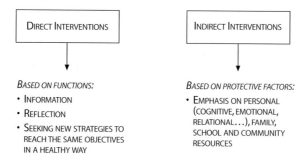

Fig. 8.1. Different types of intervention, both direct and indirect, that can be utilized in the prevention of risk behavior in adolescence.

native behavior. It must be noted that the functions of risk behavior should not be considered in a personalized way, with reference to a single adolescent, but in general terms so that every adolescent can reflect personally, alone or with others, on which functions most apply to them. Again, the objective is to help adolescents discover methods that do not compromise their physical, psychological, or social health but that aid them in developing an independent identity and achieving positive relationships with others. In order to be successful, this type of prevention requires the commitment of an adult educator and the active involvement of adolescents although the exact form it can take depends on the educational setting. In this way, adolescents themselves are called on to identify and try out other safe behavior aimed at reaching the same important goals for development. This task also requires the involvement of the peer group, as the development of individual identity and the formation of values does not occur alone but is shared with peers (Fig. 8.2).

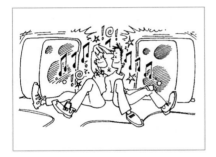 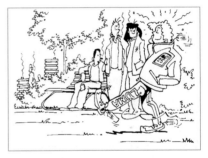

SOME YOUNG PEOPLE FEEL THAT THERE ARE DEFINITIVE ADVANTAGES TO USING CANNABIS. BUT VERY OFTEN, THESE ADVANTAGES CAN BE ACHIEVED IN ANOTHER WAY AS WELL. SOME SAY, FOR INSTANCE, THAT SMOKING HASH IS A WAY TO ESCAPE FROM THE WORLD AROUND YOU. BUT THE SAME EFFECT CAN BE ACHIEVED BY GOING TO A FILM OR BY LISTENING TO LOUD HOUSE MUSIC.

SOME YOUNG PEOPLE SEE DEFINITIVE ADVANTAGES TO SMOKING. BUT THESE ADVANTAGES CAN OFTEN BE GAINED IN A DIFFERENT WAY AS WELL. MANY BOYS FEEL THAT IT LOOKS TOUGH TO SMOKE. BUT IF YOU WANT TO LOOK TOUGH, YOU COULD ALSO WEAR A TOUGH JACKET. YOU DON'T HAVE TO START SMOKING BECAUSE YOU DON'T KNOW WHAT TO DO WITH YOUR HANDS; JUST PUT THEM IN YOUR POCKETS.

Fig. 8.2. The two vignettes are from a series of pamphlets on psychoactive substance use addressed to students in the first year of secondary school in the Netherlands (Netherlands Institute on Alcohol and Drugs, Stimulants Series, Wolters-Noordhoff, 1994). In the Netherlands, adolescents begin secondary school a year earlier than in Italy; therefore, the recipients of these pamphlets are 13- to 14-year-olds. The pamphlets are part of a coordinated prevention program that involves parents as well as teachers and that proposes various activities and topics for reflection to be carried out individually and in groups. Figures and captions are presented after some exercises in which students are asked to identify the advantages and disadvantages of smoking cigarettes and using marijuana. They are a good example of how to confront, using appropriate language and in an explicit but nonpersonalized way, the theme of functions, suggesting healthy alternatives to obtain the same personally significant advantages.

For example, the family plays a direct role in prevention when it speaks about these topics, supplies information on various types of risk behavior, and reflects - along with children - on the functions and implications of risk behavior in the short and long term. Parents' positive models and attitudes play an important role, and parents should not hesitate to voice their opinions. The school - even more so, as it is the educational setting where adolescents spend the majority of their time - can intervene directly in the prevention of risk behavior not only by supplying information but also by discussing the functions of each individual risk behavior. This task should be introduced, as much as possible, into the daily school curriculum and can involve a number of different disciplines. For example, psychoactive substance use can be covered along with scientific subjects or humanities. Even when special lessons have been prepared, such as presentations by experts from outside the school, these lessons should be coordinated and connected to the daily classroom activities in order to guarantee continuity of the educational message and to enhance the value of teachers' responsibilities as educators. We should keep in mind that teachers, like parents, also play a direct role in prevention through their behavioral models and attitudes.

The community directly affects prevention through the models and attitudes it displays, the information it communicates, and the rules for behavior that it requires. The models and values, in a pluralist society like the one we live in today, are widely varied, and we do not certainly wish that they will level off. Preventative actions aimed at dangerous behavior would require greater reflection on the broad spectrum of behavior and on the different implications and meanings that are assigned to different behavioral choices. It would also require information and attitudes that are more critical of the positive values that, for economic and market-related reasons, many types of risk behavior (such as risky driving and psychoactive substance use) hold in our society. Rules, too (for example, laws that regulate psychoactive substance use), and strict requirements to respect these rules, are also important for prevention, as they constitute a frame of reference for the adolescent in the process of choosing to act out a risk behavior, as rules are an indicator of what society approves or disapproves of. We must also work to discredit the commonly held belief that the existence of a rule does nothing but stimulate the adolescent's desire for transgression and encourage the unwanted behavior. In reality, this belief overestimates the transgressive function of risk behavior, which, as we have seen, is relevant only for certain groups at certain ages. In addition, it overlooks the role of rules and the requirement to respect these rules, which, for the vast majority of adolescents, is protective. Often, it seems that this belief serves as a convenient alibi for adults, justifying their lack of commitment to educating youth.

Indirect preventative action aims at encouraging the factors that have been shown to carry out a protective role, both on a personal and contextual level. In indirect preventative action, risk behavior is not considered specifically. Instead, this type of prevention promotes the aspects that facilitate a preference by adolescents for nondangerous behavior that is functionally equivalent.

The family carries out an indirect preventative action by offering both emotional support and open dialogue and supervision, which requires establishing rules for everyday life and seeing that these rules are respected. The combination of these elements encourages involvement in nondangerous behavior for a number of reasons: rules give adolescents a frame of reference in the process of regulating their behavior and encourage long-term planning, while dialogue and support guarantee adolescents an opportunity to talk with their parents about themselves and their futures, to develop values and shared goals, and to seek help from their parents when necessary.

The school plays an important indirect preventative role by reinforcing the personal, cognitive, and social resources that encourage the ability to commit to significant plans, to self-actualize, and to deal with personal and relational difficulties. Through their continuous daily work in normal curricular activities, teachers can improve boys' and girls' self-efficacy, their ability to resolve problems and conflicts, and their planning skills and help them to apply rules both in their school work and social lives. These cognitive, emotional, and social skills are defined by WHO, along with others (such as effective communication, empathy, critical and creative thinking, and emotion and stress management) as life skills (WHO 1999). These are closely connected competencies and abilities that allow the individual to effectively deal with the changes and requirements of daily life and are therefore tied to better adjustment and greater psychological and physical well being. These skills are acquired in daily life through relationships with adults as well as peers.

The community can carry out significant indirect preventative interventions by offering times and places where adolescents have an occasion both to act and to reflect. These opportunities allow them to assume responsibility in a protected environment, to become involved in activities that are beneficial to society, to take on meaningful but nondangerous challenges, and to gain visibility in a positive way. The prevention of psychoactive substance use, for instance, might take place through projects organized by a town or neighborhood involving youth and not only through advertising campaigns or specific courses. The results of our study show that activities that involve adolescents in projects meaningful to them on both a personal and social level are useful, as they let them escape from "empty," nonproductive use of their time. Even participation in sports, often superficially considered a sure antidote to involvement in risk, can have a preventative function but only in the presence of positive models and an educational program aimed at identity development and facilitated by adults.

Involvement in volunteer activity is worth special attention as, for some adolescents, it appears to be linked to feelings of discomfort. This is consistent with the findings presented in the literature on different motivations and different levels of adjustment in people who choose to do volunteer work (Marta et al. 1998; Marta and Pozzi 2005, in press). Precisely because of the characteristics of this period, it is essential that involvement in volunteer work is introduced into an educational program and evaluated by attentive and aware adults so that adolescents can take on tasks that encourage processes of identity construction and abilities that allow them to confront the requirements of the environment.

8.5 Which Type of Knowledge; What to Avoid

The preventative model presented here differs greatly from the cognitive approach that characterizes many of the current intervention programs both in the area of adolescent risk behavior and, more generally, in lifestyles that are harmful to the health at any age. Many prevention programs today are based on the implicit conviction that it is sufficient to explain to adolescents, or to adults, that some types of behavior are compromising to their health both in the short and long term: it is assumed that knowledge of the negative effects of certain types of behavior is able to persuade people to give up or avoid these behavior types. Unfortunately, this assumption is completely erroneous, founded on a naively intellectual concept of human action that fails to consider the emotional, affective, and social aspects that, together, motivate action. For these reasons, knowing that a behavior is harmful is certainly not enough to prevent a person from carrying it out; the well-known Italian advertising slogan "AIDS: If you know it, you'll avoid it" is completely ineffective and lacking in foundation. Human action, as we have seen, is tied to the combination of the various meanings that a person associates with that action; therefore, it is essential at any age to consider the positive functions carried out by behavior that in other respects is dangerous.

The results of our research, which are consistent with other findings presented in the literature, indicate that there is no direct relationship between knowledge of the negative effects of the numerous types of risk behavior considered here and avoidance of these types of behavior. Adolescents are generally fairly aware of the inherent risks involved in various behavior types, but this does not lead them to abstain from acting out this behavior.

It should also be noted that some risk behavior, such as smoking cigarettes, for instance, do not have immediate negative consequences. The consequences arise at a future time that, psychologically, seems distant and unreal. Despite the fact that adolescents are cognitively capable of representing the distant or hypothetical future - thanks to their newly acquired abilities of abstract thought - they are unable to grasp the personal importance and emotional significance of this representation. Thus, this knowledge remains abstract and free of value. The same behavior can, on the other hand, assume a strong positive value in the present when it carries out a number of subjectively significant functions (for instance, facilitating communication with friends, sharing a lifestyle, looking like an adult). Even when the risks involved relate to the more immediate future (as in the case of unprotected sex), strong emotional involvement and the pursuit of instant gratification can make it difficult to represent the dangers involved and can even mobilize defense mechanisms of denial and invulnerability. This sense of invulnerability, combined with a false sense of control, often comes into play in those types of behavior that pose an immediate and clearly evident risk, such as risky driving. These mechanisms make adolescents feel immune to danger and ready to take on chance when they are at the wheel of a vehicle.

Despite the previous discussion of the ineffectiveness of the cognitive approach, we can surely not conclude that knowledge of the consequences of risk behavior, especially medical consequences, should not be provided. This knowledge should be provided and reinforced but within a framework of preventative action based on functions - that is to say, by focussing on the positive meanings and advantages that adolescents find in risk behavior. As for psychoactive substances, for instance, we must go further than simply providing information on the chemical characteristics and the neuropsychological effects of different substances. Two commonly used but ineffective methods of presentation in particular should be avoided. The first concentrates on the direct effects of substances on mental activity and emphasizes the alterations to an individual's state of consciousness. The second focuses on inciting fear and exaggerating the damage that can be caused by the use of various substances, which results in a loss of credibility. Both of these methods can be completely self-defeating because, as we have seen, many types of behavior are chosen by adolescents precisely because they are dangerous and for the effects that they can produce. These substances allow adolescents to experience new sensations and states of consciousness, face danger, explore their limits, and emulate others.

In general, the psychological and social advantages that an adolescent immediately draws from a risk behavior often far outweigh the damage it can cause. Thus, knowledge about risk behavior and its consequences should be given but always in relation to the functions it serves and with the awareness that this knowledge is not enough to motivate healthy behavior. In reality, people are motivated to act based on knowledge that has significance and value and not by abstract notions with no personal relevance.

At the same time, the preventative model proposed opposes the hypotheses of legalization and decriminalization of psychoactive substances use, and marijuana use in particular. This is, in part, because greater social acceptance and legitimacy of a behavior tend to increase involvement. This can be observed in the case of cigarette smoking where we see a trend toward earlier initiation, heavier involvement, and similar patterns of involvement by both genders, which our findings confirmed. We cannot agree with this proposal, as it would mean relinquishing the responsibility to supply boys and girls with opportunities to develop other more advanced ways of dealing with the difficulties and problems they are faced with during adolescence. In this way, adults avoid having to call upon adolescents to develop the social and cognitive competencies that are necessary to successfully confront this age - more specifically, the ability to resolve problems, make long-term plans, think critically and creatively, communicate effectively, and manage emotions and stress.

In this way, the development of those competencies, which are defined as vital to a person's well-being, is obstructed. The development of these advanced abilities requires, above all, a high level of functioning and maturation in the neocortex, unaltered by substances that affect the brain's biochemical equilibrium and cerebral functioning, which are the fruit of biological evolution that has occurred over the course of millions of years. The most recent studies on this issue indicate that the brain continues to develop throughout the last years of adolescence and into early adulthood. For some time, it has been known that, even well after adolescence, the great plasticity of the human brain allows richer and more elaborate neuron connections to form in relation to the tasks an individual undertakes. In other words, the maturation and development of the brain depend greatly on environmental conditions - that is to say, the way in which we use our brain and the stimuli it is exposed to during adolescence, as in other previous and successive ages. Therefore, it is vitally important to ensure both the absence of stimuli by means of psychoactive substances that interfere with cerebral functioning, and the possibility for positive learning through the actual experience of confronting reality and its problems without escape or regression. As one of the effects of marijuana is the difficulty to deal with information and resolve complex problems, it is clear that regular users of this substance risk entering a vicious cycle, and the younger the adolescent, the greater the damage.

Thus, it seems entirely inappropriate to speak of "damage prevention" to adolescents who are either not yet users or who do not use regularly. What must be prevented is involvement in the use of the substances, especially early or habitual use, by giving boys and girls the opportunity to respond in a more productive way to the developmental tasks of this age and to fully develop their cognitive and social competencies. It is essential that adults, in their role as parents, teachers, or educators, give up the idea of escaping from their responsibilities, which would mean failing to perform an educational role and showing disinterest toward adolescents. As we have noted, it is the boys and girls who are most neglected by their parents - parents who provide no rules and no emotional support - who are most involved in marijuana and other drug use, as well as other types of risk behavior.

8.6 Conclusion

The prevention model proposed here is based on a two-part affirmation: on the one hand, the centrality of the adolescent and the adolescent's actions in the process of his or her own development; and on the other hand, the strong educational role of adults, who must not relinquish their responsibility to boys and girls who are experiencing this important transitional phase. The two aspects are certainly not contradictory, as the educational role of the adult is achieved in the first place by consciously working, within the context of the family, school, and community, to make opportunities and resources available that boys and girls can draw from in the process of constructing their identity and forming relationships with others. In a complementary way, taking on a strong educational role means making precise demands of adolescents, committing them to reflection, to a plan for self-actualization, and to meaningful actions that are both personally and socially relevant and for which they are equipped with the necessary resources to confront. In this way, adolescents' needs for personal achievement and the construction of personal identity meet with society's need to have future adults who are active, participating members.

As we have noted several times, involvement in risk behavior is significantly lower in communities where adolescents are seen as a resource that can be called upon and where they are expected to be committed and responsible than it is in communities where adolescents are seen, primarily, as a source of discomfort and disturbance. For adults, taking on a strong protective role does not mean doing something "for" adolescents or working "on" adolescents, as in a paternalistic approach, but rather working actively "with" adolescents who are applying themselves in the construction of their identities and lending meaning to their current conditions and their futures. These tasks apply not only to adolescents but to adults as well, as the development of identity is a process that unfolds over the course of one's entire existence. Throughout life, individuals must deal with changes, both inside themselves and in the surrounding world, and must find meaning in their actions and in their very existence. This continuous process is never only individual but rather coincides with others within a given culture. When faced with the present reality that is filled with contrasting and often conflictual values and a future that is in many ways uncertain, adolescents are not the only ones who find it difficult to transform the great opportunities that the modern world has to offer into significant achievements on both an individual and social level. Working with adolescents means undertaking a shared path where different generations discover that they have much in common and where both adolescents and adults can contribute reciprocally to their own development and to the development of the culture in which they live.

Introduction

The appendix includes all the questions from the questionnaire *Io e la Mia Salute* (Me and My Health) (Bonino 1995, 1996) and their related answers used in the analyses presented in this book. Here, they are not in the order in which they actually appear in the questionnaire but are grouped based on the four variable systems defined by Jessor's conceptual model (described along with the questionnaire and methodology in Chap. 2): The Social Environment System, The Personality System, The Perceived Environment System, and The Behavior System (see Fig. 2.1). Within each system, the variables are grouped in alphabetical order by theme; the variables within each theme are also in alphabetical order. Note that the variables can be based on single questions or scales (summation of the responses to multiple questions). For each variable, the following information is reported from left to right:
- Number within the theme considered
- Name of the variable
- Corresponding question or questions
- Variable's minimum and maximum values (range)
- Possible responses and score attributed to each; this column has been left blank in the case of open-ended questions - in other words, questions that did not have a series of predefined responses to choose from
- Number of subjects who responded to the question or questions
- Statistical value of Cronbach's alpha (α), used to measure the reliability of the scale
- Values ("eigen value" and "percentage of explained variance") of the component extracted from the factor analyses, which measure the dimensionality of the scale.

Within the four systems, some variables are defined as "calculated variables"; this is information that was not requested directly but was calculated based on responses to other questions (for example, repeated school years were calculated by comparing students' ages and their year in school).

After the variables related to the four systems, the so-called "constructed" variables are reported. These are typologies that were constructed by grouping different ways of responding to questions or scales; here, the method for constructing these typologies is also reported.

The "Appendix" does not include questionnaire questions that were not utilized in the analyses of the findings reported in the chapters of this book (for example, questions on adolescents' jobs or their involvement in homosexual relations).

Variable	Question/scale	Range	Answer modalities	No. of cases	Cronbach's alpha	First factor Eigen value	First factor % explained variance
1 Composition of the family unit	Mark below all of the people you are living with this year: a) mother, b) father, c) stepmother, d) stepfather, e) older brothers f) older sisters, g) younger brothers, h) younger sisters, i) foster parents, l) grandparents, m) uncles or aunts, n) your husband or your wife, o) your own children, p) alone, q) other people.	/	/	2,273	2255		
2 Father's job	More specifically, what is the name of your father's/stepfather's job?	/	/	2,045			
3 Father's occupation	Your father/stepfather	1-7	1 = working at a job full time 2 = working at a job part time 3 = out of work 4 = does he take a subsidy from the state because his factory is not working in this period? 5 = retired 6 = don't know 7 = other	2,273			

4 Gender	What sex are you?	1-2	1 = boy 2 = girl	2,266
5 Integrity of the family unit	If both your parents are alive, do they live together?	1-4	1 = yes 2 = they're separated 3 = they're divorced 4 = other	2,212
6 Mother's job	More specifically, what is the name of your mother's/stepmother's job?	/	/	2,041
7 Mother's occupation	Your mother/stepmother	1-8	1 = working at a job full time 2 = working at a job part time 3 = out of work 4 = homemaker 5 = does she take a subsidy from the state because her factory is not working in this period? 6 = retired 7 = don't know 8 = other	2,273

Variable	Question/scale	Range	Answer modalities	No. of cases	Cronbach's alpha	First factor Eigen value	First factor % explained variance
8 Parents' education level	Which is the highest grade each of your parents/stepparents completed in school? a) mother, b) father.	2-20	1 = elementary school 2 = middle school (not finished) 3 = middle school 4 = professional course 5 = high school (not finished) 6 = high school 7 = university (not finished) 8 = M.A. 9 = don't know 10 = other	2,242			
9 Place of origin	Which Italian region or foreign country are you from?	/	/	2,227			
10 Parents' place of origin	Which Italian region or foreign country are your parents from: a) mother, b) father?	/	/	2,227			
11 Parental presence	Are your parents living?	1-4	1 = neither 2 = my father 3 = my mother 4 = both	2,269			

| 12 Place of residence | Where do you live? | 1-8 | 1 = little mountain village
2 = little hill village
3 = little country village
4 = village
5 = small town
6 = town
7 = large town
8 = other | 2,263 |
| 13 School class | What grade are you in? | 1-5 | 1 = first
2 = second
3 = third
4 = fourth
5 = fifth | 2,259 |

Variable	Question/scale	Range	Answer modalities	No. of cases	Cronbach's alpha	First factor Eigen value	% explained variance
ATTITUDE TOWARD DEVIANCE							
1 **Disapproval of antisocial behavior**	How wrong is it to: 1) start a fist fight or shoving match, 2) shoplift from a store, 3) damage or mark up public or private property on purpose, 4) lie to a teacher, 5) take things that don't belong to you, 6) stay out all night without permission, 7) damage school property on purpose, 8) lie to your parents about where you have been or who you were with, 9) skip school without permission, 10) hit someone because you didn't like what they said or did, 11) be in a fight with members of a gang or a sport's group fan, 12) carry a weapon (such as a knife), 13) have a serious fight at school?	13-52	1 = not at all 2 = a little 3 = fairly 4 = very	2,191	.88	5.33	41
BODY MEASUREMENTS AND IMAGE							
1 **Height**	How tall are you?	/	/	2,250			
2 **Recent height change**	Has your height changed a lot in the past year?	1-2	1 = no 2 = yes	2,247			

3 Recent weight change	Has your weight changed a lot in the past year?	1-3	1 = it's gone down a lot 2 = it hasn't changed very much 3 = it's gone up a lot	2,263
4 Satisfaction with height	How do you feel about your height?	1-5	1 = would like to be a lot taller 2 = would like to be a little taller 3 = my height is right 4 = would like to be a little shorter 5 = would like to be a lot shorter	2,259
5 Satisfaction with weight	How do you feel about your weight?	1-5	1 = would like to gain several kg 2 = would like to gain 2-3 kg 3 = my weight is right 4 = would like to loose less than 2-3 kg 5 = would like to loose 2-3 kg	2,265
6 Weight	How much do you weight?	/	/	2,259

Variable	Question/scale	Range	Answer modalities	No. of cases	Cronbach's alpha	First factor Eigen value	First factor % explained variance
EXPECTATIONS AND SELF-PERCEPTION							
1 Believe oneself to be attractive to the opposite sex	Do you think you are attractive to the opposite sex?	1-4	1 = not at all 2 = not too 3 = fairly 4 = very	2,249			
2 Depressive feelings	In the past six months, have you: 1) just felt really down about things, 2) felt pretty hopeless about the future, 3) spent a lot of time worrying about little things, 4) just felt depressed about life in general, 5) felt alone?	5-20	1 = no 2 = a little 3 = fairly often 4 = a lot	2,253	.78	2.72	54
3 Expectations for future success	What are the chances that you will: 1) be able to own your own home, 2) have a job that you enjoy, 3) have a happy family life, 4) stay in good health, 5) be able to live wherever you want to, 6) be respected in your community, 7) have good friends you can count on?	7-35	1 = very low 2 = low 3 = about 50% 4 = high 5 = very high	2,219	.77	3.02	43
4 Expectations to continue school	What are the chances that you will: 1) graduate from high school, 2) go to university?	2-10	1 = very low 2 = low 3 = about 50% 4 = high 5 = very high	2,260	.65	1.5	76

5 **Not seeing the point in what one does**	How much do you agree with the following statement? Hardly anything I'm doing in my life means very much to me.	1–4	1 = disagree 2 = a little 3 = fairly much 4 = very much	2,241
6 **Overall satisfaction with self**	On the whole, how satisfied are you with yourself?	1–4	1 = not at all 2 = not too 3 = fairly 4 = very	2,261
7 **Perceived chances of attending university**	What are the chances that you will go to university?	1–5	1 = very low 2 = low 3 = about 50% 4 = high 5 = very high	2,260
8 **Perceived chances of obtaining a diploma**	What are the chances that you will graduate from high school?	1–5	1 = very low 2 = low 3 = about 50% 4 = high 5 = very high	2,260
9 **Perception of own academic abilities**	What do you think about your abilities to do well at school work?	1–4	1 = not too able 2 = sufficient 3 = fairly able 4 = very able	2,261

APPENDIX The Personality System

292

Variable	Question/scale	Range	Answer modalities	No. of cases	Cronbach's alpha	First factor Eigen value	First factor % explained variance
10 Positive expectations for school	How sure are you that you will: 1) get at least 7 (B) average this year, 2) be considered a bright student by your teachers, 3) be one of the best in your class, 4) be thought of as a good student by your teachers?	4-16	1 = not sure at all 2 = not too sure 3 = pretty sure 4 = very sure	2,237	.85	2.74	67
11 Positive self-perception	1) What do you think about your abilities to do well at school work? 2) How much do you think that you can deal with everyday problems? 3) Do you feel yourself able to take important decisions about your life? 4) Are you sure that you can learn new skills when you need them? 5) Do you think you are attractive to the opposite sex? 6) On the whole, how satisfied are you with yourself? 7) Can you resist peer pressure from the rest of the group?	7-28	The answers' modalities are different according to each question. The range is between 1 and 4.	2,210	.63	2.30	33
12 Satisfaction with relationships with peers	How well do you get along with others your age?	1-4	1 = not well at all 2 = not too well 3 = pretty well 4 = very well	2,268			

		Range	Scale	N			
13 Self-confidence in coping	1) How much do you think that you can deal with everyday problems? 2) Do you feel yourself able to make important decisions about your life? 3) Are you sure that you can learn new skills when you need them?	3-12	1 = never 2 = sometimes 3 = often 4 = always	2,254	.57	1.63	54
14 Self-regulatory efficacy	Can you resist peer pressure from the rest of the group?	1-4	1 = never 2 = sometimes 3 = often 4 = always	2,264			
15 Sense of alienation	How much do you agree with each of the statements below: 1) I often feel left out of things that other kids do, 2) I sometimes feel unsure about what I really am, 3) it's hard for me to know how to act if it is not clear what other people expect from me, 4) hardly anything I'm doing in my life means very much to me?	4-16	1 = disagree 2 = a little 3 = fairly much 4 = very much	2,225	.66	1.99	50

Variable	Question/scale	Range	Answer modalities	No. of cases	Cronbach's alpha	First factor Eigen value	% explained variance
	INFORMATION AND ATTITUDES TOWARD SEXUALITY, CONTRACEPTION, AND AIDS						
1 Attitude toward having sex in adolescence	How much do you agree with the following proposition? Kids my age are just too young to have sex.	1-4	1 = not at all 2 = a little 3 = fairly much 4 = very much	2,254			
2 Attitude toward having sex in adolescence and getting pregnant	How much do you agree with the following proposition? It's better not to have sex rather to risk getting pregnant.	1-4	1 = not at all 2 = a little 3 = fairly much 4 = very much	2,248			
3 Awareness of being informed on contraception	Do you think you have received sufficient information about contraceptive methods?	1-2	1 = no 2 = yes	2,227			
4 Embarrassment for buying contraceptive methods	Were you ever embarrassed buying condoms or asking for other contraceptive methods?	1-3	1 = never 2 = at first 3 = always	559			

5 General knowledge about AIDS	1) Can a person get AIDS from another person affected by the virus by a) holding hands with him/her, b) kissing him/her, c) sharing needles used to inject drugs, d) being bitten by mosquitoes, flies or other insects, e) giving blood, f) taking a blood transfusion, g) using public toilets, h) having sexual intercourse without a condom, i) being in the same class with a serum-positive student, l) drinking from the same glass, m) just looking at him/her? 2) Can a pregnant woman who has the HIV virus infect her unborn baby with the virus? 3) Is there a cure for AIDS infection? 4) Is it true that only homosexual (gay) people can get AIDS infection? 5) Can people reduce their chances of becoming infected with the HIV virus by a) not having sexual intercourse, b) using condoms during sexual intercourse, c) not having sexual intercourse with people who inject drugs, d) taking birth control pills?	18-57	1 = no 2 = not sure 3 = yes	2,065	.60	2.90	16

Variable	Question/scale	Range	Answer modalities	No. of cases	Cronbach's alpha	First factor Eigen value	First factor % explained variance
6 Interest in covering the subject of AIDS in school	Should students of your age be taught about AIDS in school?	1-3	1 = no 2 = not sure 3 = yes	2,265			
7 Knowledge of the possibility of AIDS transmission without condoms	Can a person get AIDS from another person affected by the virus by having sexual intercourse without a condom?	1-3	1 = no 2 = not sure 3 = yes	2,229			
8 Knowledge that using condoms can prevent AIDS	Can people reduce their chances of becoming infected with the HIV virus by using condoms during sexual intercourse?	1-3	1 = no 2 = not sure 3 = yes	2,245			
9 Negative attitude toward contraception	How much do you agree with each of the following statements? 1) Using birth control is just too much of a hassle. 2) It's not right to use birth control. 3) The whole idea of birth control is embarrassing to me.	3-12	1 = not at all 2 = a little 3 = fairly much 4 = very much	2,182	.65	1.78	59

				N			
10 Perceived seriousness of AIDS	How much do you agree with each of the following statements? 1) Getting AIDS isn't something teenagers of your age really have to worry about. 2) AIDS is not as big a problem as it's made out to be.	2-8	1 = strongly 2 = fairly much 3 = a little 4 = not at all	2,237	.56	1.39	70
11 Positive attitude toward contraception	How much do you agree with each of the following statements? 1) It's smart to use birth control to prevent an unplanned pregnancy. 2) It's a good idea to use condoms to protect against getting AIDS. 3) Teenagers who use birth control show they care about themselves and their future.	3-12	1 = not at all 2 = a little 3 = fairly much 4 = very much	2,210	.32	1.42	47
12 Sources of information on contraception	From whom did you receive sufficient information about contraceptive methods?	/	/	1,534			
13 Subject of AIDS already covered in school	Have you been taught about AIDS in school?	1-3	1 = no 2 = not sure 3 = yes	2,254			
14 Worry over contracting AIDS	Do you ever worry about getting AIDS yourself?	1-3	1 = never 2 = sometimes 3 = often	2,250			

Variable	Question/scale	Range	Answer modalities	No. of cases	Cronbach's alpha	First factor Eigen value	First factor % explained variance
KNOWLEDGE TOWARD HEALTH							
1 Awareness of the consequences of inactivity	Do you think not exercising regularly can have an effect on the health of young people your age?	1-4	1 = not at all 2 = mild 3 = fairly serious 4 = very serious	2,267			
2 Awareness of the consequences of irregular eating	Do you think skipping breakfast most days can have negative effects on the health of young people your age?	1-4	1 = no 2 = mild 3 = serious 4 = very serious	2,261			
3 Awareness of the consequences of being sedentary	Do you think that just sitting around a lot can have negative effects on the health of young people your age?	1-4	1 = no 2 = mild 3 = serious 4 = very serious	2,262			
4 Awareness of the consequences of unhealthy eating	Do you think eating a lot of "junk food" can have negative effects on the health of young people your age?	1-4	1 = no 2 = mild 3 = serious 4 = very serious	2,249			

5 External locus of control for health	How much do you agree with the following statements? 1) I can get sick no matter how much I try to take care of myself. 2) Kids of my age are just too young to do much about their health. 3) Staying healthy seems to be mostly a matter of luck for me. 4) People in my family just seem to get sick easily. 5) Once I'm sick, there is not much I can do to get better except wait.	5-20	1 = not at all 2 = a little 3 = fairly much 4 = strongly	2,238	.58	1.91	38
6 Internal locus of control for health	How much do you agree with the following statements? 1) If I keep a regular life (eating right, getting enough sleep, taking exercise) it's easy to stay in good health. 2) If I get sick, there are things I can do to get better. 3) I might get sick more often if I didn't take care of myself.	3-12	1 = not at all 2 = a little 3 = fairly much 4 = strongly	2,250	.43	1.43	48
PERCEPTION OF NEGATIVE CONSEQUENCES TIED TO RISKY BEHAVIOR							
1 Awareness of physical consequences of being overweight	Do you think being overweight can have negative physical effects on the health of young people your age?	1-4	1 = no 2 = mild 3 = serious 4 = very serious	2,049			

Variable	Question/scale	Range	Answer modalities	No. of cases	Cronbach's alpha	First factor Eigen value	First factor % explained variance
2 Awareness of physical risk tied to alcohol consumption	Do you think daily use of alcohol can have negative effects on the health of young people of your age? a) Physical effects.	1-2	1 = no 2 = yes	2,202			
3 Awareness of physical risk tied to cigarette smoking	Do you think smoking can have a negative effect on the health of young people of your age? a) Physical effects.	1-4	1 = almost none 2 = mild 3 = serious 4 = very serious	2,194			
4 Awareness of physical risk tied to marijuana smoking	Do you think using marijuana can have negative effects on the health of young people of your age? a) Physical effects.	1-4	1 = no 2 = mild 3 = serious 4 = very serious	2,169			
5 Awareness of psychological consequences of being overweight	Do you think being overweight can have negative psychological effects on the health of young people your age?	1-4	1 = no 2 = mild 3 = serious 4 = very serious	2,000			

#	Item	Question	Range	Coding	N			
6	Awareness of psychological risk tied to alcohol consumption	Do you think daily use of alcohol can have negative effects on the health of young people of your age? a) Psychological effects.	1-2	1 = no 2 = yes	1,939			
7	Awareness of psychological risk tied to cigarette smoking	Do you think smoking cigarettes can have a negative effect on the health of young people of your age? a) Psychological effects.	1-4	1 = almost none 2 = mild 3 = serious 4 = very serious	1,640			
8	Awareness of psychological risk tied to marijuana smoking	Do you think using marijuana can have negative effects on the health of young people of your age? a) Psychological effects.	1-4	1 = no 2 = mild 3 = serious 4 = very serious	2,053			
9	Awareness of consequences of substance use	1) Do you think daily use of alcohol can have negative effects on the health of young people your age? a) Physical effects, b) psychological effects. 2) Do you think smoking can have a negative effect on the health of young people your age? a) Physical effects, b) psychological effects. 3) Do you think using marijuana can have negative effects on the health of young people your age? a) Physical effects, b) psychological effects.	6-24	1 = no 2 = mild 3 = serious 4 = very serious	1,466	.70	2.44	41

Variable	Question/scale	Range	Answer modalities	No. of cases	Cronbach's alpha	First factor Eigen value	First factor % explained variance
10 Seriousness of negative consequences tied to alcohol consumption	Do you think daily use of alcohol can have negative effects on the health of young people of your age? a) Physical effects, b) psychological effects.	2-4	1 = no 2 = yes	2,070	.63	1.46	74
11 Seriousness of negative consequences tied to cigarette smoking	Do you think smoking cigarettes can have a negative effect on the health of young people of your age? a) Physical effects, b) psychological effects.	2-8	1 = almost none 2 = mild 3 = serious 4 = very serious	1,917	.51	1.35	67
12 Seriousness of negative consequences tied to marijuana smoking	Do you think using marijuana can have negative effects on the health of young people of your age? a) Physical effects, b) psychological effects.	2-8	1 = no 2 = mild 3 = serious 4 = very serious	2,111	.87	1.77	88

↑ VALUES

#	Variable	Item	Range	Response categories	N			
1	**Tendency toward prosocial behavior**	How much do you agree with the following proposition? I think that I should try to help when people I know are having problems.	1–4	1 = disagree 2 = a little 3 = fairly much 4 = very much	2,254			33
2	**Value on health**	How important is it to you to: 1) feel in good shape, 2) know that your weight is right about where it should be, 3) be able to play active games and sports without getting tired too quickly, 4) have a good shape, 5) not get sick when something like the flu is going around, 6) get better quickly whenever you're sick, 7) keep yourself healthy even if it takes some extra effort, 8) have good, healthy habits about eating, 9) practice physical exercise regularly?	9–36	1 = not at all 2 = not too 3 = somewhat 4 = very	2,245	.73	2.99	33
3	**Value on independence**	How important is it to you to: 1) decide by yourself how to spend your free time independently from adults, 2) choose your own clothes, 3) be free to use the money you have the way you want to, 4) make your own decisions about what movies to see or books to read?	4–16	1 = not at all 2 = not too 3 = somewhat 4 = very	2,247	.58	1.90	48

Variable	Question/scale	Range	Answer modalities	No. of cases	Cronbach's alpha	First factor Eigen value	First factor % explained variance
4 Value on religion	How important is it to you to: 1) be able to rely on religious teaching when you have a problem, 2) believe in God, 3) rely on religious belief as a guide for day-to-day living, 4) be able to turn to prayer when you're facing personal problems?	4-16	1 = not at all 2 = not too 3 = somewhat 4 = very	2,211	.85	3.10	62
5 Value on school experience	How important is it to you to: 1) get good grades this year, 2) be considered a bright student by your teachers, 3) be one of the best students of your class, 4) achieve a specialization or an M.A. after high school?	4-16	1 = not at all 2 = not too 3 = somewhat 4 = very	2,242	.59	1.90	48

Variable	Question/scale	Range	Answer modalities	No. of cases	Cronbach's alpha	First factor Eigen value	First factor % explained variance
→ FAMILY							
1 **Affection toward parents**	How close do you feel to your family?	1-4	1 = not close 2 = not too close 3 = fairly close 4 = very close	2,264			
2 **Maternal model for healthy eating habits**	How much do these people pay attention to eating a healthy diet? a) Mother.	1-4	1 = not at all 2 = a little 3 = rather a lot 4 = a lot	2,212			
3 **Maternal model for physical exercise**	How much do these people pay attention to getting enough exercise? a) Mother.	1-4	1 = not at all 2 = a little 3 = rather a lot 4 = a lot	2,204			
4 **Maternal model for regular sleeping**	How much do these people pay attention to getting enough sleep? a) Mother.	1-4	1 = not at all 2 = a little 3 = rather a lot 4 = a lot	2,208			

Variable	Question/scale	Range	Answer modalities	No. of cases	Cronbach's alpha	First factor Eigen value	% explained variance
5 Maternal model for safety belt or helmet use	How much do these people pay attention to using seat belts in a car or a crash helmet on a motorcycle? a) Mother.	1-4	1 = not at all 2 = a little 3 = rather a lot 4 = a lot	2,202			
6 Older siblings' model for cigarette smoking	This variable was constructed by combining the information drawn from two items: 1) Mark below all of the people you are living with this year: a) older brothers, b) older sisters; 2) If you have brothers or sisters, does anybody smoke cigarettes?	1-2	1 = no 2 = yes	1,479			
7 Parental control	In your family, how strict are the rules you have to follow about: 1) when and which television shows you can watch, 2) getting your homework done, 3) what time you go to sleep at night, 4) getting chores done around the house, 5) letting your family know where you're going when you go out, 6) being at home by a certain time at night, 7) going to parties, 8) dating with your partner?	8-32	1 = not at all 2 = not too 3 = fairly 4 = very	2,061	.74	2.89	36

	Question	Range	Scale	N			
8 Parental control for behavior at home	In your family, how strict are the rules you have to follow about: 1) when and which television shows you can watch, 2) getting your homework done, 3) what time you go to sleep at night, 4) getting chores done around the house?	4-16	1 = not at all 2 = not too 3 = fairly 4 = very	2,235	.58	1.90	38
9 Parental control for behavior outside the home	In your family, how strict are the rules you have to follow about: 1) letting your family know where you're going when you go out, 2) being at home by a certain time at night?	2-8	1 = not at all 2 = not too 3 = fairly 4 = very	2,235	.58	1.90	38
10 Parental control for going to parties or dates with partner	In your family, how strict are the rules you have to follow about: 1) going to parties, 2) dating with your partner?	2-8	1 = not at all 2 = not too 3 = fairly 4 = very	2,174	.60	1.43	72
11 Parental knowledge of children's smoking	Do your parents know that you smoke?	1-4	1 = neither 2 = father only 3 = mother only 4 = both	1,152			

Variable	Question/scale	Range	Answer modalities	No. of cases	Cronbach's alpha	First factor Eigen value	First factor % explained variance
12 Parental model for cigarette smoking	Does either of your parents (or stepparents) smoke cigarettes?	1-4	1 = neither 2 = father only 3 = mother only 4 = both	2,252			
13 Parental support	1) Is it easy for you to talk with your parents about personal problems, thoughts, feelings? 2) Is it easy for you to talk with your parents about problems with school?	2-8	1 = no 2 = somewhat 3 = fairly 4 = very	2,263	.64	1.48	74
14 Parents' approval of cigarette smoking	How do your parents feel about someone your age smoking cigarettes?	1-3	1 = disapprove 2 = neither approve nor disapprove 3 = approve	2,255			
15 Parents' approval of psychoactive substance use	1) How do your parents feel about someone your age smoking cigarettes? 2) How do your parents feel about someone your age drinking alcohol? 3) How do your parents feel about someone your age using marijuana?	3-9	1 = disapprove 2 = neither approve nor disapprove 3 = approve	2,202	.43	1.41	47

16 Paternal model for healthy eating habits	How much do these people pay attention to eating a healthy diet? a) Father.	1-4	1 = not at all 2 = a little 3 = rather a lot 4 = a lot	2,179
17 Paternal model for physical exercise	How much do these people pay attention to getting enough exercise? b) Father.	1-4	1 = not at all 2 = a little 3 = rather a lot 4 = a lot	2,177
18 Paternal model for regular sleeping	How much do these people pay attention to getting enough sleep? a) Father.	1-4	1 = not at all 2 = a little 3 = rather a lot 4 = a lot	2,175
19 Paternal model for safety belt or helmet use	How much do these people pay attention to using seat belts in a car or a crash helmet on a motorcycle? a) Father.	1-4	1 = not at all 2 = a little 3 = rather a lot 4 = a lot	2,172
20 Stress caused by family life	In the past six months, how much stress or pressure have you felt because of your family life?	1-4	1 = none 2 = a little 3 = rather a lot 4 = a lot	2,261

Variable	Question/scale	Range	Answer modalities	No. of cases	Cronbach's alpha	First factor Eigen value	First factor % explained variance
21 **Strictness of parents**	How strict are your parents with you?	1-4	1 = not at all 2 = not too 3 = fairly 4 = very	2,254			
↑ PEER GROUP AND FRIENDS							
1 **Attitude of friends toward psychoactive substances use**	1) How do your friends feel about someone of your age smoking cigarettes? 2) How do your friends feel about someone of your age drinking alcohol? 3) Do most of your friends approve of someone your age using marijuana?	3-9	1 = disapprove 2 = neither approve nor disapprove 3 = approve	2,206	.60	1.69	56
2 **Best-friend model for healthy eating habits**	How much do these people pay attention to eating a healthy diet? a) Best friend.	1-4	1 = no 2 = a little 3 = fairly much 4 = a lot	2,150			
3 **Best-friend model for physical exercise**	How much do these people pay attention to getting enough exercise? a) Best friend.	1-4	1= not at all 2= a little 3= rather a lot 4= a lot	2,161			

4	**Best-friend model for regular sleeping**	How much do these people pay attention to get enough sleep? a) Best friend.	1-4	1 = no 2 = a little 3 = fairly much 4 = a lot	2,143
5	**Best-friend model for safety belt or helmet use**	How much do these people pay attention to using seat belts in a car or a crash helmet on a motorcycle? a) Best friend.	1-4	1 = no 2 = a little 3 = fairly much 4 = a lot	2,119
6	**Contraceptive use by friends**	How many of your friends who have had sexual intercourse used some kind of contraceptive method?	1-5	1 = almost none 2 = some 3 = most 4 = all 5 = don't know	1,971
7	**Friends' control**	If you were going to do something people think is wrong, would your friend try to stop you?	1-4	1 = definitively would not 2 = probably would not 3 = probably would 4 = definitively would	2,247
8	**Friends' involvement in sex**	Think of all your friends: How many have had sexual intercourse with someone of the opposite sex?	1-4	1 = none 2 = some 3 = most 4 = all	1,971

Variable	Question/scale	Range	Answer modalities	No. of cases	Cronbach's alpha	First factor Eigen value	First factor % explained variance
9 Friends' model for being sedentary	Do your friends usually sit around a lot doing nothing instead of getting some exercise or practicing other kinds of activities?	1-4	1 = none 2 = some 3 = most 4 = all	2,234			
10 Friends' model for conventional behavior	How many of your friends: 1) participate in school clubs or organizations, 2) go to church pretty regularly, 3) are in a community youth group, such as boy scouts, 4) get good grades in school, 5) do volunteer work in the school community, 6) take part in organized sport groups, 7) spend a lot of time with their families?	7-28	1 = none 2 = some 3 = most 4 = all	2,195	.64	2.24	32
11 Friends' model for dropping out	Do you have any friends who have dropped out of school?	1-4	1 = none 2 = some 3 = most 4 = all	2,268			
12 Friends' model for habitual alcohol consumption	How many of your friends drink alcohol regularly?	1-4	1 = none 2 = some 3 = most 4 = all	2,254			

13 Friends' model for habitual smoking	How many of your friends smoke cigarettes on a regular basis?	1–4	1 = none 2 = some 3 = most 4 = all	2,251		
14 Friends' model for habitual marijuana smoking	How many of your friends use marijuana?	1–4	1 = none 2 = some 3 = most 4 = all	2,248		
15 Friends' model for unhealthy eating habits	How many of your friends eat a lot of "junk food" (fried, fat)?	1–4	1 = none 2 = some 3 = most 4 = all	2,226		
16 Friends' risk behavior	1) How many of your friends smoke cigarettes on a regular basis? 2) How many of your friends drink alcohol regularly? 3) How many of your friends use marijuana? 4) Think of all your friends: How many have had sexual intercourse with someone of the opposite sex?	4–16	1 = none 2 = some 3 = most 4 = all	2,049	.63	1.97 49
17 Friends' support	When you have personal problems, do you feel that your friends take care of them?	1–4	1 = never 2 = sometimes 3 = often 4 = always	2,260		

Variable	Question/scale	Range	Answer modalities	No. of cases	Cronbach's alpha	First factor Eigen value	% explained variance
18 Number of close friends	How many close friends do you have?	1-4	1 = none 2 = 1 3 = 2-3 4 = 4 or more	2,263			
19 Peer pressure to drink	Have your friends pressured you to drink or drink more than you wanted?	1-4	1 = never 2 = sometimes 3 = often 4 = all the times	2,262			
20 Peer pressure to have sex	How much do peers influence each other to have sex?	1-4	1 = not at all 2 = a little 3 = a fair amount 4 = a lot	2,249			
21 Quality of relationship with friends	How well do you get along with others your age?	1-4	1 = not well at all 2 = not too well 3 = fairly well 4 = very well	2,258			
22 Stress caused by social life	In the past six months, how much stress or pressure have you felt because of your social relationships?	1-4	1 = no 2 = a little 3 = fairly much 4 = a lot	2,259			

RELATION BETWEEN FRIENDS AND PARENTS						
1 Compatibility between friends and parents	1) Would your friends agree with your parents about what is really important in life? 2) Would your friends agree with your parents about what the kind of person you should become?	2-8	1 = not at all 2 = a little 3 = rather a lot 4 = a lot	2,198	.69	1.53	77
2 Orientation toward friends in making decisions	If you had to make a serious decision about these topics, where would you turn: a) school, b) life's choices, c) health?	3-9	1 = nobody 2 = parents most 3 = both parents and friends 4 = friends most	2,182	.33	1.30	43
3 Parental versus friends' influence	1) If you had to make a serious decision about these topics, where would you turn: a) school, b) life's choices, c) health? 2) Is your outlook on life (what is important for you) nearest to that of your friends or your parents?	4-12	1 = nobody 2 = parents most 3 = both parents and friends 4 = friends most	2,169	.48	1.43	36
4 Similarity of concept of life	Is your outlook on life (what is important for you) nearest to that of your friends or your parents?	1-4	1 = nobody 2 = parents most 3 = both parents and friends 4 = friends most	2,258			

Variable	Question/scale	Range	Answer modalities	No. of cases	Cronbach's alpha	First factor Eigen value	% explained variance
RELATIONS WITH OTHER SIGNIFICANT ADULTS							
1 Reference to other adults	1) Besides your parents, is there another adult you can talk to when you are having problems, thought, feelings? 2) Besides your parents, is there another adult you can talk to when you are having problems with school?	2-4	1 = no 2 = yes	2,248	.65	1.49	.74
SCHOOL EXPERIENCE							
1 Competition with school mates	Do you feel in competition with your mates at school about success?	1-4	1 = not at all 2 = just a little 3 = fairly much 4 = very much	2,267			
2 Meeting with school mates	Do you stay with your mates during free time?	1-4	1 = never 2 = sometimes 3 = often 4 = always	2,268			
3 Overall satisfaction with school experience	1) How do you feel about going to school? 2) Do you like your teachers? 3) Do you like your schoolmates?	3-12	1 = not at all 2 = a little 3 = fairly much 4 = very much	2,251	.46	1.46	49

4	**Parental support for doing homework**	1) If you ask your parents to help you with your homework, do they do it? 2) Do your parents ask if you've gotten your homework done?	2-8	1 = never 2 = sometimes 3 = often 4 = always	2,223	.36	1.2,2	61
5	**Peer pressure not to get good grades**	Do you agree or disagree with the statement below: I feel some pressure from my friends not to do too well in school?	1-4	1 = strongly disagree 2 = agree a little 3 = agree 4 = strongly agree	2,252			
6	**Perceived difficulty of school subjects**	Are any of your classes too hard for you?	1-4	1 = no 2 = one or two 3 = several 4 = all	2,263			
7	**Perceived future usefulness of school**	Do you agree or disagree with each of the following statements? 1) Staying in school will be important for my future. 2) Being in school helps me to become the person I'd like to be. 3) Finishing high school is not that important for what I want to do with my life.	3-12	1 = strongly disagree 2 = agree a little 3 = agree 4 = strongly agree	2,242	.43	1.48	49
8	**Perceived present usefulness of school**	Do you agree or disagree with each of the statements below? 1) I'm learning a lot from being in school. 2) Being in school makes me feel good about myself. 3) If I make good grades, I will be appreciated by many boys and girls.	3-12	1 = strongly disagree 2 = agree a little 3 = agree 4 = strongly agree	2,247	.54	1.58	53

Variable	Question/scale	Range	Answer modalities	No. of cases	Cronbach's alpha	First factor Eigen value	First factor % explained variance
9 Perceived usefulness of school	Do you agree or disagree with each of the statements below? 1) I'm learning a lot from being in school. 2) Being in school makes me feel good about myself. 3) If I make good grades, I will be appreciated by many boys and girls. 4) Staying in school will be important for my future. 5) Being in school helps me to become the person I'd like to be. 6) Finishing high school is not that important for what I want to do with my life.	6-24	1 = strongly disagree 2 = agree a little 3 = agree 4 = strongly agree	2,221	.55	2.25	38
10 Satisfaction with relationships with classmates	Do you like your classmates?	1-4	1 = not at all 2 = a little 3 = fairly much 4 = very much	2,266			
11 Satisfaction with relationships with teachers	Do you like your teachers?	1-4	1 = not at all 2 = a little 3 = fairly much 4 = very much	2,263			

12 Satisfaction with school experience	How do you feel about going to school?	1-4	1 = don't like it at all 2 = don't like it very much 3 = like it enough 4 = like it a lot	2,261			
13 Stress caused by school	In the past six months, how much stress or pressure have you felt because of school?	1-4	1 = none 2 = a little 3 = rather a lot 4 = a lot	2,264			
14 Value on academic achievement by friends	It is important to your friends that you do well in school?	1-4	1 = not at all 2 = a little 3 = fairly 4 = very	2,252			
15 Value on academic achievement by parents	It is important to your parents that you do well in school?	1-4	1 = not at all 2 = a little 3 = fairly 4 = very	2,265			
STRESS							
1 Stress	1) In the past six months, how much stress or pressure have you felt because of your social relationship? 2) In the past six months, how much stress or pressure have you felt because of school? 3) In the past six months, how much stress or pressure have you felt because of your family life?	3-12	1 = none 2 = a little 3 = rather a lot 4 = a lot	2,252	.61	1.69	56

Variable	Question/scale	Range	Answer modalities	No. of cases	Cronbach's alpha	First factor Eigen value	First factor % explained variance
↑ ACTIVITIES AFTER SCHOOL AND ON WEEKEND							
1 **Time spent watching TV on the weekend**	About how many hours do you usually spend watching TV on the weekend?	1-6	1 = none 2 = 1 hour 3 = 2-3 hours 4 = 4-5 hours 5 = 6-7 hours 6 = 8 hours or more	2,261			
2 **Time spent weekly doing nothing or listening to music**	About how many hours do you usually spend each week: 1) just sitting around doing nothing, 2) listening to music alone?	2-12	1 = none 2 = 1 hour 3 = 2-3 hours 4 = 4-5 hours 5 = 6-7 hours 6 = 8 hours or more	2,22,2	.30	1.19	60
3 **Time spent weekly exercising alone**	About how many hours do you usually spend each week: 1) working out as a part of a personal exercise program (such as running, biking)?	1-6	1 = none 2 = 1 hour 3 = 2-3 hours 4 = 4-5 hours 5 = 6-7 hours 6 = 8 hours or more	2,242			

			Range	Response scale	N			
4	Time spent weekly in a discotheque	About how many hours do you usually spend each week: 1) going to the disco?	1-6	1 = none 2 = 1 hour 3 = 2-3 hours 4 = 4-5 hours 5 = 6-7 hours 6 = 8 hours or more	2,243			
5	Time spent weekly in conventional activities	About how many hours do you usually spend each week: 1) studying and doing homework, 2) reading for fun, 3) talking on the telephone, 4) listening to music alone, 5) staying with your family?	5-30	1 = none 2 = 1 hour 3 = 2-3 hours 4 = 4-5 hours 5 = 6-7 hours 6 = 8 hours or more	2,165	.55	1.81	36
6	Time spent weekly in family activities	About how many hours do you usually spend each week: 1) staying with your family, 2) taking care of younger brothers or sisters?	2-12	1 = none 2 = 1 hour 3 = 2-3 hours 4 = 4-5 hours 5 = 6-7 hours 6 = 8 hours or more	2,141	.22	1.13	56
7	Time spent weekly in nonorganized activities	About how many hours do you usually spend each week: 1) just sitting around doing nothing, 2) staying in a pub or game room, 3) going to the disco?	3-18	1 = none 2 = 1 hour 3 = 2-3 hours 4 = 4-5 hours 5 = 6-7 hours 6 = 8 hours or more	2,211	.50	1.50	50

Variable	Question/scale	Range	Answer modalities	No. of cases	Cronbach's alpha	First factor	
						Eigen value	% explained variance
8 Time spent weekly in organized activities	About how many hours do you usually spend each week: 1) studying and doing homework, 2) reading for fun, 3) staying with family, 4) taking care of younger brothers or sisters, 5) practicing hobbies and artistic activities?	5-30	1 = none 2 = 1 hour 3 = 2-3 hours 4 = 4-5 hours 5 = 6-7 hours 6 = 8 hours or more	2,210	.45	1.61	32
9 Time spent weekly in public places	About how many hours do you usually spend each week: 1) staying in a pub or game room, 2) going to the disco?	2-12	1 = none 2 = 1 hour 3 = 2-3 hours 4 = 4-5 hours 5 = 6-7 hours 6 = 8 hours or more	2,244	.60	1.42	71
10 Time spent weekly in social activities	About how many hours do you usually spend each week: 1) meeting with friends, 2) staying alone with your partner, 3) talking on the telephone?	3-18	1 = none 2 = 1 hour 3 = 2-3 hours 4 = 4-5 hours 5 = 6-7 hours 6 = 8 hours or more	2,158	.45	1.46	49

	Question	Range	Coding	N			
11 Time spent weekly in sport-related activities	About how many hours do you usually spend each week: 1) working out as a part of a personal exercise program (such as running, biking), 2) playing pickup games (such as football, volleyball)?	2-12	1 = none 2 = 1 hour 3 = 2-3 hours 4 = 4-5 hours 5 = 6-7 hours 6 = 8 hours or more	2,206	.40	1.25	62
12 Time spent weekly playing team sports	About how many hours do you usually spend each week: 1) playing pickup games (such as football, volleyball)?	1-6	1 = none 2 = 1 hour 3 = 2-3 hours 4 = 4-5 hours 5 = 6-7 hours 6 = 8 hours or more	2,243			
13 Time spent weekly reading	About how many hours do you usually spend each week: 1) reading for fun?	1-6	1 = none 2 = 1 hour 3 = 2-3 hours 4 = 4-5 hours 5 = 6-7 hours 6 = 8 hours or more	2,242			
14 Time spent weekly sitting around doing nothing	About how many hours do you usually spend each week: 1) just sitting around doing nothing?	1-6	1 = none 2 = 1 hour 3 = 2-3 hours 4 = 4-5 hours 5 = 6-7 hours 6 = 8 hours or more	2,248			

Variable	Question/scale	Range	Answer modalities	No. of cases	Cronbach's alpha	First factor Eigen value	First factor % explained variance
15 Time spent weekly studying and reading	About how many hours do you usually spend each week: 1) studying and doing homework, 2) reading for fun?	2-12	1 = none 2 = 1 hour 3 = 2-3 hours 4 = 4-5 hours 5 = 6-7 hours 6 = 8 hours or more	2,213	.46	1.30	65
16 Time spent weekly watching TV	On an average school day, about how many hours do you usually watch TV?	1-6	1 = none 2 = 1 hour 3 = 2-3 hours 4 = 4-5 hours 5 = 6-7 hours 6 = 8 hours or more	2,265			
17 Time spent weekly with friends	About how many hours do you usually spend each week: 1) meeting with friends?	1-6	1 = none 2 = 1 hour 3 = 2-3 hours 4 = 4-5 hours 5 = 6-7 hours 6 = 8 hours or more	2,253			

	Question	Range	Response options	N
18 Time spent weekly with the family	About how many hours do you usually spend each week: 1) staying with your family?	1-6	1 = none 2 = 1 hour 3 = 2-3 hours 4 = 4-5 hours 5 = 6-7 hours 6 = 8 hours or more	2,240
AFFECTIVE RELATIONSHIPS				
1 Affective relationship	Are you dating someone fairly regularly or going steady now?	1-2	1 = no 2 = yes	2,257
2 Number of dates with someone of the opposite sex	How often in the past six months did you go out on a date with someone of the opposite sex?	1-7	1 = never 2 = once or twice 3 = 3-4 times 4 = about once a month 5 = 2-3 times a month 6 = once a week 7 = several times a week	2,257
ALCOHOL CONSUMPTION				
1 Age of initiation of alcohol consumption	Think about the first time you had an alcoholic drink. How old were you?	/	/	1,739
2 Alcohol consumption	Have you ever had a drink of beer, wine, or liquor?	1-5	1 = never 2 = only once 3 = a few times 4 = several times 5 = usually	2,258

Variable	Question/scale	Range	Answer modalities	No. of cases	Cronbach's alpha	First factor Eigen value	% explained variance
3 Frequency of alcohol consumption	Over the past six months, how often did you drink alcohol?	1-9	1 = never 2 = once or twice 3 = 3-4 times 4 = about once a month 5= 2-3 days a month 6 = once a week 7 = 2-3 days a week 8= 4-5 days a week 9 = every day	2,250			
4 Frequency of getting drunk	In the past six months, how many times have you gotten drunk?	1-4	1 = never 2 = only on particular occasions 3 = often 4 = very often	1,783			
5 Heavy alcohol consumption	Over the past six months, how many times did you drink five or more drinks of beer, wine, or liquor?	1-9	1 = never 2 = once 3 = 2-3 times 4 = 4-5 times 5 = once a month 6 = 2-3 times a month 7 = once a week 8 = twice a week 9 = more than twice a week	2,236			

#								
6	Problems caused by alcohol consumption	Over the past six months, how many times has each of the following things happened because you drank: a) got into trouble with your parents, b) had problems at school or with schoolwork, c) had problems with your friends, d) had problems with your partner, e) got into trouble with the police, f) had accidents, g) had problems with health?	7-28	1 = never 2 = once 3 = 2-4 times 4 = 5 or more times	1,721	.68	2.51	36
7	Relation context in which first consumption of alcohol occurs	Think about the first time you had an alcoholic drink: Whom were you with?	/	Your parents Your friends Alone	1,848			

Variable	Question/scale	Range	Answer modalities	No. of cases	Cronbach's alpha	First factor Eigen value	First factor % explained variance
↑ ANTISOCIAL BEHAVIOR							
1 Antisocial behavior	During the past six months, how often have you: 1) started a fist fight or shoving match, 2) shoplifted from a store, 3) damaged or marked up public or private property, 4) lied to a teacher to cover up something you did, 5) taken things that didn't belong to you, 6) stayed out all night without permission, 7) damaged school properties on purpose, 8) stayed out all night without permission, 9) skipped school without permission, 10) hit someone because you didn't like what they said or did, 11) started or got into a fight with members of a gang, 12) carried a weapon (such as a knife), 13) had a serious fight at school?	13-52	1 = never 2 = once 3 = 2-4 times 4 = 5 or more times	303	.82	3.74	29
2 Lies and disobedience	During the past six months, how often have you: 1) lied to a teacher to cover up something you did, 2) stayed out all night without permission, 3) stayed out all night without permission, 4) skipped school without permission?	4-16	1 = never 2 = once 3 = 2-4 times 4 = 5 or more times	2,244	.62	1.90	48

		Range	Response scale	N			
3 Physical aggression	During the past six months, how often have you: 1) started a fist fight or shoving match, 2) hit someone because you didn't like what they said or did, 3) started or got into a fight with members of a gang, 4) carried a weapon (such as a knife), 5) had a serious fight at school?	5-20	1 = never 2 = once 3 = 2-4 times 4 = 5 or more times	2,245	.73	2.44	49
4 Theft and vandalism	During the past six months, how often have you: 1) shoplifted from a store, 2) damaged or marked up public or private property, 3) taken things that didn't belong to you, 4) damaged school properties on purpose?	4-16	1 = never 2 = once 3 = 2-4 times 4 = 5 or more times	2,245	.63	1.92	48
CIGARETTE SMOKING							
1 Age of initiation of cigarette smoking	How old were you when first smoked a cigarette?	/	/	1,228			
2 Age of stabilization of cigarette smoking	How old were you when you started smoking on a pretty regular basis?	/	/	750			
3 Cigarette smoking	Have you ever smoked a cigarette?	1-5	1 = never 2 = once 3 = a few times 4 = several times 5 = regularly	2,262			

Variable	Question/scale	Range	Answer modalities	No. of cases	Cronbach's alpha	First factor Eigen value	First factor % explained variance
4 **Daily frequency of cigarette smoking**	During the past month, how many cigarettes have you smoked during an average day?	1-5	1 = none 2 = 1-5 3 = half a pack 4 = a pack 5 = more than a pack	2,246			
CONTRACEPTION AND PREGNANCY							
1 **Contraceptive use the first time**	That first time you had sex, did you or your partner use any kind of contraceptive method?	1-3	1 = no 2 = yes 3 = don't remember	685			
2 **Method used the first time**	If you or your partner used any kind of contraceptive method that first time you had sex, which one?	/	/	464			
3 **Pregnancy**	Have you ever been pregnant or made a girl pregnant?	1-3	1 = no 2 = once 3 = more than once	553			
4 **Pregnancy resolution**	If pregnancy occurred, what did you and your partner do about the pregnancy?	1-5	1 = had the baby and kept him/her 2 = had the baby and gave him/her up for adoption 3 = had a miscarriage 4 = had an abortion 5 = other	15			

The Behavior System 331

#	Item	Question		Response options	
5	Reasons for not using contraception	If contraception was not used, what was the reason?	/	/	211
6	Regular contraceptive use during the past year	When you had sex during the past year, did you make sure that some kind of birth control method or contraceptive was used, either by you or by the other person?	1-4	1 = never 2 = sometimes 3 = most of the times 4 = always	503
7	Sharing choice of contraception with partner	When you had sex in the past year, who usually made the decision about whether or not to use birth control?	1-3	1 = I did 2 = my partner did 3 = we both did	481
8	Type of contraceptive method used the last time	The last time you had sex, what type of birth control method or contraceptive was used?	/	/	
9	Type of contraception method usually used	What kind of contraceptive methods do you usually use?	/	condom birth control pill diaphragm/intrauterine device withdrawal Ogino-Knaus method basal temperature spermicide cream other	526

Variable	Question/scale	Range	Answer modalities	No. of cases	Cronbach's alpha	First factor Eigen value	First factor % explained variance
DIFFICULTY IN SLEEPING							
1 Difficulty in sleeping	In the past six months, have you had trouble falling asleep or staying asleep at night?	1-4	1 = never 2 = sometimes 3 = often 4 = always	2,268			
DRIVING CARS AND MOTORCYCLES							
1 Being the passenger in a vehicle driven by someone who has used psychoactive substances	In the past six months, how often did you ride in a car when a friend who had been drinking or using drugs was driving it?	1-4	1 = never 2 = once or twice 3 = 3-5 times 4 = 6 or more times	2,261			
2 Dangerous driving	During the past six months, how often did you: 1) take chances for the fun of it when driving in traffic, 2) take some risks while driving in traffic because it made driving more fun?	2-8	1 = never 2 = once or twice 3 = 3-5 times 4 = 6 or more times	1,344	.77	1.63	81

3 **Driving under the influence of alcohol**	During the past six months, how often did you: 1) drive after you had one or two drinks of wine or cans of beer, 2) drive after you had three or more drinks of wine or cans of beer?	2-8	1 = never 2 = once or twice 3 = 3-5 times 4 = 6 or more times	1,364	.89	1.81	91
4 **Driving under the influence of psychoactive substances**	During the past six months, how often did you: 1) drive after you had one or two drinks of wine or cans of beer, 2) drive after you had three or more drinks of wine or cans of beer, 3) drive after you used marijuana?	3-12	1 = never 2 = once or twice 3 = 3-5 times 4 = 6 or more times	1,327	.81	2.19	73
5 **Exceeding the speed limit**	During the past six months, how often did you: 1) drive more than 30 km/h over the speed limit, 2) drive at high speed through a school zone?	2-8	1 = never 2 = once or twice 3 = 3-5 times 4 = 6 or more times	1,346	.60	1.50	72
6 **Failing to give the right of way**	During the past six months, how often did you: 1) drive through a stop sign without coming to a full stop, 2) drive through a red light, 3) race a car on city streets?	3-12	1 = never 2 = once or twice 3 = 3-5 times 4 = 6 or more times	1,334	.72	1.92	64
7 **Failing to respect safe braking distance**	During the past six months, how often did you: 1) drive too close to the car in front of you?	1-4	1 = never 2 = once or twice 3 = 3-5 times 4 = 6 or more times	1,344			

Variable	Question/scale	Range	Answer modalities	No. of cases	Cronbach's alpha	First factor Eigen value	% explained variance
8 Fines	In the past six months, how many times have you: 1) had a traffic accident because you were driving carelessly?	1-4	1 = never 2 = once 3 = twice 4 = 3 or more times	1,354			
9 Frequency of use of safety belt and helmet when the subject is a passenger	1) When you are riding in a car or on a motorcycle that a friend is driving, do you usually use a seat belt or a crash helmet? 2) When you are riding in a car that your mother or father is driving, do you usually use a seat belt?	2-8	1 = never 2 = sometimes 3 = most of the time 4 = always	2,251	.80	1.68	84
10 Frequency of use of safety belt and helmet when the subject is driving	1) When you are driving by yourself, do you use a seat belt? 2) When you are driving with a friend in your car or on motorcycle, do you use your seat belt or your crash helmet?	2-8	1 = never 2 = once or twice 3 = 3-5 times 4 = 6 or more times	999	.68	1.51	76
11 Involvement in driving	This variable was constructed by the information drawn from the item: "Which one of these transport means have you driven in the past six months"?	/	/	2,163			

	Question	Range	Response scale	N		Mean	
12 Kilometers driven in an ordinary week	How many kilometers do you drive in an average week?	1-5	1 = 1-10 2 = 11-30 3 = 31-50 4 = 51-100 5 = more than 100	1,333			
13 Nighttime driving	In an average week, how much of your driving do you do after 8 o'clock at night?	1-4	1 = none 2 = a little 3 = some 4 = most	1,369			
14 Risky driving	During the past six months, how often did you: 1) drive after you had one or two drinks of wine or cans of beer, 2) drive more than 30 km/h over the speed limit, 3) drive through a stop sign without coming to a full stop, 4) pass a car in a no-passing zone, 5) drive after you had three or more drinks of wine or cans of beer, 6) take chances for the fun of it when driving in traffic, 7) drive too close to the car in front of you, 8) drive at high speed through a school zone, 9) drive after you had used marijuana, 10) drive through a red light, 11) race a car on city streets, 12) cut in front of another car at full speed, 13) take some risks while driving in traffic because it made driving more fun?	13-52	1 = never 2 = once or twice 3 = 3-5 times 4 = 6 or more times	1,168	.89	5.90	45

Variable	Question/scale	Range	Answer modalities	No. of cases	Cronbach's alpha	First factor Eigen value	First factor % explained variance
15 Road accidents	In the past six months, how many times have you got a ticket for speeding or any other traffic violation (not a parking ticket)?	1-4	1 = never 2 = once 3 = twice 4 = 3 or more times	1,354			
16 Traffic code offenses	During the past six months, how often did you: 1) drive more than 30 km/h over the speed limit, 2) drive through a stop sign without coming to a full stop, 3) pass a car in a no-passing zone, 4) take chances for the fun of it when driving in traffic, 5) drive too close to the car in front of you, 6) drive at high speed through a school zone, 7) drive through a red light, 8) race a car on city streets, 9) cut in front of another car at full speed, 10) take risks while you were driving in traffic because it made driving more fun?	10-40	1 = never 2 = once or twice 3 = 3-5 times 4 = 6 or more times	1,175	.87	5.12	47
17 Type of driver's license	Do you have a driving license or a learner's permit?	/	no driving license for car driving license for motorcycle learner's permit	483			

18 Use of safety belt or helmet	1) When you are driving by yourself, do you use your seat belt? 2) When you are riding in a car that your mother or father is driving, do you use your seat belt? 3) When you are riding in a car that a friend is driving, do you use your seat belt? 4) When you are driving with a friend in your car or on motorcycle, do you use your seat belt or your crash helmet? 5) When you are riding in a car or on motorcycle that a friend is driving, do you use your seat belt or a crash helmet?	5-20	1 = never 2 = sometimes 3 = often 4 = always	760	.86	3.2.2	64
19 Vehicles driven	Which one of these transportation means have you driven in the past six months?	/	a car a motorcycle a motorcycle of small cubic capacity none	2,163			
EATING HABITS **1 Being on a diet**	Are you on a diet to lose weight now?	1-3	1 = no 2 = for healthy motives 3 = for aesthetic motives	2,248			

Variable	Question/scale	Range	Answer modalities	No. of cases	Cronbach's alpha	First factor Eigen value	First factor % explained variance
2 Comfort eating	How many times do you: 1) eat even when you're not really hungry, 2) keep on eating even after you feel full, 3) eat because you're depressed, 4) eat just because you're bored?	4-16	1 = never 2 = sometimes 3 = often 4 = always	2,246	.69	2.11	53
3 Dieting	In the past six months, how many times have you started a diet to lose weight?	1-4	1 = never 2 = once 3 = 2-3 times 4 = 4 or more times	2,254			
4 Healthiness of eating habits	In your usual eating habits, how much attention do you pay to: 1) seeing if your diet is healthy, 2) keeping down the amount of salt you eat, 3) eating only as much as your body really needs, 4) keeping down the amount of fat you eat, 5) drinking enough milk (or yogurt) every day, 6) eating in healthy way even when you're with your friends, 7) eating some fresh vegetables and fruit, 8) eating a little candy, 9) eating a little fried foods?	9-36	1 = none 2 = a little 3 = some 4 = a lot	2,138	.88	4.62	51

#	Variable	Question	Range	Coding	N			
5	Purging behavior	1) In the past six months, have you ever used diet pills, laxatives, or other products to help you to lose weight or to stay thin? 2) In the past six months, have you ever made yourself throw up as a way to lose weight or to stay thin?	2-8	1 = never 2 = once or twice 3 = several times 4 = often	2,256	.51	1.34	67
6	Referent for diet	If you want to start a diet, whom would you address for advice?	1-5	1 = nobody 2 = friend or parent 3 = chemist 4 = doctor 5 = dietitian	2,215			
7	Regularity of eating habits	1) How often do you skip breakfast? 2) How often do you skip a meal? 3) How often do you eat dinner with your family? 4) How often do you snack instead of eating regular meals?	4-16	1 = always 2 = often 3 = sometimes 4 = never	2,254	.42	1.54	39
	HAVING A JOB							
1	Having a job	Do you work?	1-3	1 = no 2 = sometimes 3 = regularly	2,247			

Variable	Question/scale	Range	Answer modalities	No. of cases	Cronbach's alpha	First factor Eigen value	First factor % explained variance
MARIJUANA SMOKING AND USE OF OTHER DRUGS							
1 Accessibility of marijuana	If you wanted to get marijuana, how easy would it be for you?	1-4	1 = difficult 2 = not too easy 3 = easy 4 = very easy	2,214			
2 Age of initiation of marijuana smoking	How old were you when you first tried marijuana?	/	/	617			
3 Frequency of getting high	Have you ever been high or stoned from using marijuana?	1-4	1 = never 2 = once 3 = more than once 4 = always	635			
4 Frequency of marijuana smoking	In the past six months, how often have you used marijuana?	1-5	1 = never 2 = 1-3 times 3 = 4-5 times 4 = 1-3 times a month 5 = once a week to every day	637			
5 Marijuana smoking	Have you ever tried marijuana?	1-3	1 = never 2 = once 3 = more than once	2,264			

		Range	Coding	N		Mean	
6 Use of other drugs	Have you used one of the following drugs: 1) pills, 2) crack, 3) cocaine, 4) LSD, 5) angel dust, 6) paint, glue, or other things, 7) heroin, 8) ecstasy, 9) other?	9-18	1 = no 2 = yes	2,151		3.48	43
RELIGION							
1 Frequency of going to religious services	How many times do you go to religious services?	1-5	1 = never 2 = on the great anniversaries or special occasions 3 = 1-2 times a month 4 = once a week 5 = more than once a week	2,250			
2 Having a religion	Do you have a religion?	1-2	1 = no 2 = yes	2,241			
3 Taking part to other religious activities	Do you take part at other religious activities?	1-2	1 = no 2 = yes	2,244			
RISK-TAKING BEHAVIOR							
1 Risk-taking behavior	In the past six months, have you: 1) done something dangerous just for the thrill of it, 2) done some risky things because it was exciting, 3) taken chances with your safety when you were out at night because it was exciting?	3-12	1 = never 2 = sometimes 3 = often 4 = always	2,260	.82	2.20	74

Variable	Question/scale	Range	Answer modalities	No. of cases	Cronbach's alpha	First factor Eigen value	First factor % explained variance
SCHOOL							
1 Intentions or attempts to drop out of school	1) Have you ever thought seriously about dropping out of school? 2) Have you ever talked seriously to your parents about dropping out of school? 3) Have you ever stopped going to classes for a while because you were seriously thinking about dropping out of school? 4) Are you currently thinking about dropping out of school?	4-12	1 = never 2 = once 3 = more than once	2,258	.66	2.08	52
2 Repeated school years	This variable was constructed by combining the information drawn from two items: school grade and age.	/	/	2,243			
3 School grades	What kind of grades do you usually get?	5-8	5 = less than 5 6 = 6 7 = 7 8 = 8 or more	2,220			
SCHOOL AND COMMUNITY ACTIVITIES							
1 Belonging to a church group	Do you belong to any church youth group or to any associations (such as boy scouts)?	1-2	1 = no 2 = yes	2,255			

2 Belonging to a sport team	Do you belong to any sporting group?	1-2	1 = no 2 = yes	2,254
3 Involvement in volunteer work	Do you do any kind of volunteer work in the community?	1-3	1 = no 2 = once in a while 3 = rather often	2,257
4 Participation in informal group	Do you belong to any other group?	1-2	1 = no 2 = yes	1,672
5 Participation in political group	Do you belong to any political group?	1-2	1 = no 2 = yes	2,255
6 Participation in school group	Do you belong to any school clubs or organizations (such as sporting club, school newspaper)?	1-3	1 = no 2 = yes 3 = I'd like to, but in my school they aren't offered	2,250
SEXUAL BEHAVIOR **1 Age of initiation**	How old were you the first time you had sexual intercourse?	/	/	678

Variable	Question/scale	Range	Answer modalities	No. of cases	Cronbach's alpha	First factor Eigen value	First factor % explained variance
2 Depth of relationship with first partner	What was your relationship with your first sexual partner?	1-5	1 = other 2 = occasional meeting 3 = knew each other a little 4 = close friend 5 = going steady	673			
3 Molestation and sexual violence committed	1) Did you happen to perform sexual harassment with your peers? 2) Did you happen to oblige somebody to have sexual contacts?	2-8	1 = never 2 = some of the time 3 = most of the time 4 = always	788	.80	1.66	83
4 Number of sexual intercourses in the past year	In the past year, how many times, if any, have you had sexual intercourse?	/	/	434			
5 Number of sexual partners in the past year	In the past year, with how many people have you had sexual intercourse?	/	/	504			
6 Number of sexual partners/sexual promiscuity	In your life, how many people have you had sexual intercourse with?	/	/	654			

7	Pornography	1) In the last six months, have you ever looked at pornographic reviews or papers? 2) In the last six months, have you ever looked at a pornographic film or home video?	2-8	1 = never 2 = once or twice 3 = about once a month 4 = about once a week or more	796	.71 1.72 86
8	Sexual intercourse/sexual activity	Have you ever had sexual intercourse with someone of the opposite sex?	1-2	1 = no 2 = yes	2,245	

Typology	Items	Construction's modalities of typology
↑ CHAPTER 3 - PSYCHOACTIVE SUBSTANCE USE		
1 Typology of cigarettes smoking	1) Have you ever smoked a cigarette? 2) During the past month, how many cigarettes have you smoked on an average day?	The typology was constructed by combining the information drawn from two items: cigarettes smoking and daily frequency of cigarette smoking. Five groups of adolescents were obtained: *nonsmokers* = adolescents who have never smoked or smoked only one cigarette in their lifetime; *ex-smokers* = adolescents who have smoked several times in their life but have not smoked in the last month; *occasional smokers* = adolescents who have smoked a few or several times in their life; *moderate smokers* = adolescents who smoke habitually and in the past month smoked from 1 to 10 cigarettes a day; *heavy smokers* = adolescents who smoke habitually and in the last month smoked from half a pack to more than a pack of cigarettes a day.
2 Typology of marijuana smoking	1) Have you ever tried marijuana? 2) In the past six months, how often have you used marijuana?	The typology was constructed by combining the information drawn from two items: marijuana smoking and frequency of marijuana smoking during the last six months. Four groups of adolescents were obtained: *nonsmokers* = adolescents who have never smoked marijuana in their life or have smoked only once; *ex-smokers* = adolescents who have not smoked marijuana in the last six months; *occasional smokers* = adolescents who have smoked marijuana between one and six times in the last six months; *habitual smokers* = adolescents who have smoked marijuana from two to three times in the last six months to everyday for the last six months.

↑ CHAPTER 6 - SEXUAL BEHAVIOR, CONTRACEPTION, AND AIDS

1 Typology of sexual behavior patterns

1) Have you ever had sexual intercourse with someone of the opposite sex? 2) In your life, how many people have you had sexual intercourse with? 3) In the past year, how many people have you had sexual intercourse with?

The typology was constructed by combining the information drawn from three items: sexual involvement, total number of sexual partners, and number of sexual partners in the last year. Five groups of adolescents were obtained: *stopped* = adolescents who have stopped sexual activity during the last year; *high faithfulness* = adolescents who have had only one sexual partner in their lives; *low faithfulness* = adolescents who have had more than one sexual partner in their lives; *ex-low faithfulness - now high faithfulness* = adolescents who have had only one sexual partner in the past year but previously had more than one. Along with these four groups, another group consisting of adolescents who are not yet sexually active was also considered.

↑ CHAPTER 7 - DISTURBED EATING

1 Typology of awareness of negative consequences of being overweight

1) Do you think being overweight can have negative physical effects on the health of young people your age? 2) Do you think being overweight can have negative psychological effects on the health of young people your age?

The responses to two items referring to awareness of the physical and psychological consequences of being overweight were divided into high-level groups and a low-level groups for the aspect considered using the median (the midpoint: half the cases fall above and half fall below this value) as the threshold. The groups obtained were then crossed to form a single variable with four categories of adolescents characterized by low awareness of the physical and psychological consequences; low awareness of the physical consequences and high awareness of the psychological consequences; high awareness of the physical consequences and low awareness of the psychological consequences; and high awareness of the physical and psychological consequences.

Typology	Items	Construction's modalities of typology
2 Typology of disturbed eating behavior	1) How many times do you: a) eat even when you're not really hungry, b) keep on eating even after you feel full, c) eat because you're depressed, d) eat just because you're bored? 2) In the past six months, have you ever used diet pills, laxatives, or other products to help you to lose weight or to stay thin? 3) In the past six months, have you ever made yourself throw up as a way to lose weight or to stay thin? 4) In the past six months, how many times have you starter a diet to lose weight?	The typology was constructed by forming two groups from the scales of comfort eating and purging behavior (using the median value as the threshold) and crossing the groups obtained with involvement or non-involvement in dieting (in the last six months they either ended a diet or were currently dieting). The typology of disturbed eating divides the adolescents in five groups: not involved; involved in comfort eating only; involved in dieting only; involved in both comfort eating and dieting; involved in purging behavior only or combined with comfort eating and/or dieting.
3 Typology of healthiness and regularity of eating habits	1) How often do you skip breakfast? 2) How often do you skip a meal? 3) How often do you eat dinner with your family? 4) How often do you snack instead of eating regular meals? In your usual eating habits, how much do you pay attention to: 1) seeing if your diet is healthy, 2) keeping down the amount of salt you eat, 3) eating only as much as your body really needs, 4) keeping down the amount of fat you eat, 5) drinking enough milk (or yogurt) every day, 6) eating in healthy way even when you're with your friends, 7) eating some fresh vegetables and fruit, 8) eating a little candy, 9) eating a little fried foods?	The responses to the items that make up the scales of healthiness and regularity of eating habits were divided into high-level and low-level groups for the aspect considered using the median (the mid-point: half the cases fall above and half fall below this value) as the threshold. The groups of adolescents obtained in this way were then crossed to form a single variable with four categories of adolescents characterized by high regularity and low healthiness of eating habits, low regularity and low healthiness of eating habits, high regularity and high healthiness of eating habits, and low regularity and high healthiness of eating habits.

↑ PARENTING STYLE

1 Parenting style

1) Is it easy for you to talk with your parents about personal problems, thoughts, feelings? 2) Is it easy for you to talk with your parents about problems with school? 3) In your family, how strict are the rules you have to follow about: a) when and which television shows you can watch, b) getting your homework done, c) what time you go to sleep at night, d) getting chores done around the house, e) letting your family know where you're going when you go out, f) being at home by a certain time at night, g) going to parties, h) dating with your partner?

The typology was constructed by combining the information drawn from the following items: parental support and parental control. Four groups of parenting style were obtained: *permissive style* = adolescents who perceived little support and low control by parents; *supportive style* = adolescents who perceived high support and low control by parents; *authoritarian style* = adolescents who perceived low support and high control by parents; *authoritative style* = adolescents who perceived high support and control by parents.

REFERENCES

ADALBJARNARDOTTIR S, RAFNSSON FD (2002) Adolescent antisocial behavior and substance use. Longitudinal analyses. Addict Behav 27:227-324

ALOISE PA, GRAHAM JW, HANSEN WB (1994) Peer influence on smoking initiation during early adolescence: A comparison of group members and group outsiders. J Appl Psychol 79:281-287

ANTONOVSKY A (1979) Health, stress and coping. Jossey Bass, San Francisco

ANTONOVSKY A (1987) Unraveling the mystery of health. Jossey Bass, San Francisco

ARDONE R (1998) Il benessere-malessere nella rappresentazione di genitori e figli preadolescenti. Psicologia Clinica dello Sviluppo II 1:99-117

ATTIE I, BROOKS-GUNN J (1989) Development of eating problems in adolescent girls: A longitudinal study. Dev Psychol 25:70-79

AUNOLA K, STATTIN H, NURMI JE (2000) Parenting styles and adolescents' achievement strategies. J Adolesc 23:205-222

BAKKER AB, BUUNK BP, MANSTED ASR (1997) The moderating role of self-efficacy beliefs in the relationship between anticipated feelings of regret and condom use. J Appl Soc Psychol 27(22):2001-2014

BAKKER AB, BUUNK BP, VAN DEN EIJNDEN RJ, SIERO FW (1998) Determinants of safe sex among adult heterosexuals: Towards theory-based interventions. In: Sandfort T (ed) The Dutch response to HIV pragmatism and consensus, Taylor & Francis, London, pp 204-225

BALTES PB, LINDENBERGER U, STAUDINGER UM (1998) Life-span theory in developmental psychology. In: Damon W (ed) Handbook of child psychology, Wiley, New York, pp 1029-1144

BANDURA A (1986) Social foundation of thought and action: A social cognitive theory. Prentice Hall, Englewood Cliffs

BANDURA A (1997) Self-efficacy: The exercise of control. WH Freeman, New York

BANDURA A (1999) Moral disengagement in the perpetration of inhumanities. Pers Soc Psychol Rev (special issue on evil and violence) 3:193-209

BANDURA A, BARBARANELLI C, CAPRARA GV, PASTORELLI C (1996) Mechanism of moral disengagement in the exercise of moral agency. J Pers Soc Psychol 71:364-374

BAUMAN KE, ENNETT ST (1996) The importance of peer influence for adolescent drug use: Commonly neglected considerations. Addiction 91:185-198

BEGG DJ, LANGLEY JD (2004) Identifying predictors of persistent non-alcohol or drug-related risky driving behaviours among a cohort of young adults. Accid Anal Prev 36:1067-1071

BENARD B (1991) Fostering resiliency in kids: Protective factor in the family, school and community. Northwest Regional Education Laboratory, Oregon

BENTHIN A, SLOVIC P, SEVERSON H (1993) A psychometric study of adolescent risk perception. J Adolesc 16:153-168

BEYTH-MAROM R, FISCHHOFF B (1997) Adolescents' decisions about risks: A cognitive perspective. In: Schulenberg J, Maggs JL, Hurrelmann K (eds). Health risks and developmental transitions during adolescence. Cambridge University Press, Cambridge, pp 110-135

BINA M, BONINO S, CATTELINO E (2004) Il ruolo delle relazioni con i coetanei ed i genitori nella promozione del benessere psicologico degli adolescenti. Età Evolutiva 79:43-52

BINA M, GRAZIANO F, BONINO S (2005) Risky driving and lifestyles in adolescence. Accident Analysis and Prevention (in press)

BISHOP DL, MACY-LEWIS JA, SCHENEKLOTH CA ET AL (1997) Ego identity status and reported alcohol consumption: A study of first-year college students. J Adolesc 20:209-218

BJÖRKQVIST K, FRY DP (1997) Cultural variation in conflict resolution. Alternatives to violence. Lawrence Erlbaum, Hillsdale

BONINO S (1995; 1996) Io e la mia salute. Regione Piemonte, Torino; Regione Autonoma Valle d'Aosta, Aosta

BONINO S (2000) Relazioni tra i pari e benessere psicosociale in adolescenza. Età Evolutiva 65:71-111

BONINO S (2001) La famiglia e il benessere degli adolescenti. Età Evolutiva 69:43-96

BONINO S, CATTELINO E (2000) L'adolescenza tra opportunità e rischio. L'uso di sostanze psicoattive. In: Caprara GV, Fonzi A (eds) L'età sospesa. Giunti, Firenze, pp 121-154

BONINO S, CATTELINO E (2002) La scuola e il benessere degli adolescenti. In: G Di Stefano, R Vianello, Psicologia dello sviluppo e problemi educativi. Giunti, Firenze, pp 324-352

BONINO S, CATTELINO E, CIAIRANO S (2006) Italy. In AA.W Routledge International Encyclopedia of Adolescence. London, Routledge (in press)

BORCA G, CATTELINO E, BONINO S (2002) Insuccesso e insoddisfazione scolastica in adolescenza. Età Evolutiva 71:67-73

BORN M (1987) Jeunes déviants ou délinquants juvéniles. Mardaga, Bruxelles

BORN M (2003) Psychologie de la délinquance. De Boeck, Bruxelles

BORN M, CHEVALIER V, HUMBLET I (1997) Resilience, desistance and delinquent career of adolescent offenders. J Adolesc 20:679-694

BOSMA H, JACKSON S (eds) (1990) Coping and self-concept in adolescence. Springer, Berlin Heidelberg New York

BOSMA H, KUNNEN S (2001) Identity and emotion. Development through self-organization. Cambridge University Press, Cambridge

BOURGAULT C, DEMERS A (1997) Solitary drinking: A risk factor for alcohol-related problems? Addiction 92(3):303-312

BRAET C (1996) Emotional eating in adolescence. In: Verhofstadt-Denéve L, Kienhorst I, Braet C (eds) Conflict and development in adolescence. DSWO, Leiden, pp 153-159

BRANDSTÄDTER J (1997) Action perspectives on human development. In: Damon W (ed) Handbook of child psychology. Wiley, New York, pp 807-863

BRENDGEN M, VITARO F, BUKOWSKI WM (2000) Deviant friends and early adolescent's emotional and behavioral adjustment. J Res Adolesc 10(2):173-189

BRONFENBRENNER U (1979) The ecology of human development Experiments by nature and design. Harvard University Press, Cambridge

BRONFENBRENNER U (1986) Ecology of the family as a context for human development: Research perspectives. Dev Psychol 22:723-742

BRONFENBRENNER U, MORRIS PA (1998) The ecology of developmental processes. In: Damon W (ed) Handbook of child psychology. Wiley, New York, 993-1028

BROOKS-GUNN J, PAIKOFF RL (1993) Sex is a gamble, kissing is a game: Adolescent sexuality and health promotion. In: Millstein SG, Petersen AC, Nightingale EO (eds) Promoting the health of adolescents: New directions for the twenty-first century. Oxford University Press, New York, pp 108-208

BROOKS-GUNN J, CHASE-LANSDALE PL (1995) Adolescent parentohood. In: Bornstein MH (ed) Handbook of parenting: Vol 3. Status and social conditions of parenting. Erlbaum, Mahwah NJ pp 113-149

BROOKS-GUNN J, PAIKOFF R (1997) Sexual and developmental transitions during adolescence. In: Schulenberg J, Maggs JL, Hurrelmann K (eds) Health risks and developmental transitions during adolescence. Cambridge University Press, Cambridge, pp 190-219

BROWN PJ, BENTLEY-CONDIT VK (1998) Culture, evolution and obesity. In: Bray GA, Bouchard C, James WPT (eds) Handbook of obesity. Marcel Dekker, New York, pp 143-155

BRUNER J (1986) Actual minds, possible worlds. Harvard University Press, Cambridge-London

BRUNER J (1990) Acts of meaning. Harvard University Press, Cambridge-London

BUUNK BP, BAKKER AB, SIERO FW ET AL (1998) Predictors of AIDS-preventive behavioural intentions among adult heterosexuals at risk for HIV infection: extending current models and measures. AIDS Educ Prev 10(2):149-172

BUYSSE W (1996) Perceived conflict, internalizing and externalizing behaviour problems in adolescence. In: Verhofstadt-Denéve L, Kienhorst I, Braet C (eds) Conflict and development in adolescence. DSWO, Leiden, pp 117-125

BUZWELL S, ROSENTHAL D (1996) Constructing a sexual self: Adolescents' sexual self-perception and sexual risk taking. J Res Adolesc 6(4):489-513

BYRNE D (1983) Sex without contraception. In: Byrne D, Fisher WA (eds) Sex and contraception. Erlbaum, Hillsdale

CAMERANA PM, SARIGIANI PA, PETERSEN AC (1990) Gender-specific pathways to intimacy in early adolescence. J Youth Adolesc 19:19-32

CAPRARA GV, PASTORELLI C, BANDURA A (1995) La misura del disimpegno morale in età evolutiva. Età Evolutiva 51:18-29

CAPRARA GV, BARBARANELLI C, PASTORELLI C, CERVONE D (2004) The contribution on self-efficacy beliefs to psychosocial outcomes in adolescence: predicting beyond global dispositional tendencies. Pers Individ Dif 37:751-763

CARLSON BR, EDWARDS WH (1990) Human values and marijuana use. International Journal of Addiction 25(3):1393-1401

CATTELINO E (2000) Relazioni con i coetanei in adolescenza: il contributo degli amici e del partner nella promozione del benessere. Età Evolutiva 65:102-111

CATTELINO E (2001) Cognitive flexibility and antisocial behavior in adolescence: An indirect relation, X European Conference on Developmental Psychology, August 22-26, Uppsala

CATTELINO E, BONINO S (1999) I comportamenti a rischio in adolescenza: il ruolo delle relazioni con i genitori e con gli amici. Età Evolutiva 64:67-78

CATTELINO E, BONINO S (2000) Il fumo di sigarette in adolescenza: implicazioni per la promozione della salute. Psicologia della Salute 1:33-49

CATTELINO E, BONINO S, KIESNER J (2000) Adolescents' risky driving and lifestyles, 7th Biennial Conference of the European Association for Research on Adolescence – EARA, Jena (Germany) 31 May - 4 June

CATTELINO E, CALANDRI E, BONINO S (2001) Il contributo della struttura e del funzionamento della famiglia nella promozione del benessere di adolescenti di diverse fasce di età. Età Evolutiva 69:49-60

CATTELINO E, BEGOTTI T, BONINO S (2002) L'interazione tra il valore e le aspettative rispetto alla scuola in adolescenza. Età Evolutiva 72:5-16

CENTRO STUDI AUXOLOGICI (2004) Growing and development of the child and the adolescent. http://www.auxologia.com/centroauxologico/index.html. Cited 16 Mar 2005

CHISHOLM L, HURRELMANN K (1995) Adolescence in modern Europe. Pluralized transition patterns and their implications for personal and social risks. J Adolesc 18:129-158

CIAIRANO S (2004) Risk behaviour in adolescence: drug-use and sexual activity in Italy and the Netherlands. Stichting Kinderstudies, Groningen

CIAIRANO S, BONINO S, JACKSON S, MICELI R (2000) Rapporti affettivi, sessualità e benessere psicosociale in adolescenza. Età Evolutiva 65:90-101

CIAIRANO S, BONINO S, JACKSON S, MICELI R (2001) Stile educativo genitoriale e benessere psicosociale in adolescenza: una ricerca in due nazioni europee. Età Evolutiva 69:61-71

CIAIRANO S, BONINO S, MOLINENGO G, MICELI R (2005) Il ruolo di moderazione delle risorse individuali ed ambientali nel contrastare il rischio in ragazzi e ragazze di età adolescenziale. In: Menesini E (eds) Fattori di protezione e promozione del benessere in adolescenza e preadolescenza. Psicologia Clinica dello Sviluppo (in press)

CLAES M, LACOURSE E, BOUCHARD C, PERUCCHINI P (2003) Parental practices in late adolescence, a comparison of three countries: Canada, France and Italy. J Adolesc 26:387-399

CLAUSEN JS (1991) Adolescent competence and the shaping of the life course. AJS 96:805-842

COHEN J, COHEN P (1983) Applied multiple regression/correlation analysis for the behavioral sciences (2nd edn), Lawrence Erlbaum, Hillsdale

COLEMAN JC (1989) The focal theory of adolescence: A psychological perspective. In: Hurrelmann K, Engel U (eds) The social worlds of adolescents: International perspectives. Walter de Gruyter, Berlin, pp 43-56

COLEMAN JC, ROKER D (1998) Teenage sexuality. Harwood Academic, Amsterdam

COMPAS BE, CONDOR JK, HINDEN BR (1998) New perspective on depression during adolescence. In: Jessor R (ed) Adolescent risk behavior. Cambridge University Press, New York, pp 319-362

CROCKETT LJ (1997) Cultural, historical and subcultural contexts of adolescence: Implication for health and development. In: Schulenberg J, Maggs JL, Hurrelmann K (eds) Health risks and developmental transitions during adolescence. Cambridge University Press, New York, pp 23-53

CROCKETT LJ, SILBEREISEN RK (eds) (2000a) Negotiating adolescence in times of social change. Cambridge University Press, Cambridge

CROCKETT LJ, SILBEREISEN RK (eds) (2000b) Social changes and adolescent development: Issues and challenges. In: Crockett LJ, Silbereisen RS (eds) Negotiating adolescence in times of social change. Cambridge University Press, Cambridge, 1-13

CSIKSZENTMIHALYI M, SCHNEIDER B (2000) Becoming adult. Perseus Books, Boulder

CUZZOLARO M (1997) Disturbi del comportamento alimentare in adolescenza: anoressie e bulimie. In: Pissacroia M (ed) Trattato di psicopatologia dell'adolescenza. Piccin, Padova, pp 287-311

DEKOVIC M (1999) Risk and protective factors in the development of problem behavior during adolescence. J Youth Adolesc 28(6):667-685

DEKOVIC M, MEEUS W (1997) Peer relations in adolescence: effects of parenting and adolescents self-concept. J Adolesc 20:163-176

DEKOVIC M, WISSINK IB, MEIJER AM (2004) The role of family and peer relations in adolescent antisocial behaviour: comparison of four ethnic groups. J Adolesc 27:497-514

DEN EXTER BLOKLAND EA, ENGELS RC, HALE WW ET AL (2004) Lifetime parental smoking history and cessation and early adolescent smoking behaviour. Prev Med 38:359-368

DE WIT J, VAN DER VEER G (1991) Psychologie van de adolescentie – Ontwikkeling en hulprerlening. Uitgeverij Intro, Nijkere

DE ZWAAN M, NUTZINGER DO, SCHOENBECK G (1992) Binge eating in overweight women. Compr Psychiatry 33:256-261

DEERY HA, LOVE AW (1996a) Driving Expectancy Questionnaire Development, psychometric assessment and predictive utility among young drivers. J Stud Alcohol 57(2):193-202

DEERY HA, LOVE AW (1996b) The effect of a moderate dose of alcohol on the traffic hazard perception profile of young drink-drivers. Addiction 91(6):815-827

DISHION TJ, NELSON SE, BULLOCK BM (2004) Premature adolescent autonomy: parent disengagement and deviant peer process in the amplification of problem behaviour. J Adolesc 27:515-530

DODGE KA (1986) Asocial information processing model of social competence in children. In: Perlmutter M (ed) Minnesota Symposium on Child Psychology. Lawrence Erlbaum, Hillsdale, pp 77-125

DOGSON AJ (1990) An Introduction to Generalized Linear Models. Chapman & Hall, London

DONOVAN DM, MARLATT GA, SALZBERG PM (1983) Drinking behaviour, personality factors and high risk driving: Review and theoretical formulation. J Stud Alcohol 44:395-428

DOWDY BB, KLIEWER W (1998) Dating, parent-adolescent conflict, and behavioral autonomy. J Youth Adolesc 27(4):473-492

DUBOIS B (1995) Functions intégratrices et cortex préfrontal chez l'homme. Entretiens d'Orthophonie, pp 39-47

DURBIN M, DI CLEMENTE RJ, SIEGEL D, KRASNOVSKY F (1993) Factors associated with multiple sex partner among junior high school students. J Adolesc Health 14(3):202-207

EIBL-EIBESFELDT I (1974) Love and hate: the natural history of behavior patterns. Methuen, London

EISER JR, MORGAN M, GAMMAGE P ET AL (1991) Adolescent health behaviour and similarity-attraction: Friends share smoking habits (really) but much else besides. Br J Soc Psychol 30:339-348

ELANDER J, WEST R, FRENCH D (1993) Behavioural correlates of individual differences in road-traffic crash risk: An examination of methods and findings. Psychol Bull 113:269-274

ELLICKSON PL, TUCKER JS, KLEIN DJ, SANER H (2004) Antecedents and outcomes of marijuana use initiation during adolescence. Prev Med 39:976-984

EMLER N, REICHER S (1995) Adolescence and delinquency. Blackwell, Oxford

EMLER N, REICHER S, ROSS A (1987) The social context of delinquent conduct. J Child Psychol Psychiatry 28:99-109

ENGEL GL (1977) The need for a new medical model: A challenge for biomedicine. Science 196:129-136

ENGELS RC (1998) Forbidden fruits. Social dynamics in smoking and drinking behavior of adolescents. Universitaire Pers Maastricht, Maastricht

ENGELS RC, KNIBBE RA, DROOP MJ, DE HANN JT (1997) Homogeneity of smoking behavior in peer groups: Influence or selection? Health Educ Behav 24:801-811

ENGELS RC, KNIBBE RA (2000) Alcohol use and intimate relationships in adolescence: When loves comes to town. Addict Behav 25:435-439

ENGELS RC, VITARO F, BLOKLAND ED ET AL (2004) Influence and selection processes in friendships and adolescent smoking behaviour: the role of parental smoking. J Adolesc 27:531-544

ENNETT ST, BAUMAN KE (1994) The contribution of influence and selection to adolescent peer group homogeneity: The case of adolescent cigarette smoking. J Pers Soc Psychol 67:653-663

ERIKSON EH (1950) Childhood and society. Norton, New York

ERIKSON EH (1958) Young man Luther. A study in psychoanalysis and history. Norton, New York

ERON LD, HUESMANN LR, ZELLI A (1991) The role of parental variables in the learning of aggression. In: Pepler DJ, Rubin KH (eds) The development and treatment of childhood aggression. Lawrence Erlbaum, Hillsdale

FAIRBURN C (1995) Overcoming binge eating. Guilford, New York

FARRINGTON DP (1990) Implications of criminal career research for the prevention of offending. J Adolesc 13:93-113

FARRINGTON DP (1994) Interactions between individual and contextual factors in the development of offending. In: Silbereisen RK, Todt E (eds) Adolescence in context. The interplay of family, school, peers, and work in adjustment. Springer, Berlin Heidelberg New York, pp 367-389

FARROW J (1985) Drinking and driving behaviors of 16 to 19 year-olds. J Stud Alcohol 46:369-374

FARROW J (1987) Young driver risk taking: A description of dangerous driving situations among 16 to 19 year-old drivers. International Journal of Addiction 22(12):1255-1267

FESTINGER L (1957) A theory of cognitive dissonance. Stanford University Press, Stanford

FIELDING H (1996) Bridget Jones's diary. Picador, London

FINKEN LL, JACOBS JE, LAGUNA KD (1998) Risky driving and driving/riding decisions: The role of previous experience. J Youth Adolesc 27(4):493-511

FONZI A (2002) Star male a scuola (Nucleo monotematico). Età Evolutiva 71:53-105

FORD DH, LERNER RM (1992) Developmental system theory. Sage, London

FRĄCZEK A, STEPIEN E (1990) Kwestionariuszem: TY i ZDROWIE [Questionnaire: You and health, Polish adaptation of Jessor, Donovan, Costa, Health Behavior Questionnaire, 1989], Zaklad Psychogii Klinicznej IPiN, Warszawa

FRĄCZEK A, ZUMKLEY H (eds) (1992) Socialization and aggression. Springer, Berlin Heidelberg New York

FRYDENBERG E (1997) Adolescent coping. Theoretical and research perspectives. London: Routledge, pp 223

FURMAN W, BRADFORD BROWN B, FEIRING C (1999) The development of romantic relationships in adolescence. Cambridge University Press, Cambridge

GALAMBOS NL, EHRENBERG MF (1997) The family as risk and opportunity: A focus on divorce and working families. In: Schulenberg J, Maggs JL, Hurrelmann K (eds) Health risks and developmental transitions during adolescence. Cambridge University Press, Cambridge, pp 139-160

GARFINKEL PE, KAPLAN AS (1994) Starvation-based perpetuating mechanism in anorexia nervosa and bulimia. Int J Eat Disord 4:661-665

GARNEFSKI N, OKMA S (1996) Addiction-risk and aggressive/criminal behaviour in adolescence: Influence of family, school and peers. J Adolesc 19:503-512

GIANNOTTA F, CIAIRANO S, BONINO S, MORERO D (2004) Le funzioni dell'uso di sostanze psicoattive e dei rapporti sessuali: il punto di vista degli adolescenti. Psicologia della Salute 3 (in press)

GIANNOTTA F, MOLINAR R, RABAGLIETTI E ET AL (2005). Emozioni, contesti relazionali e benessere psicosociale in adolescenza: uno studio longitudinale. In: Menesini E (eds) Fattori di protezione e promozione del benessere in adolescenza e preadolescenza. Psicologia Clinica dello Sviluppo (in press)

GORDON RA (1990) Anorexia and bulimia. Anatomy of a social epidemic. Basil Blackwell, Oxford

GOTTFREDSON MR, HIRSHI T (1990) A general theory of crime. Stanford University Press, Stanford

GRABER JA, BROOKS-GUNN J (1996) Transitions and turning points. Navigating the passage from childhood through adolescence. Dev Psychol 32(4):768-776

GRABER JA, BROOKS-GUNN J, GALEN BR (1998) Betwixt and between: Sexuality in the context of adolescent transition. In: Jessor R (ed) New perspectives on adolescent risk behavior. Cambridge University Press, Cambridge, pp 270-316

GRAHAM JW, MARKS G, HANSEN WB (1991) Social influence processes affecting adolescent substance use. J Appl Psychol 79:291-298

GRUENEWALD PJ, MITCHELL PR, TRENO AJ (1996) Drinking and driving: Drinking patterns and drinking problems. Addiction 91(11):1637-1649

GUAL D, COLOM J (1997) Why has alcohol consumption declined in countries of southern Europe? Addiction 92 (Suppl 1):21-31

HAGELL A, NEWBORN T (1996) Family and social context of adolescent re-offenders. J Adolesc 19:5-18

HALL GS (1904) Adolescence. Appleton, New York

HARAKEH Z, SCHOLTE R, VERMULST A ET AL (2004) Parental factors and adolescents' smoking behavior: an extension of the theory of planned behaviour. Prev Med 39:951-961

HAVIGHURST RJ (1952) Developmental tasks and education, Davis Mc Kay, New York

HAVIGHURST RJ (1953) Human development and education. Longman, New York

HEATHERTON TF, BAUMEISTER RF (1991) Binge eating as a way to escape self-awareness. Psychol Bull 110:86-108

HEINZ WR (2002) Self-socialization and post-traditional society. Advances in Life Course Research 7:41-64

HELSEN M, VOLLEBERGH W, MEEUS W (2000) Social support from parents and friends and emotional problems in adolescence. J Youth Adolesc 29:319-335

HENDERSON-KING D, HENDERSON-KING E (1997) Media effects of women's body-esteem: Social and individual difference factors. J Appl Soc Psychol 27:399-417

HENDRY LB, KLOEP M (2002) Life-span development: Challenges, resources and risks. Thomson, London

HERMAN CP, POLIVY J, LANK CN, HEATHERTON TF (1987) Anxiety, hunger and eating behaviour. J Abnorm Psychol 96:264-269

HOLLAND J, THOMPSON R (1998) Sexual relationships, negotiation and decision making. In: Coleman J, Roker D (eds) Teenage sexuality. Harwood Academic, Amsterdam, pp 59-79

HORNE JA, REINER LA (1995) Driver sleepiness. J Sleep Res 4 (Suppl 2):23-29

IRWIN CE, MILLSTEIN SG (1986) Biopsychosocial correlates of risk-taking behaviors during adolescence. J Adolesc Health Care 7:82S-96S

ISRAEL AC, IVANOVA MY (2002) Global and dimensional self-esteem in preadolescent and early adolescent children who are overweight: Age and gender differences. Int J Ead Disord 31:424-429

ISTAT (1997) Rapporto annuale 1996. La situazione del Paese

ISTAT (1998) Statistica degli incidenti stradali. Anno 1997

ISTAT (2001a) La mortalità per causa nelle regioni italiane. Anni 1997-1999

ISTAT (2001b) Classificazione delle professioni, Metodi e norme – nuova serie n 12

ISTAT (2002) Italia in cifre, Anno 2001

ISTAT (2004) Annual report. The situation of the country 2003. http://www.istat.it. Cited 16 Mar 2005

ISTAT/ACI (2001) Statistica degli incidenti stradali. Anno 2000

IVERSEN H (2004) Risk-taking attitudes and risky driving behaviour. Transportation Research F7:135-150

JACK MS (1989) Personal fable: A potential explanation for risk-taking behavior in adolescents. J Pediatr Nurs 4:334-338

JACKSON S (1989) L'aide aux jeunes en difficulté: le rôle de l'école. L'Orientation Scolaire et Professionnelle 4:337-350

JACKSON S, BOSMA H (1990) Coping and self-concept: Retrospect and prospect. In: Bosma H, Jackson S (eds) Coping and self-concept in adolescence. Springer, Berlin Heidelberg New York, pp 203-222

JACKSON S, BORN M, JACOB M (1997) Reflections on risk and resilience in adolescence. J Adolesc 20:609-616

JACKSON S, BIJSTRA J, OOSTRA L, BOSMA H (1998) Adolescents' perceptions of communication with parents relative to specific aspects of relationships with parents and personal development. J Adolesc 21:305-322

JACOBSON KC, CROCKETT LJ (2000) Parental monitoring and adolescent adjustment: an ecological perspective. J Res Adolesc 10(1):65-97

JESSOR R (1992) Health behavior questionnaire, Institute of Behavioral Science, University of Colorado, Boulder

JESSOR R (ed) (1998) New perspectives on adolescent risk behavior. Cambridge University Press, New York

JESSOR R, JESSOR SL (1977) Problem behavior and psychosocial development: A longitudinal study of youth. Academic Press, New York

JESSOR R, DONOVAN JE, COSTA FM (1991) Beyond adolescence – Problem behaviour and young adult development. Cambridge University Press, New York

JESSOR R, TURBIN MS, COSTA FM (1997) Predicting developmental change in risky driving: The transition to young adulthood. Dev Sci 1(1):4-16

JOHNSTON LD, O'MALLEY PM, BACHMAN JG (1994) National survey results on drug use from the monitoring the future study 1975-1993. National Institute of Drug Abuse, Rockville

JONAH BA (1990) Age differences in risky driving. Health Educ Res 5:139-149

JONAH BA, THIESSEN R, AU-YEUNG E (2001) Sensation seeking, risky driving and behavioral adaptation. Acc Anal Prev 33:679-684

JUANG LP, SILBEREISEN RK (1999) Supportive parenting and adolescent adjustment across time in former East and West Germany. J Adolesc 22:719-736

JUANG LP, SILBEREISEN RK (2001) Family transitions for young adult females in the context of a changed Germany: timing, sequence and duration. Special issue: Family and adolescent development: Germany before and after unification. Am Behav Sci 44:1899-1917

JUANG LP, SILBEREISEN RK (2002) The relationships between adolescent academic capability beliefs, parenting and school grades. J Adolesc 25:3-18

JUBY H, FARRINGTON DP (2001) Disentangling the link between disrupted families and delinquency sociodemography, ethnicity and risk behaviours. Br. J Criminol 41:22-40

JULIEN RM (2005) A primer of drug action. WH Freeman, New York

KANDEL DB (1978) Antecedents of adolescent initiation into stages of drug use: A developmental analysis. In: Kandel DB (ed) Longitudinal research on drug use. John Wiley, New York

KANDEL DB (1986) Processes of peer influences in adolescence. In: Silbereisen RK, Eyferth K, Rudinger G (eds) Development as action in context. Problem behaviour and normal youth development. Springer, Berlin Heidelberg New York

KANDEL DB, LOGAN AJ (1984) Patterns of drug use from adolescence to early adulthood. Periods of risk for initiation, stabilization and decline in drug use from adolescence to adulthood. Am J Public Health 74:260-266

KAPLAN HB (1980) Deviant behavior in defense of self. Academic Press, New York

KAUFFMAN SA (1993) The origins of order: Self organization and selection in evolution. Oxford University Press, New York

KERR M, STATTIN H (2000) Parenting of adolescents: Action or Reaction? In: Croute AC, Booth A (eds) Children's influence on family dynamics: The neglected side of family relationships. Lawrence Erlbaum, Mahwah (NJ), pp 121-151

KIESNER J, KERR M (2004) Families, peers, and contexts as multiple determinants of adolescent problem behavior. J Adolesc 27:493-495

KINZL JF, TRAWEGER C, TREFALT E ET AL (2001) Binge eating disorders in females: A population-based investigation. Cambridge University Press, New York

KOOPS W (1996) Historical developmental psychology of adolescence. In: Verhofstadt-Denève L, Kienhorst I, Braet C (eds) Conflict and development in adolescence. DSWO, Leiden, pp 1-12

KOOPS W, OROBIO DE CASTRO B (2004) The development of aggression and its linkages with violence and youth delinquency. European Journal of Developmental Psychology. 1(3):241-269

KROGER J (2000) Identity development. Adolescence through adulthood. Sage, Thousand Oaks

LABORIT H (1987) Dieu ne joue pas aux dés. Grasset, Paris

LABOUVIE EW (1986) The coping function of adolescent alcohol and drug use. In: Silbereisen RK, Eyferth K, Rudinger G (eds) Development as action in context. Problem behaviour and normal youth development. Springer, Berlin Heidelberg New York, pp 229-240

LAM LT (2003) A neglected risky behavior among children and adolescents: Underage driving and injury in New South Wales, Australia. Journal of Safety Research 34:315-320

LARSON R (1994) Youth organizations, hobbies, and sports as developmental context. In: Silbereisen RK, Todt E (eds) Adolescence in context. The interplay of family, school, peers, and work in adjustment. Springer, Berlin Heidelberg New York, pp 47-65

LAVERY B, SIEGEL AW (1993) Adolescent risk-taking: An analysis of problem behaviors in problem children. J Exp Child Psychol 55:277-294

LERNER RM (1998) Theoretical models of human development. In: Damon W (ed) Handbook of child psychology, vol 1. Wiley, New York

LEVITT MZ, SELMAN RL, RICHMOND JB (1991) The psychosocial foundations of early adolescents' high-risk behavior: Implications for research and practice. J Res Adolesc 1(4):349-378

LEWIS MD, FERRARI M (2001) Cognitive-emotional self-organization in personality development and personal identity. In: Bosma HA, Kunnen SE (eds) Identity and emotion. Cambridge University Press, Cambridge, pp 177-198

LLOYD B, LUCAS K (1998) Smoking in adolescence. Images and identities. Routledge, London New York

LO COCO A, PACE U, ZAPPULLA C (2000) Autonomia emotiva in adolescenza e benessere psicologico. Età Evolutiva 65:76-81

LO COCO A, INGOGLIA S, ZAPPULLA C, PACE U (2001) Condizioni di stress genitoriale, autonomia emotiva e adattamento psicologico durante l'adolescenza. Età Evolutiva 69:88-94

LOEBER R (1990) Disruptive and antisocial behavior in childhood and adolescence: Development and risk factors. In: Hurrelmann K, Losel F (eds) Health hazards in adolescence. Walter de Gruyter, Berlin New York, pp 233-257

LOEBER R, FARRINGTON DP (2000) Young children who commit crime: Epidemiology, developmental origins, risk factors, early interventions, and policy implications. Dev Psychol 12:737-762

LOEBER R, STOUTHAMER-LOEBER M (1986) Family factors as correlates and predictors of juveniles conduct problems and delinquency. In: Morris N, Tonry M (eds) Crime and justice, vol 7. University of Chicago, Chicago, pp 29-149

LOEBER R, FARRINGTON DP, STOUTHAMER-LOEBER M, VAN KAMMEN WB (1998) Antisocial behavior and mental health problems. Explanatory factors in childhood and adolescence. Lawrence Erlbaum, Mahwah

Loeber R, Drinkwater M, Yin Y et al (2000) Stability of family interaction from ages 6 to 18. J Abnorm Child Psychol 28:353-369

Lucidi F, Devoto A, Braibanti P, Bertini M (1998) Una ricerca intervento per la prevenzione delle "stragi del sabato sera". Psicologia della Salute 1:77-86

Lyon J (1996) Adolescents who offend. J Adolesc 19:1-4

Määttä S, Stattin H, Nurmi JK (2002) Achievement strategies at school: Types and correlates. J Adolesc 25:31-46

Magnusson D, Stattin H (1998) Person-context interaction theories. In: Damon W (ed) Handbook of child psychology. Wiley, New York, pp 685-759

Magnusson D, Stattin H, Allen VA (1986) Differential maturational among girls and its relevance to social adjustment: A longitudinal perspective. In: Featherman DL, Lerner RM (eds) Life-span development and behavior. Academic Press, New York, pp 135-172

Mahoney JL, Stattin H (2000) Leisure activities and adolescent antisocial behavior: The role of structure and context. J Adolesc 23:113-127

Marcia JE (1980) Identity in adolescence. In: Adelson J (ed) Handbook of adolescent psychology. Wiley, New York

Marcia JE (1996) The importance of conflict for adolescent and life span development. In: Verhofstadt-Denève L, Kienhorst I, Braet C (eds) Conflict and development in adolescence. DSWO, Leiden, pp 13-19

Marcoen A, Goossens L (1993) Loneliness, attitude towards aloneness, and solitude: Age differences and developmental significance during adolescence. In: Jackson S, Rodriguez-Tomé H (eds) Adolescence and its social worlds. Lawrence Erlbaum, Hove, pp 197-227

Marta E (1997) Parent-adolescent interactions and psychosocial risk in adolescents: An analysis of communication, support and gender. J Adolesc 20:473-487

Marta E, Pozzi M (2005) Young volunteers, family and social capital: from the care of family bonds to the care of community bonds. In: Hofer M, Sliwka A, Diedrich M (eds) Citizenship education: youth theory, research and practice. Waxmann, New York (in press)

Marta E, Rossi G, Boccacin L (1998) Youth, solidarity and civic commitment in Italy: An analysis of the personal and social characteristics of volunteers and their organizations. In: Youniss J, Yates M (eds) Community service and civic engagement in youth: International perspectives. Cambridge University Press, Cambridge, pp 73-96

Mayew DR, Simpson HM (1990) New to the road, young drivers and novice drivers: Similar problems and solutions? Traffic Injury Research of Canada, Ottawa

Mc Cullagh P, Nelder JA (1983) Generalized Linear Models, Chapman & Hall, New York

McDonald K, Thompson, JK (1992) Eating disturbance, body image dissatisfaction, and reasons for exercising: Gender differences and correlational findings. Int J Eat Disord 11(2):289-292

McKenna FP (1993) It won't happen to me: Unrealistic optimism or illusion of control? Br J Psychol 84:39-50

McNair B (1996) Mediated sex pornography and postmodern culture. Arnold, London

Mead M (1928) Coming of age in Samoa. William Morrow, New York

Meeks BS, Hendrick SS, Hendrick C (1998) Communication, love and relationship satisfaction. J Soc Pers Relat 15(6):755-773

Meeus W (1994) Adolescentie. Wolters-Noorkhoff, Groningen

Meeus W, Helsen M, Vollebergh W (1996) Parents and peers in adolescence: From conflict to connectedness – Four studies. In: Verhofstadt-Denève L, Kienhorst I, Braet C (eds) Conflict and development in adolescence. DSWO, Leiden, pp 103-115

Meeus W, Oosterwegel A, Vollebergh W (2002) Parental and peer attachment and identity development in adolescence. J Adolesc 25:93-106

Mendelson BK, White DR (1985) Development of self-body-esteem in overweight youngsters. Dev Psychol 21:90-96

Mitchell K, Wellings K (1998) Risks associated with early sexual activity. In: Coleman J, Roker D (eds) Teenage sexuality. Harwood Academic, Amsterdam, pp 81-100

Moffitt T (1993) Adolescence-limited and life-course-persistent antisocial behavior: A developmental taxonomy. Psychol Rev 100:674-701

Moffitt T, Caspi A, Rutter M, Silva P (2001) Sex differences in antisocial behaviour. Cambridge University Press, Cambridge

Molinar R, Ciairano S, Bonino S et al (2004) Il ruolo della scuola nella prevenzione dell'uso di sostanze psicoattive. Psicologia della Salute 3 (in press)

Molinengo G, Ciairano S, Bonino S, Miceli R (2004) I rapporti sessuali come transizione verso l'adultità: le emozioni e le motivazioni nella prospettiva degli adolescenti. In: Aleni Sestito L (ed) Processi di formazione dell'identità in adolescenza. Liguori, Napoli, pp 175-211

Montgomery MJ, Sorell GT (1998) Love and dating experience in early and middle adolescence: grade and gender comparisons. J Adolesc 21:677-689

Moore S, Gullone E (1996) Predicting adolescent risk behavior using a personalized cost-benefit analysis. J Youth Adolesc 25(3):343-359

Mroziak B, Frączek A (eds, 1999) Sense of Coherence (SOC) and psychological-adjustment. Polish Psychol Bull 30:4

Nelder JA, Wedderburn RWM (1972) Generalized Linear Models. Journal of Royal Statistic Society 135:370-380

NETHERLANDS INSTITUTE ON ALCOHOL AND DRUGS (NIAD) (1994) Stimulants Series. Wolters-Noordhoff, Groningen

NOACK P, KRACKE B (1997) Social change and adolescent well-being: Healthy country, healthy teens. In: Schulenberg J, Maggs JL, Hurrelmann K (eds) Health risks and developmental transitions during adolescence. Cambridge University Press, New York, pp 55-84

NOACK P, HOFER M, YOUNISS J (eds) (1995) Psychological responses to social change. Walter de Gruyter, Berlin

NOACK P, KERR M, OLAH A (1999). Family relations in adolescence. J Adolesc 22:713-717

NURMI JE (1997) Self-definition and mental health during adolescence and young adulthood. In: Schulenberg J, Maggs JL, Hurrelmann K (eds) Health risks and developmental transitions during adolescence. Cambridge University Press, New York, pp 395-419

OETTING ER, BEAVAIS F (1986) Peer cluster theory: Drugs and the adolescent. J Couns Dev 65:17-22

OLWEUS D (1993) Bullying at school. What we know and what we can do. Blackwell, Oxford

PALMONARI A (ed) (1997) Psicologia dell'adolescenza. Il Mulino, Bologna

PALMONARI A (2000) Prefazione. In: Emler N, Reicher S (eds) Adolescenti e devianza. Il Mulino, Bologna, VII-XXI

PALMONARI A, RUBINI M (1995) Orientamenti verso le autorità formali e partecipazione politica degli adolescenti. Giornale Italiano di Psicologia, XXII, 5, pp 757-774

PALMONARI A, RUBINI M (1998) Adolescenti, scuola e rapporto con le autorità istituzionali. In: Colucci FP (ed) Il cambiamento imperfetto. Unicopli, Milano

PALMONARI A, CARUGATI F, RICCI BITTI PE, SARCHIELLI G (1979) Identità imperfette. Il Mulino, Bologna

PALMONARI A, POMBENI ML, KIRCHLER E (1989) Peer groups and evolution of the self-system in adolescence. J Psychol 1:3-15

PALMONARI A, POMBENI ML, KIRCHLER E (1993) Developmental tasks and adolescents' relationship with their peer and their family. In: Jackson S, Rodriguez-Tomé H (eds) Adolescence and its social words. Lawrence Erlbaum, Hove, pp 145-167

PARSONS JT, SIEGEL AW, COUSINS JH (1997) Late adolescent risk-taking: Effects of perceived benefits and perceived risks on behavioral intentions and behavioral change. J Adolesc 20:381-392

PASTORELLI C, STECA P, GERBINO M, VECCHIO G (2001) Il ruolo delle convinzioni di efficacia personale e genitoriale rispetto alle condotte delinquenziali e all'uso di sostanze nel corso dell'adolescenza. Età Evolutiva 69:80-87

PATERNOSTER R, BRAME R (1997) Multiple routes to delinquency? A test of developmental and general theories of crime. Criminology 35(1):49-80

PATTERSON GR (1982) A social learning approach, vol 3, Coercive family process. Castalia, Eugene

PATTERSON GR, REID JB, DISHION TJ (1992) A social learning approach. Antisocial boys, vol 4. Castalia, Eugene

PETERSEN AC (2000) Adolescents in the 21st century: Preparing for an uncertain future. In: Crockett LJ, Silbereisen RK (eds) Negotiating adolescence in times of social changes. Cambridge University Press, Cambridge, pp 294-298

PIAGET J (1964) Six études de Psychologie. Gonthier, Paris

PIAGET J (1972) Intellectual evolution from adolescence to adulthood. Human Development 15:1-12

PIAGET J (1975) L'équilibration des structures cognitives. PUF, Paris

PIERCE JW, WARDLE J (1997) Cause and effects beliefs and self-esteem in overweight children. J Child Psychol Psychiatry 38:645-650

PIKO BF, VAZSONYI AT (2004) Leisure activities and problem behaviours among Hungarian youth. J Adolesc 27:717-730

PINHAS L, TONER B, ALI A ET AL (1999) The effects of the ideal of female beauty on mood and body satisfaction. Int J Eat Disord 25:223-226

PLANT M, PLANT M (1992) Risk-takers: Alcohol, drugs, sex and youth. Routledge, New York

RABAGLIETTI E, BONINO S, CATTELINO E, CIAIRANO S (2005) Violazione dei diritti propri e dell'altro e pornografia: una ricerca sulla violenza sessuale tra gli adolescenti. In: Petrillo G (ed) Diritti dei minori in contesto: significati sociali, responsabilità e ruoli educativi. Franco Angeli, Milano (in press)

REICHER S, EMLER N (1986) The management of delinquent reputations. In: Beloff H (ed) Getting into life. Methuen, London

REISS AJ (1998) Co-offending and criminal careers. In: Tonry M, Morris N (eds) Crime and justice: A review of research, vol 10. University of Chicago Press, Chicago, pp 1-33

RODRIGUEZ-TOMÉ H, BARIAUD F (1990) Anxiety in adolescence: Sources and reactions. In: Bosma H, Jackson S (eds) Coping and self-concept in adolescence. Springer, Berlin Heidelberg New York, pp 169-188

ROGGERO A, MOLINENGO G, RABAGLIETTI E, CIAIRANO S (2005) Il ruolo delle emozioni e delle conoscenze nei comportamenti a rischio degli adolescenti: quali aspetti sono più importanti? In: Mauri A, Tinti C (eds) Psicologia della salute. Applicazioni e metodi. UTET, Torino (in press)

ROSENBERG F, SIMMONS R (1975) Sex differences in the self-concept in adolescence. Sex Roles 1:147-159

RUTTER M (1985) Family and school influences on behavioural development. J Child Psychol Psychiatry 26:249-368

RUTTER M (1987) Psychosocial resilience and protective mechanisms, Am J Orthopsychiatry 57:316-331

RUTTER M (1990) Psychosocial resilience and protective mechanisms. In: Rolf J et al (eds) Risk and protective factors in the development of psychopathology. Cambridge University Press, Cambridge

RUTTER M (1993) Resilience: Some conceptual considerations. J Adolesc Health 14:626-631

RUTTER M (1996) Psychosocial adversity: Risk, resilience and recovery. In: Verhofstadt-Denève L, Kienhorst I, Braet C (eds) Conflict and development in adolescence. DSWO, Leiden, pp 21-33

RUTTER M, RUTTER M (1992) Developing minds. Challenge and continuity across the life span. Penguin, London

RUTTER M, GILLER H, HAGELL A (1998) Antisocial behavior by young people. Cambridge University Press, New York

SAVADORI L, RUMIATI R (1996) Percezione del rischio negli adolescenti italiani. Giornale Italiano di Psicologia 1:85-106

SCABINI E (1995) Psicologia sociale della famiglia. Sviluppo dei legami e trasformazioni sociali. Bollati Boringhieri, Torino

SCABINI E, LANZ M, MARTA E (1999) Psychosocial adjustment and family relationships: a typology of Italian families with a late adolescent. J Youth Adolesc 28(6)633-644

SCABINI E, MARTA E, LANZ M (2005) Transition to adulthood and family relationships: An intergenerational perspective. Psychology Press/Routledge, London (in press)

SCHACTER DL (1996) Searching for memory. The brain, the mind and the past. Basic Books, New York

SCHAFFER HR (2000) The early experience assumption: Past, present and future. Int J Behav Dev 24(1)5-14

SCHNEIDER BH (1998) Tra rischio e disadattamento. Il ruolo trascurato dei fattori protettivi. Età Evolutiva 60:81-86

SCHULENBERG J, MAGGS JL, HURRELMANN K (1997) Negotiating developmental transitions during adolescence and young adulthood: Health risks and opportunities. In: Schulenberg J, Maggs JL, Hurrelmann K (eds) Health risks and developmental transitions during adolescence. Cambridge University Press, Cambridge, pp 1-19

SEIFFGE-KRENKE I (1990) Developmental processes in self-concept and coping behaviour. In: Bosma H, Jackson S (eds) Coping and self-concept in adolescence. Springer, Berlin Heidelberg New York, pp 51-68

SEIFFGE-KRENKE I (1995) Stress, coping, and relationships in adolescence. Lawrence Erlbaum, Mahwah

SEIFFGE-KRENKE I, SHULMAN S (1993) Stress, coping and relationships in adolescence. In: Jackson S, Rodriguez-Tomé H (eds) Adolescence and its social worlds. Lawrence Erlbaum, Hove, pp 169-196

SETTANNI M, GIANNOTTA F, CIAIRANO S (2005) Gli aspetti positivi dei comportamenti a rischio in adolescenza e un'introduzione all'approccio delle life skills. In: Mauri A, Tinti C (eds) Psicologia della salute. Applicazioni e metodi. UTET, Torino (in press)

SHAPIRO R, SIEGEL AW, SCOVILL LC, HAYS J (1998) Risk-taking patterns of female adolescents: What they do and why. J Adolesc 21:143-159

SILBEREISEN RK (1998) Lessons we learned: Problems still to be solved. In: Jessor R (ed) New perspectives on adolescent risk behavior. Cambridge University Press, New York, pp 518-543

SILBEREISEN RK, KASTNER P (1986) La prevenzione della droga negli adolescenti. Prospettive teorico-evolutive. Età Evolutiva 24:6-22

SILBEREISEN RK, KRACKE B (1997) Self-reported maturational timing and adaptation in adolescence. In: Schulenberg J, Maggs JL, Hurrelmann K (eds) Health risks and developmental transitions during adolescence. Cambridge University Press, New York, pp 85-109

SILBEREISEN RK, NOACK P (1988) On the constructive role of problem behavior in adolescence. In: Bolger A, Caspi A, Dolwney G, Moorhose M (eds) Person in context: Development process. Cambridge University Press, Cambridge, pp 152-180

SILBEREISEN RK, NOACK P (1990) Adolescents' orientation for development. In: Bosma H, Jackson S (eds) Coping and self-concept in adolescence. Springer, Berlin Heidelberg New York, pp 111-127

SILBEREISEN RK, TODT E (1994a) Adolescence in context. The interplay of family, school, peers, and work in adjustment. Springer, Berlin Heidelberg New York

SILBEREISEN RK, TODT E (1994b) Adolescence-A matter of context. In: Silbereisen RK, Todt E (eds) Adolescence in context. The interplay of family, school, peers, and work in adjustment. Springer, Berlin Heidleberg New York, pp 3-21

SILBEREISEN RK, EYFERTH K, RUDINGER E (1986) Development as action in context. Problem behaviour and normal youth development. Springer, Berlin Heidelberg New York

SILBEREISEN RK, SCHÖNPFLUG U, ALBRECHT HT (1990) Smoking and drinking: Prospective analyses. In: Hurrelmann K, Lösel F (eds) Health hazards in adolescence. Walter de Gruyter, Berlin, pp 167-191

SILBEREISEN RK, NOACK P, VON EYE A (1992) Adolescents' development of romantic friendship and change in favourite leisure contexts. J Adolesc Res 7:80-93

SKOWRONSKI J, CARLSTON D (1989) Negativity and extremity biases in impression formation. Psychol Bull 105:131-142

SMITH PK, SHARP S (1994) School bullying: Insights and perspectives. Routledge, London

SMITH TW (1994) Attitudes towards sexual permissiveness: Trends, correlates, and behavioral connection. In: Rossi AS (ed) Sexuality across the life course. University of Chicago Press, Chicago, pp 63-97

SPIJKERMAN R, VAN DEN EIJNDEN R, VITALE S, ENGELS RC (2004) Explaining adolescents' smoking and drinking behavior: The concept of smoker and drinker prototypes in relation to variables of the theory of planned behaviour. Addict Behav 29:1615-1622

SPRUIJT-METZ D (1999) Adolescence, affect and health. Psychology Press, Hove

STATTIN H, KERR M (2000) Parental monitoring: a reinterpretation. Child Devel 71(4):1072-1085

STATTIN H, MAGNUSSON D (1996) Antisocial development: A holistic approach. Devel Psychopath 5:541-566

STEINBERG L, AVENEVOLI S (1998) Disengagement from school and problem behavior in adolescence: A developmental-contextual analysis of the influences of family and part-time work. In: Jessor R (ed) New perspectives on adolescent risk behavior. Cambridge University Press, New York, pp 392-424

STERN D (1985) The interpersonal world of the infant Basic Books, New York

SUMMALA H, MIKKOLA T (1994) Fatal accidents among car and truck drivers: Effects of fatigue, age and alcohol consumption. Hum Factors 36:285-297

TONOLO G (1999) Adolescenza e identità. Il Mulino, Bologna

TSCHANN JM, ADLER NE (1997) Sexual self-acceptance, communication with partner, and contraceptive use among adolescent females: A longitudinal study. J Res Adolesc 7(4):413-430

TURRISI R, JACCARD J, KELLY SQ, O'MALLEY CM (1993) Social psychological factors involved in adolescent's efforts to prevent their friends from driving while intoxicated. J Youth Adolesc 22(2)147-169

TYSZKOWA M (1990) Coping with difficult school situations and stress resistance. In: Bosma H, Jackson S (eds) Coping and self-concept in adolescence. Springer, Berlin Heidelberg New York, pp 189-202

VAN GEERT P (1994) Dynamic systems of developments: Change between order and chaos. Prentice Hall/Harvester Wheatsheaf, New York

VAN GEERT P (2001) Fish, foxes and talking in the classroom: Introducing dynamic systems concept and approaches. In: Bosma HA, Kunnen SE (eds) Identity and emotion. Cambridge University Press, Cambridge, pp 64-88

VANDEREYCKEN W (1996) Multidimensional treatment of patients with eating disorders. In: Verhofstadt-Denève L, Kienhorst I, Braet C (eds) Conflict and development in adolescence. DSWO, Leiden, pp 147-152

VAVRIK J (1997) Personality and risk-taking: A brief report on adolescent male drivers. J Adolesc 20:461-465

VERHOFSTADT-DENÈVE L, KIENHORST I, BRAET C (eds) (1996) Conflict and development in adolescence. DSWO, Leiden

WADE TD, LOWES J (2002) Variables associated with disturbed eating habits and overvalued ideas about the personal implications of body shape and weight in a female adolescent population. Int J Eat Disord 32:39-45

WALLACE JM, WILLIAMS DR (1997) Religion and adolescent compromising behavior. In: Schulenberg J, Maggs JL, Hurrelmann K (eds) Health risks and developmental transitions during adolescence. Cambridge University Press, Cambridge, pp 445-468

WEICHOLD K, SILBEREISEN RK, SCHMITT-RODERMUND E (2003) Short-term and long-term consequences of early vs late physical maturation in adolescents. In: Hayward C (ed) Gender differences at puberty. Cambridge University Press, Cambridge, pp 241-276

WERNER EE (1990) Antecedents and consequences of deviant behavior. In: Hurrelmann K, Losel F (eds) Health hazards in adolescence. Walter de Gruyter, Berlin, pp 219-231

WERNER H (1940) Comparative psychology of mental development. International University Press, New York

WEST R, ELANDER J, FRENCH D (1993) Mild social deviance, type-A behavior pattern and decision-making style as predictors self-reported driving style and traffic accident risk. Br J Psychol 84:207-219

WEST R, WILDING J, FRENCH D, KEMP R, IRVING A (1993) Effect of low and moderate doses of alcohol on driving hazard perception latency and driving speed. Addiction 88:527-532

WIESNER M, SILBEREISEN RK (2003) Trajectories of delinquent behaviour in adolescence and their covariates: relations with initial and time-averaged factors. J Adolesc 26:753-771

WILLIAMS AF (1998) Risky driving behavior among adolescents. In: Jessor R (ed) New perspectives on adolescent risk behavior. Cambridge University Press, Cambridge, pp 221-237

WILLIAMS AF, LUND AK, PREUSSER DF (1986) Drinking and driving among high school students. International Journal of Addiction 21:643-655

WORLD HEALTH ORGANIZATION (WHO) (1946) Preamble to the Constitution of the World Health Organization. Official Record 2. World Health Organization Library

WORLD HEALTH ORGANIZATION (WHO) (1999) Partners in life-skills education. Conclusions from a United Nations inter-agency meeting. World Health Organization, Department of Mental Health, Geneva

YOUNISS J, SMOLLAR J (1990) Self through relationship development. In: Bosma H, Jackson S (eds) Coping and self-concept in adolescence. Springer, Berlin Heidelberg New York, pp 130-148

YZER MC, SIERO FW, BUUNK BP (2000) Can public campaigns effectively change psychological determinants of safer sex? An evaluation of three Dutch campaigns. Health Educ Res 15(3):339-352

ZANI B (1993) Dating and interpersonal relationships in adolescence. In: Jackson S, Rodriguez-Tomé H (eds) Adolescence and its social world. De Gruyter, Berlin, pp 95-120

ZAZZO B (1966) Psychologie différentielle de l'adolescence. PUF, Paris

ZIMBARDO PG, KEOUGH KA, BOYD JN (1997) Present time perspective as a predictor of risky driving. Personal Individual Differences 23(6):1007-1023

ZUCKERMAN M (1983) A biological theory of sensation seeking. In: Zuckerman M (ed), Biological bases of sensation seeking, impulsivity, and anxiety. Lawrence Erlbaum Associates, Hillsdale, NJ, pp 37-76